Regulatory Biology

Genetics and Biogenesis of Mitochondria and
Chloroplasts
5–7 September 1974
C. W. Birky, Jr., P. S. Perlman, and T. J. Byers

Regulatory Biology
4–6 September 1975
J. C. Copeland and G. A. Marzluf

Analysis of Ecological Systems
29 April–1 May 1976
D. J. Horn, G. R. Stairs, and R. D. Mitchell

EDITED BY JAMES C. COPELAND AND

GEORGE A. MARZLUF

Regulatory Biology

OHIO STATE UNIVERSITY PRESS: COLUMBUS

Library of Congress Cataloguing in Publication Data

Copeland, J C
  Regulatory biology.

  (Ohio State University biosciences colloquia)
  Includes index.
    1. Cellular control mechanisms. I. Marzluf, G. A.,
joint author. II. Title. III. Series: Ohio. State
University, Columbus. Ohio State University biosciences
colloquia.
QH604.C66   574.8'76   77-2256
ISBN 0-8142-0262-4

Contents

Preface

Regulatory biology is one of the most central and important topics of modern biological investigation—and rightly so, in view of the presence and crucial role of regulatory events in all living organisms. Control mechanisms can be detected in the simplest organisms known, the small single-stranded RNA phage, which possess only enough genetic material to encode three proteins. At the other extreme of the biological spectrum, the complex process of differentiation and development of vertebrates appears to be primarily dependent upon regulatory phenomena, particularly selective gene expression. It now appears that all of the significant activities of living cells are subject to regulation, which explains the fascination and importance of regulatory biology.

The objective of the Ohio State University Biosciences Colloquium on Regulatory Biology was to examine a variety of regulatory phenomena, which control widely divergent cellular activities. To provide perspective and to illustrate the unity of regulatory principles, the presentations ranged from control of transcription and DNA replication in coli phage lambda to development in *Dictyostelium* and in amphibians. Between these far-spaced limits, other equally exciting and informative control processes were analyzed, namely, the lac operon, guanosine tetraphosphate control, autogenous control of gene expression, the cell cycle, chromosomal replication, and fungal gene expression. The presentation of contributed papers on related topics served very well to strengthen and broaden the inquiry into, and our appreciation of, regulatory biology.

The colloquium was attended by more than three hundred persons from all parts of the United States and from Canada. We were most pleased by the enthusiastic response. We are grateful to Dean Richard Böhning and Associate Dean Richard Moore of the College of Biological Sciences for their support and encouragement. Our appreciation also goes to the speakers, the Colloquium Series Committee, our students, and to the many others who contributed to the colloquium in so many ways.

Second Annual Biosciences Colloquium
College of Biological Sciences
Ohio State University
4–6 September 1975

REGULATORY BIOLOGY

Organizers

James C. Copeland, Associate Professor of Microbiology, Ohio State University

George A. Marzluf, Professor of Biochemistry, Ohio State University

Speakers

Suzanne Bourgeois, Salk Institute for Biological Studies, San Diego

Michael Cashel, Section on Regulatory Cell Physiology, Laboratory of Molecular Genetics, National Institute of Child Health and Human Development, National Institutes of Health

James C. Copeland, Department of Microbiology, Ohio State University

Robert Dottin, Department of Biology, Johns Hopkins University

Robert F. Goldberger, Laboratory of Biochemistry, National Cancer Institute, National Institutes of Health

Thomas Humphreys, Department of Biochemistry, Kewalo Marine Laboratory, University of Hawaii

George A. Marzluf, Department of Biochemistry, Ohio State University

Waclaw Szybalski, McArdle Laboratory for Cancer Research, University of Wisconsin

Erik Zeuthen, Biological Institute, Carlsberg Foundation, Copenhagen

Jonathan King, Department of Biology, Massachusetts Institute of Technology (paper does not appear in this volume)

OHIO STATE UNIVERSITY BIOSCIENCES COLLOQUIA

Regulatory Biology

WACLAW SZYBALSKI

Initiation and Regulation of Transcription and DNA Replication in Coliphage Lambda

1

INTRODUCTION

It has been said that the decades of the 1950s and 1960s were the age of simplification. I cannot recall whether this statement pertained to science or politics, but there is little doubt in my mind that in the complex field of regulatory biology the early, very basic concepts of the operon and its control elements, the promoter and operator, were actually simplifications. In this contribution, an updated and expanded summary of my previous reviews, I shall outline the intricate network of transcriptional controls active during development of the *Escherichia coli* bacteriophage λ and discuss current models for the structure and function of the promoters, operators, terminators, the origin of DNA replication, and other regulatory recognition sites. It will be apparent that the age of simplification is over since, even for as simple a virus as λ, the developmental controls are quite complex.

The references in this review will be mainly to studies published after 1973; earlier references are contained in previous reviews from our laboratory (Szybalski, 1969, 1970, 1971, 1972, 1974a,b,c; Szybalski et al., 1969, 1970) and others (Dove, 1968; Echols, 1971a,b, 1972; Eisen and Ptashne, 1971; Herskowitz, 1974; Kourilsky, Bourguignon, and Gros, 1971; Maniatis et al., 1975; Ptashne, 1971; Ptashne et al., 1976).

BACTERIOPHAGE λ

Coliphage λ is a conventional phage of medium size; the head contains a linear DNA molecule of 31.8×10^6 daltons, corresponding to 48,000 nucleo-

McArdle Laboratory for Cancer Research, School of Medicine, University of Wisconsin, Madison, Wisconsin 53706.

tide pairs (Davidson and Szybalski, 1971). Upon phage infection λ DNA is injected into the *Escherichia coli* host cell through the flexible phage tail. After entering the bacterial cell, the linear DNA molecule is converted into a circular form (fig. 1a,b) by the covalent joining of its two single-stranded cohesive ends, each composed of 12 complementary deoxynucleotides, employing the DNA ligase of the host.

Depending on the phage strain and the physiological state of the bacterial host, λ infection may evoke either a lytic or a lysogenic response. In the *lytic* response λ functions become sequentially expressed, λ DNA replicates, heads and tails are synthesized, and ultimately a new crop of mature phage progenies is produced, culminating in death and lysis of the host cell. In the *lysogenic* response the lytic cycle is interrupted, the host cell survives, and the circular λ genome is linearized while inserted into the bacterial genome, as depicted in figure 1 (c + d = e). This is possible because the Int enzyme, a λ gene product, mediates the insertion of the phage genome, and because λ can elicit synthesis of the *repressor,* the product of gene *c*I, which blocks all the

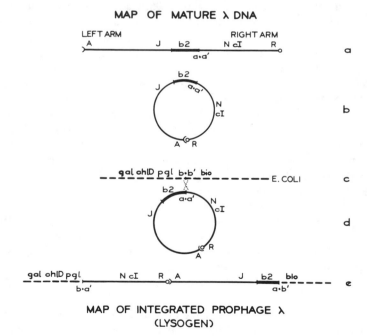

Fig. 1.   Campbell's model for the integration (a→e) and excision (e→a) of the coliphage λ genome. Symbols *a.a'* and *b.b'* represent the attachment site on the viral (solid lines) and bacterial (broken lines) genomes, respectively (modified from Szybalski *et al.*, 1969).

lytic λ functions. The lysogenic response can occur if the repressor is produced early enough to block lytic development and hence to prevent death of the infected host cell.

In the lysogenic state the integrated phage genome, now denoted *prophage*, can be considered as a cluster of genes comprising about 1% of the host DNA. Since the λ prophage is an integral part of the bacterial genome, it is vertically inherited by all the bacterial progeny cells, a very efficient and harmless form of symbiotic propagation of the viral genome. Obviously, prophage propagation by this means would be terminated in the event of death of the lysogenic host cell. To ensure its survival, the λ prophage evolved a mechanism for sensing impending demise of the host and for entering the lytic cycle, which leads to production of a crop of *mature phage* particles. Conversion from the lysogenic (prophage) state into the lytic cycle is denoted *induction*, and its first step is the inactivation of the λ repressor protein.

Below I shall describe first the transcriptional controls in the repressed λ prophage and then the chain of events following induction of the lysogenic cell. A simplified genetic and transcriptional map of phage λ DNA is shown in figure 2.

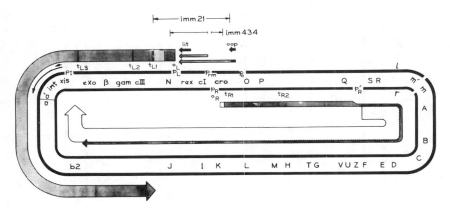

Fig. 2. Simplified genetic and transcriptional map of bacteriophage λ DNA. The leftward and rightward transcriptions are indicated by the arrows (see fig. 3). Five major termination-antitermination controls are represented: the major (1) leftward and (2) rightward transcriptions, initiated by the p_L and p_R promoters and prematurely terminated at the t_{L1} and t_{R1} terminators, respectively, are extended by the action of the N product; the (3) *oop* and the (4) *int* leader RNAs, initiated by the p_o and p_1 promoters and prematurely terminated at the t_o and t_1 terminators, respectively, are extended by the concerted action of the cII and cIII products, to code for genes cI and *int*, respectively; (5) the 198-nucleotide RNA originated at the p_R promoter is elongated into the major late RNA by the action of the Q product. A detailed description of the various genes and recognition sites was compiled by Szybalski (1974b,c, 1976).

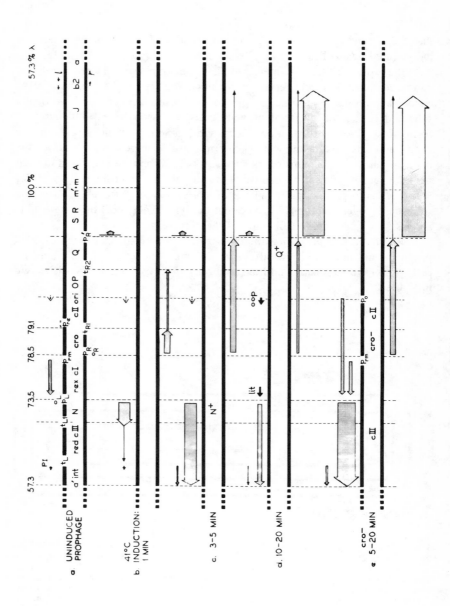

THE PROVIRUS STATE

To establish a provirus state (also denoted prophage or lysogenic state) two conditions must be met: (1) the expression of viral genes that code for products harmful to the host must be curtailed; and (2) the replication of the provirus genome must be carefully controlled and coordinated with that of the host. Under normal circumstances the λ prophage satisfies condition (1) by directing the synthesis of the repressor protein, the product of λ gene cI, which blocks directly the major leftward and rightward viral transcriptions and indirectly the autonomous λ DNA replication. Condition (2) is met by linear insertion of λ DNA into the host genome, which places the replication of the prophage entirely under the host DNA replication controls.

In other systems different means are known or could be imagined to satisfy conditions (1) and (2). For example, to meet condition (1) the repressor might be elaborated by the host, instead of by the virus; or the viral attachment site (symbol $a.a'$; fig. 1) might be located between the lytic viral genes and their promoter, with linear insertion of the provirus leading to "split" and thus inactivation of the viral operon. Condition (2) can often be satisfied by formation of an intricately controlled *plasmid,* rather than by integration. Even λ mutants that have lost the capacity to integrate (λN^-, λdv) can enter a fairly stable plasmid state, thanks to their capacity for autogenous regulation of the genes that control replication of the plasmid. This autogenous regulation is attributed to the product of gene *cro* (or *tof*), a second repressor of λ, whereas the repressor produced by gene cI is dispensable for maintenance of the plasmid state. The replication of such a plasmid cannot be either too rapid, since it would then outgrow and kill the host, or too slow, which would cause it to be progressively lost by dilution.

Fig. 3 (opposite).   Schematic representation of the temporal sequence of transcriptional events in prophage λ. The leftward transcripts are coded by the *l* strand and drawn above λ DNA; the rightward transcripts are coded by the *r* strand and drawn below λ DNA. (a) Transcription in the uninduced prophage. The cI-*rex* transcripts correspond to 80–90% of the total prophage RNA. (b) Immediate-early transcription after induction. (c) Delayed-early transcription. (d) Late transcription. (e) Decontrolled transcription in an induced *cro⁻* mutant of λ. The prophage maps are not drawn to scale, with the immunity region expanded. The numbers in the top line indicate the positions of various sites in respect to the left end (0 %λ) and right end (100 %λ) of mature λ DNA (on the prophage map the 0 and 100 %λ termini are fused and represented by the 100 %λ point; see fig. 1a): *att* (57.3 %λ), p_1 promoter (about 60.3 %λ; S. Hu, W. Szybalski and A. Campbell, unpublished data), t_{LI} (about 71.1 %λ; J. Salstrom and W. Szybalski, unpublished), s_L-$p_L o_L$ region (about 73.5 %λ), p_{rm}-$p_R o_R$ region (about 78.5 %λ), t_{RI} (about 79.1 % λ), p_o (about 80.2 % λ), *oop* RNA (79.9 to 80.1 % λ), *ori* site (about 81 %λ), t_{R2} site(s) (84 to 89 %λ), p_R' (or p_Q) (92 to 93 %λ). The width of the arrows is a measure of the rate of transcription. In the case of the 198 nucleotide 6 S RNA transcribed early (p_R'; figs. 3a–c), it was found by Dahlberg and Blattner (1973) that *in vitro* synthesis provides 10 to 20 times more of the 5'-proximal 15 nucleotide sequence (represented by the verical line in a-c) than of the total 6 S RNA (arrow under p_R'). Thus, p_R' is the strongest λ promoter but is immediately followed by strong termination signals that could apparently be overcome by the Q product, with resulting synthesis of late RNA (drawing d) (modified from Szybalski, 1974a).

TRANSCRIPTION IN THE PROPHAGE STATE

In the prophage state, in which the λ genome exists as an innocuous or even beneficial component of the bacterial chromosome, only one major operon of λ is transcribed. The host RNA polymerase recognizes the p_{rm} promoter and synthesizes the mRNA for genes cI and *rex,* copying the l strand of λ DNA (fig. 3a). The cI-*rex* mRNA is translated into the λ repressor protein (cI product) and the *rex* product. The repressor interacts with the o_L and o_R operators and blocks expression of all the major λ genes. Thus in the prophage state only about 4% (map position 74.3–78.4%λ; fig. 3a) of the prophage genome is transcribed. The λ repressor confers immunity against infection by λ phage, whereas the *rex* function blocks the development of certain mutants of the unrelated coliphages T1, T4 and T5. In this manner prophage λ pays tribute to the host by offering limited protection against several phages, a factor of possible evolutionary significance. The *rex* gene function might also be of some importance for efficient phage propagation or lysogenization under certain adverse conditions (Campbell and Rolfe, 1975), and it was even reported that a λ lysogen can have a selective advantage over nonlysogens by reproducing more rapidly (Edlin, Lin, and Kudrna, 1975). As described later, the *rex* product could also facilitate the natural induction.

The cI-*rex* transcription corresponds to about 90% of the total λ prophage transcription, with the remainder assigned to a few other sites, including the *oop* (traces of an about 78-nucleotide RNA) and *int* leader RNAs on the l strand and a 198-nucleotide RNA in the p_R' region on the r strand. However, these very minor transcriptions (also some in the b2 region; fig. 3a) appear to be of no physiological importance to the maintenance of the prophage state. As will be discussed later, the p_{rm}-promoted cI-*rex* transcription is controlled in both a positive and negative fashion.

INACTIVATION OF THE REPRESSOR PROTEIN

To induce phage development, it is necessary first to inactivate the λ repressor. To simplify this task, especially since *natural* (or *indirect*) induction is a slow and asynchronous process, many λ mutants have been isolated in which the cI protein is thermosensitive (ts). Heating these λcIts lysogens to about 41°C inactivates the repressor but does not otherwise interfere with phage development. Since the active repressor has an oligomeric structure, its inactivation is probably associated with dissociation into cI subunits. This *direct* method of inactivation of the repressor is commonly practiced in the laboratory because it results in synchronous and almost instantaneous induction.

The *indirect* (or *natural*) method of prophage induction is based on the fact that transient interference with the host DNA synthesis by, e.g., irradiation, base analogs, or mitomycin treatment, results in a chain of events leading to the appearance of "special structures" (gaps; R. Sussman, personal communication) in the DNA that have acquired a low affinity for the ind^+ repressor of λ. The repressor is competitively scavenged from the o_L and o_R operators (Sussman and Ben Zeev, 1975), and, in addition, it is enzymatically cleaved (Roberts and Roberts, 1975). This indirect process requires over a half-hour and is inoperative if the bacteria carry mutations like *rec* A or *lex,* or if the phage has an ind^- mutation in gene cI. Apparently the *rec*A and *lex* products are involved in the creation of the "special structures" in the total DNA of the lysogen, and the ind^- mutation abolishes the repressor affinity for these structures. The indirect route of repressor inactivation is prevalent among many kinds of lysogenic strains as found in nature and, as already mentioned, is probably of evolutionary significance because it permits rescue of the prophage from a sickly or dying host cell by conversion into mature and infective phage particles.

Induction can also occur during conjugation when the prophage is transferred from the lysogen into a repressor-free receptor cell. This phenomenon is called *zygotic* induction.

TRANSCRIPTION AFTER INDUCTION OR INFECTION

The major events after λ prophage induction or after phage infection are (1) initiation of p_L and p_R promoted transcription (fig. 3b), (2) extension of this *immediate-early* transcription beyond the t terminators (*delayed-early transcription;* fig. 3c) and (3) appearance of a high level of p_R'-promoted *late* RNA (fig. 3d). Both the positive and negative controls of these events will be discussed. The immediate turnoff of the p_{rm}-cI-*rex* transcription after induction, the appearance of the new short *oop* and *lit* transcripts, and the turn-on of the cII-cIII-dependent immunity transcription will be described next. The cII-cIII-dependent *immunity-establishment* transcription (see the longest leftward p_o-*oop*-cII-cI-*rex* arrow in figure 4) is characteristic of the lysogenic response after infection, and is then replaced by the p_{rm}-promoted *immunity-maintenance* cI-*rex* transcription (fig. 3a). After induction, the immunity-establishment type of transcription is observed only in special (cro^-) mutants (fig. 3e).

As will be discussed later, this scheme is the first approximation of the actual events, which are really more complex as to be well in tune and quite responsive to the ever changing natural environment. However, we shall first present an idealized picture of the chain of transcriptional events that follow λ prophage induction. Subsequently, we plan to discuss some of the events in more detail and describe the molecular mechanisms underlying the initiation, termination and antitermination processes.

IMMEDIATE-EARLY TRANSCRIPTION AFTER PROPHAGE INDUCTION

Inactivation of the λ repressor and its removal from the o_L and o_R operators permits the host RNA polymerase to initiate the leftward and rightward transcriptions at the p_L and p_R promoters (fig. 3b). The leftward transcription, however, does not proceed very far (about 2%λ), the bulk of it being terminated at the t_{L1} terminator. Similarly, most of the rightward transcription is blocked at the t_{R1} terminator, with only about an 0.5%λ length being transcribed, and the remainder of the t_{R1} readthrough is probably stopped at the t_{R2} terminator (fig. 3b). The host factor denoted *rho* (ρ) is instrumental in blocking transcription at the t sites. Immediate-early leftward transcription yields mRNA for gene *N*, and the bulk of the immediate-early rightward mRNA codes for the product of gene *cro* (or *tof*).

DELAYED-EARLY TRANSCRIPTION

The product of gene *N* acts as the antitermination factor. As will be outlined below, it interacts with the host RNA polymerase and abolishes the *rho*-imposed termination at the t sites. In this manner the leftward transcription extends from the p_L site to gene *int*, and the rightward transcription, which originates at p_R, covers genes *cro, O, P. Q*, and beyond (fig. 3c).

LATE TRANSCRIPTION

Although the p_R-initiated delayed-early transcription appears to extend beyond gene Q, it yields very little mRNA that codes for the head and tail genes *A* to *J*, barely enough to produce protein components for one phage particle per cell. To amplify the transcription in the *S-R-A-J* region, a special regulatory mechanism is provided. The product of gene Q permits the RNA polymerase to override the strong termination signals after the 15th and 198th nucleotide and to extend the p_R'-initiated minor rightward RNA, with a resulting massive rightward transcription of the *S-J* region (fig. 3d). Thus enough products are provided for about 100 or more phage particles per cell.

This orderly and sequential chain of transcriptional events results in expression of all the λ genes and should lead to production of a healthy crop of progeny phage. However, additional controls are required to make the process more efficient and more responsive to environmental factors. In the following three sections I shall outline the interplay of genes *cro*, *c*I, and *N* in controlling the transcription promoted by p_L, p_R, and p_{rm}, the three modes of the immunity region transcription, and the role of transcription in the initiation of λ DNA replication.

REGULATION OF EARLY TRANSCRIPTION

The genome of λ codes for two repressor proteins, the products of genes *c*I and *cro*, and it is responsive to their action. As already mentioned, the *c*I product has three direct effects: it very efficiently blocks the transcriptions promoted by p_L and p_R, and has both a positive and a weak negative effect on the p_{rm}-*c*I-*rex* transcription. The product of gene *cro*, the "second repressor" or "antirepressor," also has three effects: it blocks quite effectively the p_{rm} and p_L-promoted transcriptions (Ai and Tof functions, respectively), and it depresses the p_R-promoted early rightward transcription (Tor function). These three functions of the gene *cro* product are shown schematically in figure 3. The Ai (=anti-immunity) function results in the disappearance of the *c*I-*rex* transcription (fig. 3a versus 3b-d), and the Tof and Tor functions depress the p_L-*N*-*int* and p_R-*cro*-*Q* transcription, respectively (thinner arrows in figure 3d than in figure 3c). Figure 3e schematically represents the decontrolled transcription in the induced *cro*⁻ lysogen.

Since the p_L-promoted *in vivo* transcription is quite powerful and several of its products are toxic to the host and required only early in λ development, the Tof controlling mechanism is quite beneficial to an orderly replication and high λ yields. The Tor effect on the p_R-initiated rightward transcription is an example of an autorepression (autogenic control), since the *cro* protein is the product of the p_R-promoted operon and it regulates its own expression. This phenomenon might be quite important for λ DNA replication since genes *O* and *P*, which control λ DNA replication, are a part of the same operon. For instance, λ*N*⁻*c*I⁻ (or its p_R-*O*-*P* fragments, denoted λdv), can persist as autonomous plasmids and replicate in concert with the host. Autogenous control of the λ replication genes by the Tor function is probably the mechanism that (1) keeps λ replication in check during the lysogenic response, so as to allow effective lysogenization without killing the host cell, and which (2) in special cases permits establishment of a stable plasmid-carrier state by maintaining a precise and self-regulating balance between the replication of the λ plasmids and that of the carrier cells.

The negative regulation by the *cro* product is actually more complex than summarized above. It was shown recently that the *cro* product efficiently represses the leftward transcription of gene *N* only when RNA is synthesized by the *N*-modified RNA polymerase. (Hu, Salstrom, and Szybalski, 1975).

The possible mechanisms of this phenomenon will be discussed, and it will be shown how it fits into the general network of transcriptional controls.

CONTROL OF LEFTWARD TRANSCRIPTION IN THE IMMUNITY REGION

There are several alternative modes of transcription within the cI-*rex* region, one of which leads to low-level and the other to high-level synthesis of the λ repressor.

Maintenance Mode

This mode of cI expression is operational in the prophage state. As already described, the cI-*rex* transcription is initiated at the p_{rm} promoter and is carried out by the host RNA polymerase (fig. 4). It appears that this transcrip-

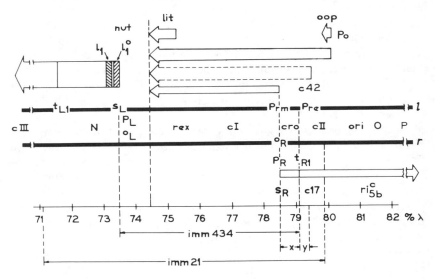

Fig. 4. Physical, genetic and transcriptional map of the immunity and neighboring regions of coliphage λ. For designations of the genes see Szybalski (1974b,c). The open arrows indicate the leftward and rightward transcripts. Three modes of immunity region transcription are shown: (1) maintenance mode p_{rm}-cI-*rex*, (2) establishment mode p_o-*oop*-*y*-*x*-cI-*rex*, i.e., the cII-cIII antiterminated extension of the *oop* transcript (the earlier concept of the establishment mode of the immunity transcription is represented by the dashed-line arrow; Reichardt, 1975a), and (3) late immunity transcription *lit*, which appears to depend on the p_o promoter and *oop* transcription (see fig. 5). The sequences of the $p_L o_L$-s_L and $p_R o_R$-s_R regions are shown in figures 10 and 11. The sequences of the $l_1°$ and l_1 segments of the p_1-N RNA are specified in figure 14. The *cis*-dominant mutation *nut* (*N ut*ilization) abolishes *N* recognition for the leftward transcription (Salstrom and Szybalski, 1976). The *cis*-dominant mutation $c42$ blocks the establishment mode of transcription. The *cis*-dominant *ori⁻* mutations ($p_o⁻$) abolish λ DNA replication, establishment mode of immunity transcription, and *oop* and *lit* RNA synthesis. Mutations $c17$ and $ri_{5b}{}^c$ create new rightward promoters (Dove et al., 1971).

tion is autogenously regulated by the cI product (Reichardt, 1975b), which at lower concentrations stimulates, and at higher concentrations depresses, the cI-*rex* transcription (Meyer, Kleid, and Ptashne, 1975). This cI-*rex* expression is also quite susceptible to repression by the Ai function of the *cro* gene product. Translation of the cI gene from the p_{rm}-cI-*rex* RNA is inefficient since this mRNA does not have the ribosomal binding site (Ptashne et al., 1976).

Establishment Mode

Since immediately after phage infection there is no repressor present, the p_{rm}-promoted maintenance mode of cI-*rex* expression is not fully operational in λ cro$^+$ phage because it depends on stimulation by the preexisting cI product. In this case the establishment mode of repressor synthesis takes over. It was once believed that in this case the transcription originated at the p_{re} promoter located between genes *cro* and cII (Fig. 4), and required two products coded by λ genes cII and cIII to act as cofactors for the host RNA polymerase (Reichardt, 1975a). At present it is far from certain whether the "repressor establishment" mode of transcription (1) really originates at the p_{re} site between genes *cro* and cII, with initiation being dependent on the cII and cIII products, or (2) rather that it is the extension of the *oop* transcript (see the longest p_o-*oop*-cI-*rex* arrow in figure 4), which originates between genes cII and O, with the cII and cIII products acting as antiterminating factors (Honigman et al., 1976). Thus the *oop* RNA might have a double role, acting as primer for the initiation of λ DNA replication, as will be discussed later, and as leader for the cI-*rex* transcription. The third possibility is that both the p_{re} promotion and *oop* extension modes for the establishment of cI-*rex* expression are operational. The establishment mode of cI-*rex* transcription is positively controlled, as already mentioned, by the cII and cIII products, and negatively controlled by the *cro* product. The *cro* control appears to be both (1) indirect, because it depresses transcription of both the cIII and cII genes (Echols, 1972), and (2) direct, since after induction no establishment mode of cI-*rex* transcription is observed in *cro*$^+$ prophages, even at the time when genes cIII and cII are efficiently transcribed. It is also possible that the *rex* product, which is always present in lysogens, inhibits the establishment pathway, thus facilitating natural induction. It might be significant that natural induction is inefficient in lysogens lacking the *rex* gene, e.g., λ*imm*434. As already mentioned, only after induction of *cro*$^-$ lysogens is the establishment mode of cI-*rex* transcription observed (see fig. 3e), even in *dnaE*$^-$ hosts defective in DNA replication (unpublished data of Hayes and Szybalski; Honigman et al. [1976]).

Late Mode

Still another mode of leftward transcription in the immunity region is observed at times later than 5 minutes after infection or thermal induction of λ*cro⁺*, when a short RNA molecule denoted *lit* (*l*ate *i*mmunity *t*ranscription; fig. 3d) is synthesized from the promoter-distal segment of the *rex* gene (Hayes and Szybalski, 1973a). Its synthesis is coordinate with the *oop* RNA, and depends on several phage and host functions (fig. 5), as will be discussed in the next section. It is not known whether the *lit* RNA is of any significance for λ development.

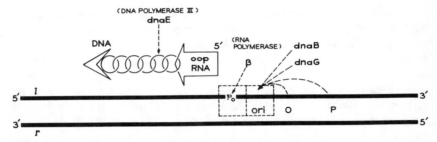

Fig. 5.   Control of *oop* RNA synthesis and a model for its role as a primer for initiation of λ DNA synthesis. The *oop* RNA synthesis starts to the left of the *ori* site. The *ori⁻* mutants are *cis*-defective for *oop* synthesis and behave as if the "activator" region of p_o, the possible site of action of the products of λ genes *O* and *P* and host genes *dnaB* and *dnaG*, was defective. Synthesis of *oop* requires, in addition, the rifampicin-sensitive RNA polymerase component. This model of the replicative complex or "replisome" postulates that the 3'OH terminus of the *oop* RNA is extended by the host DNA polymerase III, the product of the gene *dnaE* (Hayes and Szybalski, 1973b). Alternatively, *oop* RNA is used as a leader for synthesis of the *c*I-*rex* RNA (Honigman et al., 1976).

All these factors exemplify the complexity of the immunity controls, with three or perhaps even more modes of expression of the genes within the *c*I-*rex* region, all being under the positive and negative controls of several already-specified factors like the products of genes *cI*, *cII*, *cIII*, *N*, and *cro*, and also several other phage and host factors, most of them involved in DNA replication.

TRANSCRIPTION AS RELATED TO THE INITIATION OF λ DNA REPLICATION

There appear to be two major phases of λ DNA synthesis: (1) early bidirectional replication of λ DNA circles (theta structures) and (2) late predominantly leftward replication leading to formation of long λ DNA concatemers (sigma structures or recombination-promoted oligomers), which have to contain at least two *cos* sites so as to allow cutting by the Ter function and packaging into the phage heads (Skalka, 1974; Stahl and Stahl, 1974). The present discussion, however, will be directed mainly to the mechanisms of initiation of λ DNA replication.

Replication of λ DNA starts 3 to 4 minutes after thermal induction at the site designated *ori* (*ori*gin of DNA replication) and is bidirectional. Its initiation requires the λ products *O* and *P* and the intact *ori* site (fig. 4). It also requires host products coded by genes *dnaB, dnaE,* and *dnaG* but not by *dnaA, C,* and *F* (Hayes and Szybalski, 1973b). Moreover, for the initiation of the λ DNA replication fork, two kinds of RNA transcription appear to be required: rightward RNA transcription in the *ori-O* region, dependent on the p_R or other auxiliary promoter, and a strong augmentation of the synthesis of the *oop* RNA (fig. 3d). Synthesis of *oop* RNA depends on the λ elements, p_o, *ori, O,* and *P,* and on the products of the host genes *dnaB* and *dnaG,* but not on *dnaE* (fig. 5; Hayes and Szybalski, 1973b). It is very significant, as will be discussed later, that the product of host gene *dnaE* (DNA polymerase III) is required for λ DNA replication but not for *oop* RNA synthesis, which is even more efficient in induced $dnaE^-$ lysogens, when only one prophage copy is present, than in dna^+ lysogens.

How could all these facts contribute to understanding the mechanism of the initiation of λ DNA replication? We shall discuss the elements of a working hypothesis that could possibly account for the experimental facts.

Elements of the Replication-Initiation Hypothesis

The host DNA polymerase III, the product of gene *dnaE*, is known to be unable to initiate DNA replication on double-stranded λ DNA, since it requires the 3'-OH terminus of a *primer* DNA strand and a complementary *template* strand to perform this task (see e.g., Gefter, 1975; Dressler, 1975). A short DNA or RNA molecule could conceivably serve as a primer by supplying its 3'-OH end. The *oop* RNA is a logical candidate for such a primer. A strong indication that *oop* RNA may be a component of a machinery for the initiation of DNA replication is the dependence of *oop* synthesis on many λ replication functions, including the products of λ genes *O* and *P* and the *E. coli* genes *dnaB* and *dnaG* (fig. 5). The most compelling evidence is that mutations in the *ori* region of λ, which are thought to represent *cis*-dominant defects in the "origin" site where λ DNA synthesis starts (Dove, Inokuchi, and Stevens, 1971; Rambach, 1973), also block *oop* RNA synthesis, acting as if they were *cis*-dominant mutations in the p_o promoter complex for *oop* transcription (Hayes and Szybalski, 1973b, 1975). One might postulate either that (1) the *ori* site and the p_o promoter are the same entity or, more likely, that (2) the *ori* site, located upstream from p_o, acts as an *activator* site (see fig. 5), somewhat analogous to the cAMP-CAP-dependent activator sites in the *lac* or *gal* promoter regions. It appears, therefore, that a concerted action of many phage and host functions is required for synthesis of the *oop* RNA, the 3'-OH end of which would then be used to prime DNA synthesis carried out by the DNA polymerase III (fig. 5). This complex DNA replication apparatus, which is composed of many host and phage proteins, can be designated as the replicative complex or "replisome" (fig. 5 and 6c).

We would like now to make a specific proposal, apparently not considered before (Gefter, 1975; Dressler, 1975), to explain how the *oop* RNA primes the *double-strand* initiation of DNA synthesis at the unique *ori* site in conjunction with "transcriptional activation" (Dove et al., 1971). The separate

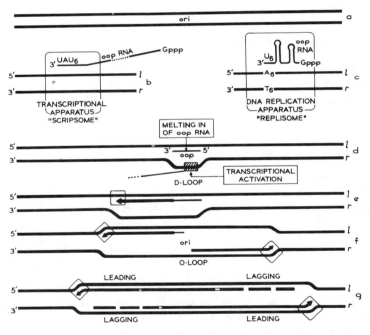

Fig. 6.   Initiation of λ DNA replication. (a) Unreplicated double-stranded DNA near the *ori* site, (b) *cis* mode of interaction between newly synthesized *oop* RNA and DNA, (c) *trans* mode of primary interaction between the U_6 sequence in *oop* RNA and $dA_6 \cdot dT_6$ in DNA, leading to the formation of a triple helical structure stabilized by a replicative complex, (d) Melting-in of *oop* RNA leading to the formation of the D-loop, and aided by active transcription of the *r* strand (transcriptional activation) by RNA polymerase (cross-hatched rectangle). (e) Initiation of DNA synthesis (*double-strand initiation*) employing the 3'OH end of *oop* RNA as primer and the *l* strand as template. (f) *Single-strand initiation* of DNA synthesis on the *r* strand leading to the formation of the O-loop. (g) Formation of Okazaki fragments along the "lagging" segments of the *l* and *r* strands. Very heavy lines represent DNA strands; thinner lines represent RNA; squares in drawings (e)-(g) represent DNA polymerase III.

problem of the *single-strand* initiation, as required for initiation of the Okazaki fragments or of the complementary strand on the ϕX174 or M13 template (see Gefter, 1975; Dressler, 1975; Kornberg, 1975) will be considered subsequently.

It is not clear whether the *oop* RNA acts in the *cis* or *trans* manner to prime initiation of DNA replication on the double-stranded template (fig. 6a). One could postulate that in the *cis* mode, DNA polymerase III "captures" the *oop* RNA by replacing the transcriptional enzymatic complex arrested at the $dA_6 \cdot T_6$ site on λ DNA when the *oop* RNA is still associated with the DNA template (fig. 6b). In the *trans* mode, the displaced *oop* RNA may either interact first with the DNA polymerase or with the *oop* site on DNA by, e.g., utilizing its 3'-terminal U_6 sequence to form a triple-stranded complex with the $dA_6 \cdot T_6$ site, where it was synthesized (fig. 6c). Theoretically, such a triple-stranded complex could be formed with any other $dA_n \cdot T_n$ sequence in DNA, when n is at least 4 or 5, and could lead to DNA synthesis initiation without completion of the subsequent step 6d, which depends on the D-loop formation. The triple-stranded complex could be further stabilized by components of the DNA replication apparatus.

The *oop* RNA, when associated with the site of its synthesis by either the 6b or 6c mechanism, could now convert this site to a so-called D-loop, in which the whole *oop* RNA or its 3'-proximal part would form a double-stranded helix with the complementary sequence on the *l* strand DNA, whereas the corresponding single-stranded region of the *r* strand would loop out (fig. 6d). This displacement reaction would be favored in the superhelical circular configuration of DNA, and it is known that λ DNA replication is initiated in such structures. By electron microscopy using a model system, we have observed D-loops formed by partial (with "whiskers" of RNA protruding) or complete "melting in" of RNA into λ DNA (M. Fiandt and W. Szybalski, unpublished).

Furthermore, such "melting in" of the *oop* RNA *in vivo* might be favored by temporary dissociation of the *r* strand during the act of active rightward transcription passing through or initiated near the *ori* site. Indeed, Dove et al. (1971) observed the dependence of λ DNA replication on the rightward transcription, a phenomenon that was termed "transcriptional activation." They considered two general mechanisms for this phenomenon, one depending on the "changing of DNA structure" in the *ori* region, and the other invoking its translocation into a site within the cell (e.g., the membrane) "where it can be acted upon". In our model of double-strand initiation we tend to favor the first mechanism, depending on either the *r*-strand transcription (promoted upstream from *ori*) or binding of the transcriptional complex initiated at the new ri^c promoters close to the *ori* region. Both events would tie up the *r* strand and favor the annealing of *oop* RNA to the *l* strand, leading to D-loop formation. However, the second mechanism of Dove et al. (1971) is not excluded, since it might also favor "melting in" of the *oop* primer.

In the following event, the 3'-OH end of *oop* RNA would be utilized as a primer by the DNA polymerase, resulting in leftward synthesis of the new *l*-complementary strand of λ DNA, which thus would be covalently linked to the *oop* RNA. Indeed, such covalent linkage between DNA and *oop* RNA was observed by Hayes and Szybalski (1975). As a consequence of DNA synthesis the D-loop would be enlarged (fig. 6e).

The next step in the initiation of λ DNA replication would be the synthesis of an Okazaki-type fragment on the unpaired *r* strand within the D-loop (fig. 6f). This is thermodynamically a much easier process than double-strand initiation since it does not require prior separation of the DNA strands. This type of initiation was extensively studied by Okazaki et al. (1973) (see also Gefter, 1975). Once this second kind of initiation occurs, the initiation structure becomes a fully symmetrical O-loop, demonstrating that the actual DNA replication is an inherently bidirectional process. To convert it back to a unidirectional mode would require some additional functions to block one of the two divergent replication forks. Further migration of the replication forks in either direction away from the *ori* site requires initiation of multiple Okazaki-type fragments (Okazaki et al., 1973) on the "lagging" strand (fig. 6g) and their subsequent fusion by mechanisms now reasonably well understood (Alberts, 1973; Gefter, 1975).

Summary of the Replication-Initiation Model

Our simplified model of the initiation of λ DNA replication, as discussed above, depends on (1) synthesis of the *oop* primer RNA, which requires the p_o promoter (activation of which is abolished by *ori⁻* mutations), the λ products *O* and *P*, the *E. coli* genes *dnaB* and *dnaG*, and RNA polymerase components (fig. 5), among others, (2) primary interaction between *oop* RNA and *oop* DNA (fig. 6a–c) leading to (3) D-loop formation with the active participation of (4) transcriptional (*r* strand) activation (fig. 6d), and finally resulting in (5) initiation of leftward DNA synthesis by the DNA polymerase, utilizing the 3'-OH end of the *oop* RNA primer (fig. 6e). Steps subsequent to this *double-strand initiation* would include (6) enlarging of the D-loop by migration of the replication fork (fig. 6e), (7) initiation of the first Okazaki-type DNA fragment on the now unbonded *r* strand within the D-loop in the *ori* region, which leads to (8) rightward *single-strand initiation*, and consequently to (9) bidirectional λ DNA replication, associated with divergent migration of both forks along the leading strands (*ori→c* I copying the *l* strand and *ori→*

P copying the r strand; fig. 6f), and (10) initiation of Okazaki-type fragments and their fusion on the lagging strands (fig. 6g), and (11) emergence of the classical Θ (theta) form of the replicating DNA molecule.

Additional Factors

Unfortunately, there remain many unexplained details and apparent inconsistencies that might require altering some elements of this composite model. These will be briefly outlined.

1. Not only the *oop* RNA but also the short *lit* RNA, transcribed from a site about 2,000 base pairs downstream from *oop,* depends for its synthesis on the same p_o promoter, which is deactivated by *ori*⁻ mutations (fig. 4). The role of the *lit* RNA is obscure, especially since it is transcribed in the dispensable region of λ (Blattner et al., 1974). Its synthesis, however, depends on all the same functions as *oop* transcription. Moreover, *lit* synthesis, and by implication also *oop* synthesis, depend in a *cis* fashion on the *O* product (Hayes and Szybalski, 1975). Thus *ori, O,* and *oop* are required in *cis,* and *P* in *trans* for *lit* synthesis.

2. Complementation experiments indicate that the *O* product acts in *trans* (see Dove et al., 1971), with the exception of some specialized experiments performed under N^- conditions (Kleckner, 1974). To reconcile the *trans* effects of the *O* product on phage replication, with its *cis* effect on *lit* (and presumably *oop*) RNA synthesis, both under N^+ conditions, one could adapt a simple model; the product of gene *O* is required in *cis* for *oop* synthesis and, in turn, *oop* acts in *trans* to prime λ DNA synthesis (Hayes and Szybalski, 1975). This hypothesis, however, does not appear to be fully consistent with some experimental results. For instance, the defective *ori*⁻ lysogens, which should not produce *oop,* can nevertheless supply the O^+ function in *trans,* albeit not in a very efficient manner (Rambach, 1973).

3. The mechanism of transcriptional activation, as postulated in our *oop* RNA priming model (fig. 6d), is strictly hypothetical. For instance, one might postulate that transcriptional activation is continuously required for the stimulation of *oop* synthesis. However, this is unlikely, since after transient thermal induction of the λcI857 lysogen, the high induced level of *oop* synthesis persists for well over 15 minutes after the p_L- and p_R-promoted transcriptions have been blocked by renaturation of the repressor (Hayes and Szybalski, 1973b).

4. It was observed by Rosenberg et al. (1975) and by Smith and Hedgpeth (1975) that *oop* RNA (fig 7a) may carry oligo(A) sequences added

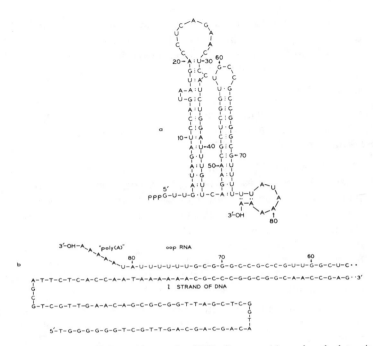

Fig. 7.   Sequence of *oop* RNA and its template DNA. Sequence (a) was largely determined by Dahlberg and Blattner (1973) with corrected sequence for the nucleotides 47–51, as determined by Rosenberg et al. (1975), and further corrections by Scherer et al. (1976). The *oop* RNA often contains an oligo(A) sequence following the 3′-terminal U₆AU sequence (Rosenberg et al., 1975; Smith and Hedgpeth, 1975) and is optimized for base pairing. The sequence (b) of the λ DNA *l* strand that codes for the 3′-proximal region of *oop* RNA was determined by Kleid et al. (1976) with correction at positions 113–14 by G. Scherer, G. Hobom, and H. Kössel (personal communication). This sequence indicates that the 3′-terminal oligo(A) in *oop* RNA is not coded by DNA.

post-transcriptionally to its 3′-end (fig. 7b). At present it is not obvious whether these sequences would enhance or block the postulated priming activity of the *oop* RNA. One could even speculate that when *oop* RNA is annealed to the *l* strand, the oligo(A) tail might turn around so as to anneal to the T₆ sequence on the *r* strand and prime the rightward DNA synthesis (fig. 8).

5. It could be argued that no special factors are required for *oop* RNA synthesis because it was observed in *in vitro* experiments (Blattner and Dahlberg, 1972). However, these low levels of *oop* produced *in vitro*, and the very low constitutive levels observed *in vivo* (fig. 2a–c), do not reflect the physiologically significant high levels of *oop* synthesis stimulated by the *O, P,* and other products when the phage is derepressed.

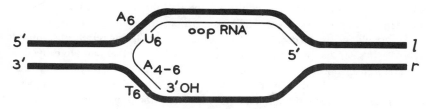

Fig. 8. Hypothetical structure formed by melting-in the *oop* RNA, carrying an oligo(A) sequence on its 3' end, into DNA containing the $A_6 \cdot T_6$ sequence.

6. *In vitro* dependence of λ DNA replication on the *oop* RNA was reported by Hayes and Szybalski (1975). Their conclusion, however, can no longer be considered valid since it has been found by E. C. Rosenvold and W. Szybalski (unpublished data) that the pancreatic nuclease heated to 100°C for 10 minutes, which was present in the *oop* RNA preparations, still possessed enough nucleolytic activity to account for the 10- to 20-fold stimulation of DNA synthesis from the λ DNA template. In these experiments the extract produced from the induced λ*gam*$^+$*N*$^+$*c*I857 lysogens had almost no DNA synthesizing activity directed by the added λ DNA template unless heat-inactivated pancreatic DNAse (with or without *oop* RNA) or only traces of nonheated DNAse were added. Although this result can at present be considered trivial, it might be interesting to note that extracts from nonlysogens, noninduced lysogens (Hayes and Szybalski, 1975), or *gam*$^-$ lysogens, but not from induced *gam*$^+$ lysogens, all direct rather high DNA synthesis from the added λDNA template. This result implies that an important factor might be nicking the λ template by the *recBC* nuclease (E. C. Rosenvold and W. Szybalski, unpublished), an enzyme inhibited by the *gam* product (Sakaki et al., 1973). Traces of pancreatic DNAse activity (which remained unsuspected in the heated *oop* preparations) would thus replace the *gam*-suppressed *recBC* nuclease activity.

It should be emphasized that the demise of the purported *in vitro* system for demonstrating the priming activity of *oop* RNA in no way weakens the hypothesis of an *in vivo* priming role for *oop* RNA. In fact it is strengthened, since some previous inconsistencies observed in the "*in vitro* system", e.g., dependence on polymerase I and lack of template specificity (Hayes and Szybalski, 1975), can now be disregarded. If our model is correct, a successful *in vitro* system for demonstrating *oop* RNA priming might require a superhelical circular template and very critical conditions for "melting-in" the primer, including perhaps active rightward transcription and other factors. Any possible role of *oop* RNA as the "leader" for the establishment mode of cI-*rex* transcription (see preceding section) might be independent or complementary to the role of *oop* RNA as a primer for DNA replication.

To conclude, we could say that the minimal conditions required to initiate DNA synthesis on perfectly double-stranded DNA in λ or λ-like systems include transcription of *both* strands in the *oop-ori* region, with one short transcript from the *l* strand, which preferably would self-terminate at its oligo(Py) sequence, and a second complementary transcriptional event that would temporarily engage the opposing DNA *r* strand, so as to assist the short primer transcript in assuming the proper configuration along the *l* strand conducive for the 3'-OH primed initiation of DNA synthesis by DNA polymerase III. One should realize, however, that different routes of priming and initiation of DNA synthesis employing various enzymatic elements could be employed in different systems (see Kornberg, 1976).

INITIATION OF TRANSCRIPTION

Jacob and Monod (1961) have proposed the concept of the *operon*, "a genetic regulatory mechanism in the synthesis of proteins." In conjunction with the subsequent notion of the promoter, the classical operon represented a block of protein-coding genes coordinately controlled by one *promoter,* where transcription is initiated, and one *operator,* where the repressor binds (see discussion of Szybalski et al., 1970). With the realization that some transcriptional units in phage λ are much more complex, may not code for proteins, and involve several new control elements, the original definition of the operon was expanded to include all kinds of transcriptional units, even those not specifying proteins, but principally defined by a *single autonomous promoter* (or rather by that part of the promoter which we call the *entry site,* i.e., the site of the first specific interaction between the RNA polymerase and the DNA template). To emphasize this expanded concept of the operon, an alternative designation, the *scripton,* was proposed for any transcriptional unit (Szybalski et al., 1970). For instance, a transcriptional unit as bizzare as that composed of the *oop* and *lit* transcripts (fig. 4) could be considered a single scripton, since synthesis of both RNAs, which most probably do not code for any proteins, appears to be initiated by only one promoter p_o and controlled by the same phage and host functions (Hayes and Szybalski, 1973a). It might be confusing to call such a unit an operon.

To understand the structure and function of the sites for the initiation and control of λ transcripts, it was soon realized that the complete nucleotide sequences of the promoter and operator regions would have to be determined. The first attempt to sequence the 5'-proximal regions of four transcripts synthesized *in vitro* from the λ DNA template was undertaken in our labora-

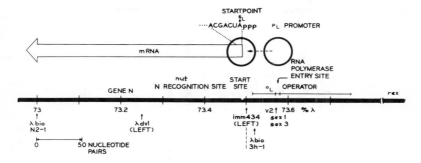

Fig. 9.   Physical map of the beginning of the p_L operon. RNA polymerase (circle) first interacts with DNA at the *entry site*, and then moves (indicated by dashed arrow) to the *start site*, where it strongly binds to DNA and is ready to initiate RNA synthesis at the *startpoint*, which corresponds to the 5'-terminal purine triphosphate of the transcript. The *N*-modified RNA polymerase is activated by the *N* recognition site, which is inactivated by the *nut* mutations (see fig. 4) mapping just downstream from the startpoint (Salstrom and Szybalski, 1976, and unpublished). Mutations *sex*1 and *sex*3 inactivate the promoter function while *v*2 decreases the operator function and increases the promoter function (modified from Blattner et al., 1972, 1974; and Szybalski, 1974a; see also fig. 10).

tory by Blattner and Dahlberg (1972). As shown soon thereafter by Lozeron et al. (1972, 1976), the *in vitro* initiation sequences for all four transcripts are identical to the *in vivo* initiation sequences, establishing the fidelity and biological significance of the *in vitro* transcription. Unfortunately, it soon became apparent (Blattner et al., 1972) that the promoter and operator sequences, as defined by *cis*-dominant promoter and operator mutations, are *not* transcribed into RNA, indicating that the transcripts sequenced by Blattner and Dahlberg (1972) and Dahlberg and Blattner (1973, 1975) did not include the promoter and operator. The crucial contribution of our early study was to show that the site of initiation of transcription is more complex (see figure 9) than hitherto suspected, and the structures involved consist of (1) the *entry site,* where the RNA polymerase makes the first effective contact with the DNA template and where known promoter mutations are located, (2) the *start site,* where the RNA polymerase binds and receives a signal for the initiation of RNA synthesis, and (3) the *startpoint,* which corresponds to the 5'-terminal triphosphate of the transcript (Blattner et al., 1972). For the p_L promoter region there is a definite distance between the entry site and the startpoint, which was somewhat overestimated in the early study of Blattner et al. (1972) and subsequently shown to correspond to about 30 nucleotide pairs (Blattner et al., 1974; Maniatis et al., 1975). From subsequent studies also carried out in our laboratories, but principally in the laboratories of M. Ptashne, V. Pirrotta, and H. G. Khorana, the total sequence of the p_L and p_R (and adjoining p_{rm}) promoter regions was determined, as shown in figs. 10

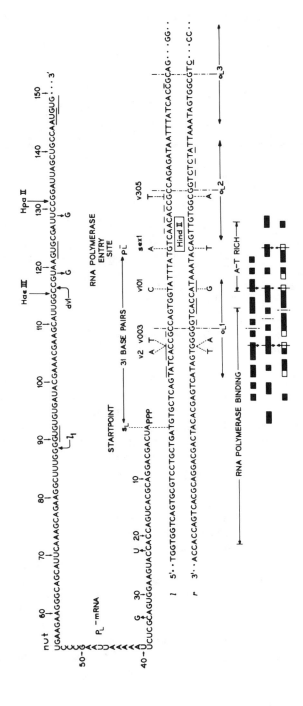

and 11 (Dahlberg and Blattner, 1975; Kleid, Agarwal and Khorana, 1975; Kleid et al., 1975; Maniatis et al., 1975, Meyer et al., 1975; Pirrotta, 1975; Walz and Pirrotta, 1975). Several relevant aspects of these structures will be discussed separately for the p_L and $p_{rm}-p_r$ regions.

Initiation at the p_L Promoter

The sequences of λ DNA, both upstream and downstream from the startpoint s_L, controlling initiation of the synthesis of the p_L mRNA are shown in figure 10. The upstream sequence, which is not transcribed into mRNA and which represents the promoter-operator region, will be discussed first.

The $p_L o_L$ region. The principal structural features of this region were discussed by Maniatis et al. (1975). There appear to be three operator sites, $o_L 1$, $o_L 2$ and $o_L 3$, with progressively decreasing affinity for the repressor. Each site is 17 base pairs long with the central axis of symmetry for imperfect inverse palindromes. For instance, the symmetry of the $o_L 1$ site can be represented as follows:

TAoCACoGo

oGoCACoAT

with symbols "o" indicating nonsymmetrically distributed bases. Thus in the $o_L 1$ site 12 base pairs participate in the inverse palindromic symmetry. There appear to be similar base pair arrangements in the $o_L 2$ and $o_L 3$ operator sites but the degree of symmetry is reduced (fig. 10). Most of the known operator mutations (designated v for virulence) are in the $o_L 1$ site, with only one weak v mutation found in the $o_L 2$ site. They all decrease the degree of symmetry in the $o_L 1$ or $o_L 2$ inverse palindromes.

Fig. 10 (opposite). DNA and RNA sequences in the N-s_L-$p_L o_L$ region. The p_L-mRNA was sequenced by Dahlberg and Blattner (1975) and the s_L-$p_L o_L$ DNA sequence is reported by Maniatis et al. (1975) and Meyer et al. (1975); part of this sequence was determined indirectly by RNA transcript analysis reported by Dahlberg and Blattner (1975). The elements of symmetry in respect to the central axes (dash-dot lines) in the $o_L 1$, $o_L 2$, and $o_L 3$ sites are indicated by horizontal bars. Three alternative inverted partial palindromes are indicated by the shaded rectangles below the $o_L 1$ segment. The arrows pointing down indicate decreases in symmetry, and the arrows pointing up (and open rectangles) increasing symmetries caused by the $v2$, $v101$ and $sex1$ mutations. Mutation $sex1$ partially inactivates the p_L promoter, and the v mutations are partially constitutive (the $v2$ mutation is also an up-promoter mutation; Hu et al., 1975). A few sites are indicated for the restriction endonucleases *Hind*II, *Hpa*II, and *Hae*III. The four indicated base changes in the p_L-mRNA were observed in $\lambda imm434$ (Lozeron et al., 1976). For dv1 and l_1 endpoints see figures 9 and 14 (Blattner et al., 1974; Lozeron et al., 1976). Position of nut^- mutations was determined by M. Rosenberg in collaboration with J. S. Salstrom and W. Szybalski (unpublished data).

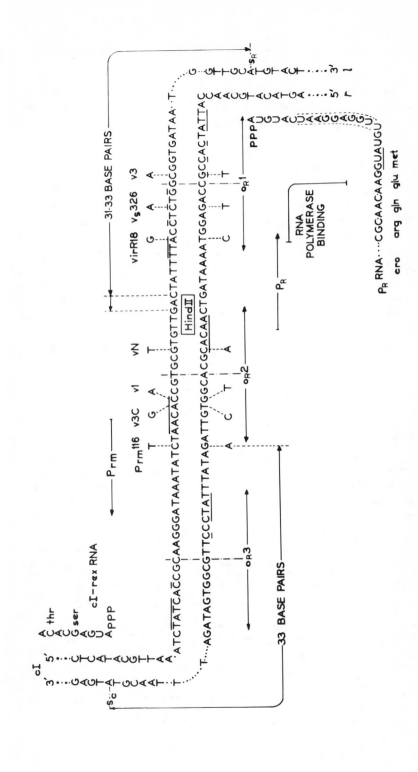

The promoter or entry site for the RNA polymerase appears to be located between o_L1 and o_L2 since the known promoter mutation *sex*1 is located there. The entry site seems to be associated with a twelve base pair segment containing ten AT pairs (fig. 10). It might be significant that the *sex*1 mutation changes the lone GC pair within the AT stretch into an AT pair. After first interacting with the DNA at the entry site, the RNA polymerase is translocated to a strong binding site that is centered near the s_L point and extends for about 40 base pairs. It is significant that the entry (promoter) site is not covered by the strongly bound RNA polymerase, which at this stage is ready to initiate mRNA synthesis (fig. 10).

There are two other features of the $p_L o_L$ region worthy of mention: (1) the entry site is associated with the recognition site for the *Hind*II restriction endonuclease; (2) there are at least two more symmetries in the o_L1 region as indicated by the solid rectangles below o_L1 in figure 10. They may have no significance, or they may indicate the site of interaction between λ DNA and other controlling proteins known to act in this region, as e.g., the product of gene *cro*. The known *v* mutations decrease the symmetries in two inverse palindromes, but the *v*2 and *v*101 mutations actually increase the degree of symmetry in the third palindrome (see figure 10; open rectangles). One might speculate that the second palindrome specifies the site of the Tof function (*cro* product binding) and the third palindrome some component of the p_L promoter function, since the *v*2 mutation, which was reported to decrease the Tof effect (Sly, Rabideau and Kolber, 1971), increases the strength of the p_L promoter (Hu et al., 1975). However, more careful examination shows that the *sex*1 mutation, which decreases the strength of the p_L promoter, also increases the symmetry of the third inverted palindrome (see figure 10; open rectangles).

Beginning of the s_L-N operon. The sequence of the RNA synthesized from this operon, as specified in figure 10, was discussed by Dahlberg and Blattner (1975). The following major features could be deduced from this sequence. (1) Although there are eight AUG and GUG codons (fig. 10), many of them are followed by an in-phase terminator. The GUG codon at position 90 is the first likely initiator of *N* protein synthesis, especially since it is preceded by the AGAAGG purine-rich sequence, which could form five base pairs with the 3′ end of the 16 S ribosomal RNA (Shine and Delgarno, 1974; see discussion of the s_R-*cro* operon). Another possibility is the UUG initiator at

---

Fig. 11 (opposite).   DNA and RNA sequences in the cI-p_{rm}-$p_R o_R$-*cro* region. The startpoint s_c for the cI-*rex* RNA and the amino-terminal of the *cro* protein are only of speculative nature. For various designations compare figures 4, 10, and 12. The DNA sequences are those reported by Maniatis et al. (1975), Pirrotta (1975), Walz and Pirrotta (1975), and Meyer et al. (1975 and personal communication). The p_R RNA sequence was determined by D. Steege and J. Steitz (personal communication) and partially by Blattner and Dahlberg (1972 and unpublished data).

position 85, activated by the AUG and GUG initiators at positions 24 and 30 followed by the in-phase UGA terminator at position 54 (see Miller, 1974), which is a part of the UGAAGAAGG sequence able to form 6 or 7 base pairs with the 3'OH-AUUCCUCCA end of the 16 S ribosomal RNA. (2) The long sequence between the s_L and the possible initiator codon for the N protein shows that the p_L mRNA has a long "leader" sequence in analogy to the *trp* operon (Bronson, Squires, and Yanofsky, 1973). As will be discussed later, the site of the N product recognition, which subsequently leads to the t_L antitermination, resides in this leader sequence. (3) Four point mutations, which do not display any obvious phenotype, were observed in the leader sequence at positions 22(23), 34, 119 and 129 (fig. 10). They probably indicate minor nonhomologies between phages λ and 434 in this region, since they were found in phage λ*imm*434. (4) The sequence reveals the sites of restriction cuts by the *Hae*III (115/116) and *Hpa*II endonucleases (131/132). (5) The left terminus of the λdvl plasmid was found to start with base 116. (6) As will be discussed later, the sites of processing of the p_L RNA by RNaseIII were determined. (7) The comparison of the p_L sequences synthesized both *in vivo* and *in vitro* provided for the first time proof that RNA polymerase-mediated *in vitro* RNA synthesis could be initiated with complete fidelity (Lozeron et al., 1972, 1976).

Initiation at the p_R and p_{rm} Promoters

As shown in figures 11 and 12, the p_{rm} and p_R promoters are very close to each other and overlap the o_R operator site. The sequences and a large part of the following discussion are derived from the papers of Maniatis et al. (1975), Meyer et al. (1976), Pirrotta (1975), and Walz and Pirrotta (1975). The sequence of the p_R promoter region was also studied by G. R. Smith and J. Hedgpeth (personal communication), and of the p_R RNA by Blattner and Dahlberg (1972 and unpublished data) and by D. Steege and J. Steitz (personal communication).

The p_R o_R region. The sequence of the p_R o_R region shows a close analogy to that of the $p_L o_L$ region, with three similar o_R1, o_R2 and o_R3 inverse palindromes representing three repressor-binding operator sites. The 12 base pair AT-rich sequence, which must correspond to the p_L (RNA polymerase entry) site, contains ten AT pairs and is located between the o_R1 and o_R2 sites. Some p_R^- mutations inactivate the *Hin*dII recognition site (at the left edge of the AT-rich segment), and thus are positioned outside the RNA polymerase strong binding site, which is centered at the s_R startpoint (fig. 11). There is one less element of symmetry in o_R1 than in o_L1 and one more in o_R2 than in o_L2. If this confers a more equivalent repressor binding on o_R1 and o_R2, it

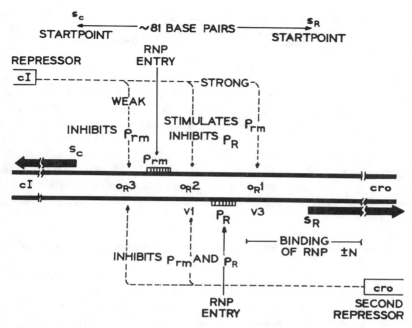

Fig. 12. Reciprocal autogenic regulation of the immunity maintenance and major rightward transcriptions by the cI and cro products. The cI product blocks the p_R transcription and at low levels stimulates the p_{rm}-promoted transcription (probably by binding to the o_R1 and/or o_R2 sites, upstream from p_{rm}), whereas at higher levels it inhibits the p_{rm} transcription (probably binding to the weakest o_R3 operator site downstream from p_{rm}) (based on Meyer et al., 1975). The cro product strongly inhibits the p_{rm}-promoted transcription and weakly its own transcription (i.e., the p_R transcription).

should not be surprising that the frequencies of v mutations in o_R1 and o_R2 appear to be similar (see figure 11). These sites probably correspond to the $virR$ and $virC$ loci, respectively (Horiuchi et al., 1969; see also figure 11).

Beginning of the s_R-cro operon. The p_R RNA sequence is shown in figure 11. It is tempting to speculate that the AUG triplet at position 19 corresponds to the initiation of the cro protein, especially since this site is preceded by the pppAUG initiation codon (position 1), the in-phase UAA termination codon (position 7), and the overlapping purine-rich AAGGAGGU sequence; starting with position 7, this RNA sequence is perfectly complementary to the 3' end of the 16 S rRNA (3'OH-AUUCCUCCA-5'), as postulated by Shine and Delgarno (1974) and as pointed out by D. Steege and J. Steitz (personal communication). The presumed amino end of the cro protein is specified in figure 11. It is not surprising that the p_R RNA has a rather short leader sequence, since the cro protein has to fit within the very limited space between the p_R

site and the right end of the *imm*434 region, as mapped and discussed by Hayes and Szybalski (1973a).

The p_{rm} region and the s_c-cI operon. The p_{rm}^- mutation (p_{rm} 116) corresponds to the change of the lone CG pair to the TA pair in a 12 base pair AT region located between the o_R3 and o_R2 operator sites (Meyer et al., 1976). The s_c-cI RNA (*cI-rex* RNA) starts at the thirty-third base pair to the left of the p_{rm}116 site, in partial analogy to the p_L *(sex)*-s_L distance of 31 base pairs.

Regulation of transcription promoted by p_R and p_{rm}. The scheme of such regulation is depicted in figure 12. As shown by the dashed arrows above the λ DNA molecule, the λ repressor (product of gene cI) inhibits initiation of the rightward transcription promoted by p_R. There is one strong binding sequence, o_R1, downsteam from the RNA polymerase entry site, and two, o_R2 and o_R3, upstream from p_R (Maniatis et al., 1975). According to the data of Meyer et al. (1976) and in agreement with the previous *in vivo* results (see e.g., Reichardt, 1975b), the λ repressor has two effects on its own transcription promoted by p_{rm}: at low concentrations it stimulates the synthesis of the s_c-cI RNA, probably acting upstream from p_{rm} at the o_R2 (and/or o_R1) site, whereas at increasing concentrations it inhibits this cI expression, probably binding at the weakest operator site, o_R3, downstream from p_{rm}.

A complementary system of controls is provided by the product of gene *cro,* the second repressor, which represses strongly the s_c-cI transcription and weakly the s_R-*cro* transcription. As shown by the dashed arrows below λ DNA (fig. 12), the most logical candidate for the site of strong p_{rm} inhibition by the *cro* product (anti-immunity, or Ai, effect) is the o_R3 or some other site downstream from p_{rm}, whereas binding of the *cro* product at the same site or at o_R2 should have a weaker effect on the p_R-promoted rightward transcription. Thus the cI and *cro* products represent a very interesting pair of reciprocally acting autogenous regulators. Superimposed over the transcriptional controls is a translational control, since the s_c-cI RNA has no ribosomal binding site, with translation originating at the 5'-terminal pppAUG triplet (fig. 11), whereas the p_o-cI mRNA, also coding for the cI protein, has a ribosomal binding site (Ptashne et al., 1976).

Comparison of the p_L, p_R and p_{rm} Regions

Examination of Figures 10 and 11 brings out several analogies between these three promoter regions. (1) Maniatis et al. (1975) pointed out the similarities between the inverted palindromes representing the six o_L and o_R operator sites. Positions 4(C:G), 6(C:G) and 8(A:T), counted from the symmetry axis (position 1), appear immutable, and positions 2, 5, and 9 change rarely. All the *v* mutations disrupt the symmetries (underlined in figures 10 and 11) present in the wild-type operator sites. (2) Promoter mutations are always located in the 12 base pair AT-rich segments between two operator sites (figs. 10, and 11; Walz and Pirrotta, 1975; Maniatis et al., 1975; Meyer et al., 1976). (3) The 31–33 base pair distance between p_L (*sex* 1) and s_L appears to be the same for the other two promoter regions, although not all evidence is direct, as yet (figs. 10 and 11). If confirmed, this observation might argue for the RNA polymerase being somehow able to measure the distance between its entry site and the startpoint where RNA synthesis is initiated. In all cases it appears that the RNA polymerase, when strongly bound at the startpoint site, does not cover its original entry site. This was determined by digesting with pancreatic DNase the DNA outside the zone protected by the strongly bound RNA polymerase (Maniatis et al., 1975). However, the bound RNA polymerase still protects the entry sites from endonucleolytic cuts by the *Hin*dII restriction nuclease (see figures 10 and 11).

Main features of the p_o-promoter region, including one operator-like site, are in good agreement with the above-discussed properties of promoter regions (Scherer et al., 1976).

TERMINATION OF TRANSCRIPTION AND THE ANTITERMINATION FUNCTIONS

As discussed in section 7, there are special termination sites, t_L and t_R, that, in conjunction with the host *rho* factor, block the early transcription initiated at the p_L and p_R promoters (fig. 3b). Moreover, there are natural termination sites depending on the U_6A-OH sequence at the end of the p_R'-promoted 6 S

Fig. 13 (following). Hypothetical mechanisms of transcription termination and antitermination. (a) The *rho* factor interacts with the C-rich sequence of the mRNA in the nontranslated regions (which are not protected by ribosomes beyond nonsense triplets represented here by AAU, i.e., UAA) and then moves along the RNA in the 5′-to-3′ direction (see b) using the ATPase reaction (ATP→ADP+P) as energy source. (b) When transcription by the RNA polymerase (RNAP) complex is temporarily arrested at a slowdown signal t (represented here by a Pu·Py sequence, dA·dT), which follows the GC-rich region (see eleven GC near the 3′ end of the *oop* RNA; see fig. 7), the *rho* factor catches up with the RNA polymerase resulting in the termination of transcription. (c) Antitermination could be explained by including the *N* product in the transcriptional complex (RNAP+N→RNAP-N), which results in either (1) blocking the interaction between the *rho* factor and the RNA polymerase, or (2) insensitivity of the RNAP-N complex to the transcriptional slowdown signals. Another possibility (3) is that the *N* product permits the ribosomes to protect mRNA beyond the nonsense codon, and thus interfere with *rho*-mRNA interaction. Drawing c depicts also the fact that the product of *cro* inhibits the *N* region transcription only in the presence of the *N* product (Hu et al., 1975). One might imagine that entry of the nonmodified RNA polymerase (RNAP) is inhibited only by the *c*I product bound to the o_{cI} operator(s), whereas a change in conformation of the *N*-modified RNA polymerase (RNAP-N) results in interference with its entry by both the *c*I product (at o_{cI}) and the *cro* product (at o_{cro}). Figs. (d–f) represent alternative mechanisms of termination and antitermination. The *rho* factor does not have to move along the mRNA, but simply (d) become modified by interaction with C-rich RNA and then (e) react with RNA polymerase and cause the termination. The temporary arrest of RNA polymerase at the slowdown signal increases the efficiency of *rho* termination but is not obligatory. The interaction between the *N* protein and RNA polymerase could occur at the *nut* site, as shown in (f).

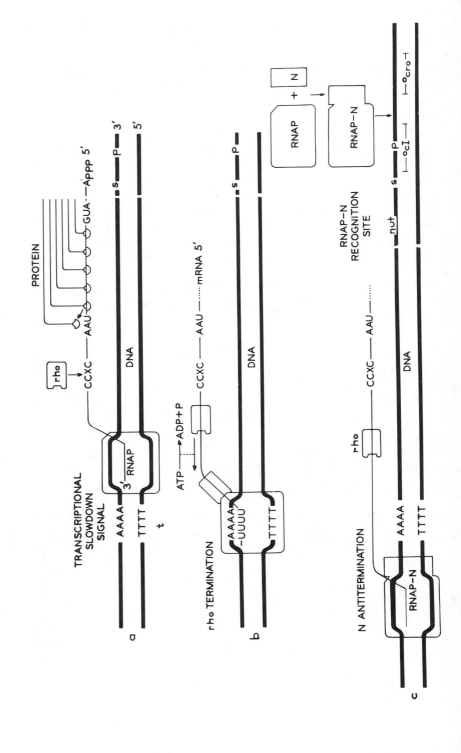

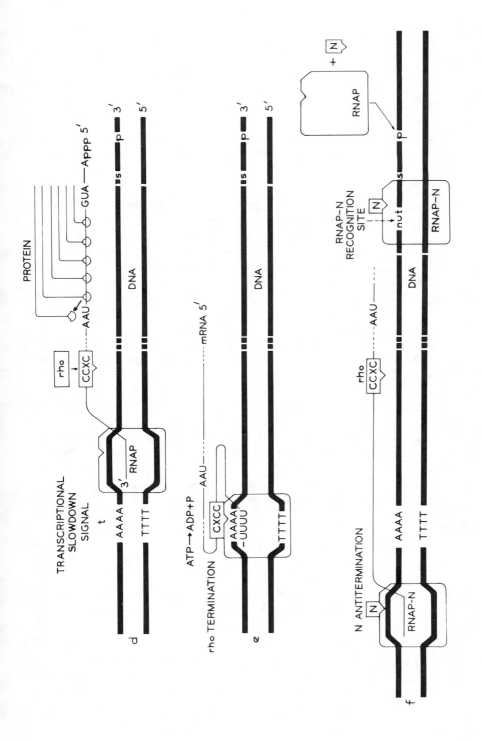

RNA and p_o-promoted *oop* RNA (figs. 3,7) (Leibowitz, Weissman, and Radding, 1971; Dahlberg and Blattner, 1973). Termination of the *oop* RNA is also assisted by the host *rho* factor with the modification of the terminal sequence to U_6AUA_n-OH (see figure 7b). I shall first discuss the possible mechanisms of the RNA termination and then consider the antitermination effects by the *N* and other products.

Termination by the rho Factor

The hypothetical mechanisms for the *rho*-effected termination are shown in figure 13. They follow the proposals emanating from the laboratories of M. Gottesman, S. Adhya, and B. de Crombrugghe, and of J. P. Richardson, as based on the following facts: (1) the *rho* factor is an ATPase, the activity of which depends on C-containing RNA; (2) the *rho* factor is coded by gene *su*A (Richardson et al., 1975); (3) there exist natural transcriptional slowdown signals on DNA, probably dPu · dPy sequences, which cause a delay in the progress of RNA synthesis (Darlix and Fromageot, 1972). The mechanism of termination could be imagined to consist of the following elements: (1) During the process of transcription RNA is being synthesized. (2) Those portions of the RNA that are utilized as a template for protein synthesis are densely covered by ribosomes and unable to interact with the *rho* factor. (3) The *rho* factor interacts only with nontranslated, unfolded parts of RNA, preferably those that contain C residues, and (4) utilizes the energy derived from hydrolysis of ATP to move along the RNA in the 5'-to-3' direction so as to catch up and interact with the RNA polymerase leading to transcription termination. (5) This is efficient only if the RNA polymerase slows down or temporarily stops at the natural termination signals of the dPu · dPy type (Szybalski et al., 1969; Darlix and Fromageot, 1972). One could speculate that (a) the frequency of C clusters in terminator-proximal untranslated RNA, (b) the length of untranslated RNA, (c) the absence of strong secondary structures in this RNA region, and (d) the strength of the slowdown signals in DNA, all independently contribute to the efficiency of a given terminator. Nonsense mutations or insertions of long stretches of untranslated DNA (e.g., IS insertions) would potentiate termination mainly for the above reasons (b) and (d). Figures 13b and e represent two alternative mechanisms leading to the interaction between *rho* and RNA polymerase.

Antitermination by the N Product

There is mounting evidence that the *N* product modifies the RNA polymerase (Epp and Pearson, 1976), probably interacting with its β subunit (Ghysen and Pironio, 1972; Georgopoulos, 1971a,b). The *N* modified polymerase has the new property of recognizing only specific signals located downstream from the p_L and p_R promoters and disregarding the corresponding terminators. The recognition of the p_L-s_L region by the N-modified RNA polymerase (but not by the normal RNA polymerase) can be abolished by the nut_L mutations, which map just downstream from s_L (Salstrom and Szybalski, 1976 and unpublished). The N modified RNA polymerase acquires other new properties like sensitivity to the Tof effect (Hu et al., 1975) and insensitivity to the *rho*-mediated termination (Greenblatt, 1973). The possible mechanisms of the N-mediated antitermination are schematically outlined in figure 13c and f. These include (1) changes in the N-modified RNA polymerase that cause its insensitivity to either (a) the *rho* factor or (b) slowdown signals on the DNA, or, more unlikely, (2) interaction of the N product with ribosomes so as to permit them to travel beyond the termination codon and protect RNA from interaction with the *rho* factor. At the *nut* site, the RNAP-N complex is either formed (fig. 13f) or its conformation is modified (fig. 13c). Alternatively, the N-ribosome interaction occurs at the *nut* sequence on mRNA. Figure 13c also shows schematically the possible overlap between the entry site for N-modified RNA polymerase (RNP-N) and the operator site, o_{cro}, that binds the *cro* product, whereas entry of the smaller normal RNA polymerase (RNAP) would not be impaired by the *cro* product, explaining the results of Hu et al. (1975).

Other Termination Events and Antitermination Factors

There are three other obvious candidates for the antitermination mechanism of transcription: the Q-mediated late transcription and the *c*II-*c*III–mediated immunity and *int* transcriptions. As already discussed, the 6 S minor rightward RNA (Leibowitz et al., 1971; Blattner and Dahlberg, 1972) initiated by the p_R' promoter is probably extended into the late RNA, which possibility was recognized as soon as the position of this RNA was first determined (Blattner and Dahlberg, 1972; Dahlberg and Blattner, 1973; Szybalski, 1972). The recent data on the sequencing of the p_R'-proximal region of the late RNA lend credence to this notion (S. M. Weissman, personal communication). Actually the events appear to be even more complex. Dahlberg and Blattner (1973) found in their *in vitro* study that the p_R' promoter is more active than all the other promoters, but there is a strong termination barrier after the 15th nucleotide that results in synthesis of 10 to 20 times more 5′-proximal 15-nucleotide fragments than 6 S RNA. The Q product apparently permits RNA polymerase to overcome barriers both at the 15th and 198th nucleotide (fig. 3).

The proposal that the *c*II and *c*III products act at the *cy* site and antiterminate the *oop* transcript and lead to the establishment mode of *c*I-*rex* transcription (Honigman et al., 1976) was already discussed in section 11 (fig. 4). Similarly, A. Honigman, S.-L. Hu, and W. Szybalski (unpublished results) find that a very short leader RNA initiated at the p_1 promoter and terminated at the t_1 terminator, both located near gene *xis,* can be extended into the *int* region under the effect of the *c*II and *c*III products (figs. 2 and 3).

PROCESSING AND DEGRADATION OF λ RNA

Processing and degradation of λ RNA proceeds according to a rather complex program. Lozeron et al. (1972, 1976) studied the degradation of the major leftward RNA, which is initiated at the p_L promoter and terminates about 7,500 nucleotides downstream, somewhere in the *J-att* region (figs. 2 and 3c). Up to half of this transcript can be recovered as about 36 S RNA while the rest is comprised of fragments from about a half and a quarter or less that size down to 4-5 S pieces. A 5′-terminal fragment $l_1{}^o$ (up to 71 bases long) and the following rather stable l_1 (4.5 S) RNA were isolated and sequenced (fig. 14). Since these fragments are not produced in RNaseIII-deficient hosts (Lozeron and Anevski, 1975), one may conclude that they are products of processing the p_L RNA by RNaseIII according to the scheme shown in figure 14.

The interpretation of these results is that the p_L-RNA is first transcribed as one large mRNA molecule, over 7,500 bases long for λN^+ and about 800 bases long for λN^-. These transcripts are then processed endonucleolytically

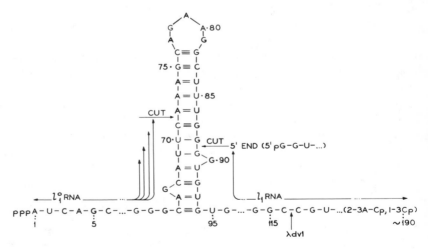

Fig. 14.   Processing of the 5′-proximal region of the p_L RNA, the sequence of which is shown in figure 10. The $l_1{}^o$ and l_1 fragments are the products of endonucleolytic cleavage of the p_L RNA, probably by RNase III (Lozeron and Anevski, 1975). The top of the hairpin loop, from position 72 to 88, is absent in the 4-5 S fraction. The 5′ end of l_1 appears to be complementary to its 3′ end, possibly accounting for the stability of the l_1 fragment. The 3′ ends of $l_1{}^o$ are staggered (''shaggy'' ends), as if they were partially degraded by a 3′→5′ exonuclease (adapted from Lozeron et al., 1976).

to produce smaller fragments. The *N* region RNA is processed to 4-5 S fragments that, with the exception of the so-called 4.5 S l_1 RNA fragment, are rapidly degraded, probably by a 3'-to-5' exonuclease.

Other examples of perhaps analogous post-transcriptional controls were studied by Ray and Pearson (1974) for the *A-J* region of λ. They observed that the late RNA is rather evenly distributed throughout the whole *A-J* region, but there are up to 1,000-fold differences in the amounts of various proteins coded by this region. One interpretation may be that the RNA corresponding to a particular cistron is processed soon after the RNA is synthesized, and thus becomes inactive as a template for protein synthesis.

CONTROL NETWORKS

To simplify the description of the control mechanisms, most of the regulatory elements were treated as separate entities in a somewhat idealized manner. The truth is that the products of λ and the host genes undergo complex interactions, and thus a change in one element results in modification of many regulatory circuits. Moreover, the recognition sites for several proteins do overlap (figs. 10, 11), as already discussed. These multiple interactions between various regulatory circuits point to both great economy in the control apparatus and intrinsic modes for autoregulation with sensitive response to environmental impulses. However, the detailed presentation of such an interlocking control network is rather difficult and will not be attempted in this general review. Thomas (1971, 1973) has explored the possibility of expressing such interlocking interactions in Boolean algebraic form.

The control networks could either be described as provided in nature, which places this kind of study in the realm of *descriptive biology,* or the research approach could be directed toward their redesign either introducing mutational or recombinational changes, or by removing or inserting selected DNA fragments, employing the novel techniques of genetic engineering. These include fragmentation by restriction endonucleases and sealing in DNA fragments either synthesized in the laboratory or obtained from λ and other organisms.

The latter approach places the study of λ in the realm of *synthetic biology* or genetic engineering, which is an open-ended field of endeavor, in contrast to purely descriptive biology.

FUTURE AIMS

Descriptive versus Synthetic Biology

The descriptive phase of the study of the transcriptional control network in λ is still far from finished. We even do not know how the RNA polymerase recognizes the promoter, its entry and start sites, and the terminator. The $p_L o_L$, $p_R o_R$, and *nut* regions have been sequenced (figs. 10 and 11), but it is not entirely clear which parts of the sequence represent the actual recognition sites for RNA polymerase and the N product. Still much less is known about the structure, function, and recognition sequences for other controlling factors, like the products of genes Q, cII and cIII. What we seem to understand now are only very general concepts of transcriptional regulation.

In addition to more fundamental understanding of the molecular basis of existing control mechanisms, future research should be directed toward the design of alternative control circuits, modified regulatory proteins, and synthetically prepared recognition sequences. This new field of *synthetic biology* offers unlimited possibilities and in some cases could provide a true teleological design instead of the normal haphazard mode of Darwinian evolution. One might, on the one hand, propose that evolution of the human brain would sometimes be able to short-circuit the normal evolutionary process; but on the other hand, one might argue that the human brain and its product, genetic engineering, are all regular elements of a Grand Plan for evolution.

Practical Aspects of Future Research: Construction of Efficient and Safe Vectors

In addition to trying to understand the natural λ phage and constructing new "better λ phages," future research should be directed toward more practical goals. For instance, mutants of λ are being constructed to serve as better vectors (or vehicles) for carrying and studying various segments of foreign DNAs and to serve as efficient templates for synthesis of new gene products. By restructuring the phage, it should be possible to easily insert and select for λ vectors that carry any desired DNA fragments from various organisms, including even human DNA, to propagate them in large quantities, and to produce the required gene products using either their natural promoters or λ promoters. Thus it should be possible to synthesize in large quantities any human protein or polypeptide, many of great medical importance. Furthermore, by directed mutagenesis many new variants of human proteins could easily be constructed and tested for the desired pharmacological activities. This is an area of great opportunity.

Since there is a general, perhaps sometimes justified, fear of the release into nature of a vector that carries some potentially harmful cloned foreign gene, effort is being directed toward the development of safer λ vectors. The design of such a vector must take into account all of its possible primary and secondary routes of escape. One should first realize that the phage vector and host combination is a two-component system, in which each component alone is essentially safe, since the bacterial host does not carry the cloned fragment, and the phage vector is unable to propagate by itself. The principal routes of escape are as follows: (1) formation of a stable lysogen or plasmid carrier in the laboratory host followed by escape of this self-replicating system; (2) escape of the phage itself, which then has to find in nature a suitable host, infect it, and either replicate or form a stable phage-host system.

Route (1) can be blocked by the *att⁻ int⁻ c*I⁻ and *vir* mutations in the phage and the *att* deletion in the laboratory host, a design that blocks the formation of stable lysogens, and by the *cro⁻*, *c*17, *ri*ᶜ, *nin*R and some *vs* mutations, which prevent the establishment of plasmids. To further reduce the danger of formation of stable lysogens or plasmid carriers, the laboratory host should carry some conditional mutations that would block its propagation in nature. Moreover, the routine treatment of the lysate with chloroform eliminates practically all surviving bacteria, including lysogens and plasmid carriers.

The successful escape of the phage particles (route 2) is by itself a very improbable event, since phage particles are quite sensitive to dessication, cannot survive the acidity of the stomach in case of accidental ingestion, and have a low chance to encounter sensitive hosts in nature. The chance of survival in nature can be further reduced by introducing mutations that (a) permit the phage to retain its integrity and to propagate only in very special laboratory media, e.g., at high putrescine concentrations, and that (b) eliminate the tail genes with resulting production of only heads packed with noninfectious DNA. When required, such heads can be made infectious but only under special laboratory conditions by adding separately prepared tails. This design practically eliminates the possibility for the packaged DNA to infect any host in the natural environment and then secondarily transmit the cloned DNA in the form of a prophage, plasmid, or even a recombinant phage, if the susceptible host encountered in the natural environment carries a lambdoid prophage. There are also many other designs possible to further enhance the safety of the λ vector, but one should always keep in mind that they must not reduce the capacity of the phage to propagate and produce a maximum yield of the desired DNA in a minimum volume, since handling of large volumes introduces additional hazards.

Another practical application may be the use of specially designed λ lysogens in a simple test for detection of potential carcinogens and other products that react with DNA and thus induce λ prophage. Induction of a lysogen in which the *lac* operon is coupled to the p_L promoter would result in production of β-galactosidase, which could be easily detected with chromogenic indicators. A very simple test could be devised that would consist of mixing (1) a lyophylized lysogen of λ*trp-lac c*I⁺, (2) lyophylized liver homogenate (to metabolically activate some carcinogens), (3) reconstitution medium containing XG (5-bromo-4-chloro-3-indoyl-β-D-galactoside) and ONPG (orthotonitrophenyl-β-D-galactoside), and (4) a putative carcinogen. Weak induction would result in production of a blue color from the XG indicator, which would progressively turn green, as higher production of induced β-galactosidase would split ONPG to a yellow product. Other genes could be coupled to the $\lambda\, p_L$ or p_R promoters and other sensitive techniques could be devised for the detection of the products of these genes. Many suitable genetic modifications could also be tried in the induction pathway of the host and in the λ gene cI, as to improve the sensitivity of the test.

These are only a few hints of future basic and practical developments in this field, for the advent of genetic engineering permits unlimited projections governed only by the imagination and ingenuity of the experimenter.

ACKNOWLEDGMENTS

The author is greatly indebted to all his former and present associates who made crucial contributions to this field, namely Fred Blattner, Kjell Bøvre, Karin Carlson, Randall Chase, Mike Fiandt, Arabinda Guha, Sid Hayes, Alik Honigman, Zdenka Hradecna, Shiu-Lok Hu, Bob Iyer, Gary Kayajanian, Henryk Kubinski, Sushil Kumar, Homer Lozeron, Sister Veronica Mary Maher, Vance Makin, K.-K. Mark, N. Murata, John Nijkamp, Zofia Opara-Kubinska, Erik Rosenvold, John Salstrom, Peter Sheldrick, Willem Stevens, Bill Summers, Elizabeth Szybalski, the late Maciej Tabaczynski, Karol Taylor, and Barbara Westmoreland (listed alphabetically) during the years of 1965–75. Collaboration with the laboratories of John Abelson, Sankar Adhya, Ekke Bautz, Peter Besmer, Enrico Calef, Rich Calendar, Allen Campbell, Jim Dahlberg, Norman Davidson, Bill Dove, David Friedman, Peter Geiduschek, Max Gottesman, Ira Herskowitz, Fumio Imamoto, Dick Jaskunas, Gobind Khorana, Art Landy, Yvonne Lanni, Peggy Lieb, Mike Malamy, Bob Miller, Ena Mosharrafa, Musuyatsu Nomura, Hans Ris, Ethan Signer, Ann Skalka, Mark Shulman, Peter Starlinger, René Thomas, Bob Weisberg, and Jim Zissler on these and related subjects, which led to joint notes or publications, is also acknowledged with gratitude. I am also thankful for permission to include the yet unpublished data of Mark Ptashne, Dennis Kleid, Barbara Meyer, Marty Rosenberg, Debbie Steege, Joan Steitz, Shiu-Lok Hu, Alik Honigman, John Salstrom, and Eric Rosenvold. Special thanks for editing this review are due to E. Szybalski.

The work leading to this review was supported in part by National Cancer Institute Grant CA-07175.

REFERENCES

Alberts, B. 1973. Studies on the replication of DNA. *In* B. A. Hamkalo and J. Papaconstantinou, eds. Molecular cytogenetics. Pp. 233–51. Plenum Press, New York.

Blattner, F. R. and J. E. Dahlberg. 1972. RNA synthesis startpoints in bacteriophage λ: Are the promoter and operator transcribed? Nature New Biol. 237:227–32.

Blattner, F. R., J. E. Dahlberg, J. K. Boettiger, M. Fiandt, and W. Szybalski. 1972. Distance from a promoter mutation to an RNA synthesis startpoint on bacteriophage λ DNA. Nature New Biol. 237:232–36.

Blattner, F. R., M. Fiandt, K. K. Hass, P. A. Twose, and W. Szybalski. 1974. Deletions and insertions in the immunity region of coliphage lambda: Revised measurements of the promoter-startpoint distance. Virology 62:458–71.

Bronson, M. J., C. Squires, and C. Yanofsky. 1973. Nucleotide sequence from tryptophan messenger RNA of *Escherichia coli:* The sequence corresponding to the amino-terminal region of the first polypeptide specified by the operon. Proc. Nat. Acad. Sci. USA 70:2335–39.

Campbell, J. H., and B. Rolfe. 1975. Function of the *rex* gene of phage lambda, p. 49. *In* Biology of temperate phage. 5th Internat. Conf., Airlie House, VA.

Dahlberg, J. E., and F. R. Blattner. 1973. *In vitro* transcription products of lambda DNA: Nucleotide sequences and regulatory sites. *In* C. F. Fox and W. S. Robinson, eds. Virus research. Pp. 533–43. Second I.C.N.-U.C.L.A. Symposium on Molecular Biology. Academic Press, New York.

Dahlberg, J. E., and F. R. Blattner. 1975. Sequence of promoter operator proximal region of the major leftward RNA of bacteriophage lambda. Nuc. Acids Res. 2:1441–58.

Darlix, J. L., and P. Fromageot. 1972. Discontinuous *in vitro* transcription of DNA. Biochimie 54:47–54.

Davidson, N., and W. Szybalski. 1971. Physical and chemical characteristics of lambda DNA. *In* A. D. Hershey, ed. The bacteriophage lambda. Pp. 45–82. Cold Spring Harbor Laboratory, Cold Spring Harbor, N.Y.

Dove, W. F. 1968. The genetics of lambdoid phages. Ann. Rev. Genet. 2:305–40.

Dove, W. F., H. Inokuchi, and W. F. Stevens. 1971. Replication control in phage lambda. *In* A. D. Hershey, ed. The bacteriophage lambda. Pp. 747–71. Cold Spring Harbor Laboratory, Cold Spring Harbor, N.Y.

Dressler, D. 1975. Recent excitement in the DNA growing point problem. Ann. Rev. Microbiol. 29:525–59.

Echols, H. 1971a. Regulation of lytic development. *In* A. D. Hershey, ed. The bacteriophage lambda. Pp. 247–70. Cold Spring Harbor Laboratory, Cold Spring Harbor, N.Y.

Echols, H. 1971b. Lysogeny: Viral repression and site-specific recombination. Ann. Rev. Biochem. 40:827–54.

Echols, H. 1972. Developmental pathways for the temperate phage: Lysis vs. lysogeny. Ann. Rev. Genet. 6:157–90.

Edlin, G., L. Lin, and R. Kudrna. 1975. λ lysogens of *E. coli.* reproduce more rapidly than non-lysogens. Nature 255:735–37.

Eisen, H., and M. Ptashne. 1971. Regulation of repressor synthesis. *In* A. D. Hershey, ed. The bacteriophage lambda. Pp. 239–45. Cold Spring Harbor Laboratory, Cold Spring Harbor, N.Y.

Epp, C., and M. H. Pearson. 1976. Association of bacteriophage lambda N gene protein with *E. coli* RNA polymerase. *In* R. Losick and M. Chamberlin, eds., RNA polymerase. Pp. 667–91. Cold Spring Harbor Laboratory, Cold Spring Harbor, N.Y.

Friedman, D. I., G. S. Wilgus, and R. J. Mural. 1973. Gene *N* regulator function of phage λ*imm*21: Evidence that a site of *N* action differs from a site of *N* recognition. J. Mol. Biol. 81:505–16.

Gefter, M. L. 1975. DNA replication. Ann. Rev. Biochem. 44:45–78.

Georgopoulos, C. P. 1971a. Bacterial mutants in which the gene *N* function of bacteriophage lambda is blocked have an altered RNA polymerase. Proc. Nat. Acad. Sci. USA 68:2977–81.

Georgopoulos, C. P. 1971b. A bacterial mutation affecting *N* function. *In* A. D. Hershey, ed. The bacteriophage lambda. Pp. 639–45. Cold Spring Harbor Laboratory, Cold Spring Harbor, N.Y.

Ghysen, A., and M. Pironio. 1972. Relationship between the *N* function of bacteriophage λ and host RNA polymerase. J. Mol. Biol. 65:259–72.

Greenblatt, J. 1973. Regulation of the expression of the *N* gene of bacteriophage lambda. Proc. Nat. Acad. Sci. USA 70:421–24.

Hayes, S., and W. Szybalski. 1973a. Control of short leftward transcripts from the immunity and *ori* regions in induced coliphage lambda. Molec. Gen. Genet. 126:275–90.

Hayes, S., and W. Szybalski, 1973b. Synthesis of RNA primer for lambda DNA replication is controlled by phage and host. *In* B. A. Hamkalo and J. Papaconstantinou, eds. Molecular cytogenetics. Pp. 277–83. Plenum Press, New York.

Hayes, S., and W. Szybalski. 1975. Role of *oop* RNA primer in initiation of coliphage lambda DNA replication. *In* M. Goulian, P. Hanawalt, and C. F. Fox, eds. DNA synthesis and its regulation. Pp. 486–512. W. A. Benjamin, Menlo Park, Calif.

Herskowitz, I. 1974. Control of gene expression in bacteriophage lambda. Ann. Rev. Genet. 7:289–324.

Honigman, A., S.-L. Hu, R. Chase, and W. Szybalski. 1976. The 4 S *oop* RNA is a leader sequence for the immunity-established transcription in coliphage lambda. Nature, 262:112–16.

Horiuchi, T., H. Koga, H. Inokuchi, and J. Tomizawa. 1969. Lambda phage mutants insensitive to temperature-sensitive repressor. I. Isolation and genetic analysis of weak-virulent mutants. Molec. Gen. Genet. 104:51–58.

Hu, S., J. S. Salstrom, and W. Szybalski. 1975. Role of gene *N* and the *v*2 mutation in the Tof function and leftward transcription in coliphage lambda. Abstr. Ann. Meeting Am. Soc. Microbiol. 75:234.

Jacob, F., and J. Monod. 1961. Genetic regulatory mechanisms in the synthesis of proteins. J. Mol. Biol. 3:318–56.

Kleckner, N. E. 1974. Plasmid formation by bacteriophage lambda. Ph.D. thesis, M. I. T., Cambridge, Mass.

Kleid, D. G., K. L. Agarwal, and H. G. Khorana. 1975. The nucleotide sequence in the promoter region of the gene *N* of bacteriophage λ. J. Biol. Chem. 250:5574–82.

Kleid, D., Z. Humayun, A. Jeffrey, and M. Ptashne. 1976. Novel properties of a restriction endonuclease isolated from *Haemophilus parahaemolyticus*. Proc. Natl. Acad. Sci. USA 73:293–97.

Kornberg, A. 1976. RNA priming of DNA replication. *In* R. Losick and M. Chamberlin, eds., RNA polymerase. Pp. 331–52. Cold Spring Harbor Laboratory. Cold Spring Harbor, N.Y.

Kourilsky, P., M.-F. Bourguignon, and F. Gros. 1971. Kinetics of viral transcription after induction of prophage. *In* A. D. Hershey, ed. The bacteriophage lambda. Pp. 647–66. Cold Spring Harbor Laboratory, Cold Spring Harbor, N.Y.

Leibowitz, P., S. M. Weissman, and C. M. Radding. 1971. Nucleotide sequence of a ribonucleic acid transcribed *in vitro* from λ phage deoxyribonucleic acid. J. Biol. Chem. 246:5120–39.

Lozeron, H. A., and P. J. Anevski. 1975. Identification of p_L-initiated RNA at the 5'-terminal end of the *N*-mediated RNA-transcript in bacteriophage λ and $\phi 80imm$ λ. Abstr. Ann. Meeting Am. Soc. Microbiol. 75:234.

Lozeron, H. A., J. E. Dahlberg, and W. Szybalski. 1976. Processing of the major leftward mRNA of coliphage lambda. Virology 71:262–77.

Lozeron, H. A., M. L. Funderburgh, J. E. Dahlberg, B. P. Stark, and W. Szybalski. 1972. Identity of *in vitro* and *in vivo* initiation of phage lambda mRNA: Analysis of *in vivo* cleavage products. Abstr. Ann. Meeting Am. Soc. Microbiol. 72:237.

Maniatis, T., M. Ptashne, K. Backman, D. Kleid, S. Flashman, A. Jeffrey, and R. Maurer. 1975. Recognition sequences of repressor and polymerase in operators of bacteriophage lambda. Cell 5:109–13.

Meyer, B., D. Kleid, and M. Ptashne. 1975. λ repressor turns off transcription of its own gene. Proc. Natl. Acad. Sci. USA 72:4785–9.

Miller, J. F. 1974. GUG and UUG are initiation codons in vivo. Cell 1:73–76.

Okazaki, R., A. Sugino, S. Hirose, T. Okazaki, Y. Imae, R. Kainuma-Kuroda, T. Ogawa, M. Arisawa, and Y. Kurosawa. 1973. The discontinuous replication of DNA. *In* R. D. Wells and R. B. Inman, eds. DNA synthesis *in vitro*. Pp. 83–106. University Park Press, Baltimore.

Pirrotta, V. 1975. Sequence of the o_R operator of phage λ. Nature 254:114–17.

Ptashne, M. 1971. Repressor and its action. *In* A. D. Hershey, ed. The bacteriophage lambda. Pp. 221–37. Cold Spring Harbor Laboratory, Cold Spring Harbor, N.Y.

Ptashne, M., K. Backman, M. Z. Humayun, A. Jeffrey, R. Maurer, B. Meyer, and R. T. Sauer. 1976. Autoregulation and function of a repressor in bacteriophage lambda. Science 194: 156–61.

Rambach, A. 1973. Replicator mutants of bacteriophage λ: Characterization of two subclasses. Virology 54:270–77.

Ray, P. N., and M. L. Pearson. 1974. Evidence for post-transcriptional control of the morphogenetic genes of bacteriophage lambda. J. Mol. Biol. 85:163–75.

Reichardt, L. F. 1975a. Control of baceriophage lambda repressor synthesis after phage infection: the role of the *N, c*II, *c*III anc *cro* products. J. Mol. Biol. 93:267–88.

Reichardt, L. F. 1975b. Control of bacteriophage lambda repressor synthesis: Regulation of the maintenance pathway by the *cro* and *c*I products. J. Mol. Biol. 93:289–309.

Richardson, J. P., C. Grimley, and C. Lowery. 1975. Transcription termination factor rho activity is altered in *Escherichia coli* with *suA* gene mutations. Proc. Nat. Acad. Sci. USA 72:1725–28.

Roberts, J. F., and C. W. Roberts. 1975. Proteolytic cleavage of bacteriophage lambda repressor in induction. Proc. Natl. Acad. Sci. USA 72:147–51.

Rosenberg, M., S. Weissman, and B. deCrombrugghe. 1975. Termination of transcription in bacteriophage λ. Heterogeneous 3'-terminal oligo-adenylate addition and the effects of ρ factor. J. Biol. Chem. 250:4755–64.

Sakaki, Y., A. E. Karu, S. Linn, and H. Echols. 1973. Purification and properties of the γ-protein specified by bacteriophage λ: An inhibitor of the host *rec* BC recombination enzyme. Proc. Natl. Acad. Sci. USA 10:2215–19.

Salstrom, J. S., and W. Szybalski. 1976. Phage lambda *nut* L mutants unable to utilize *N* product for leftward transcription. Fed. Proc. 35:1538.

Scherer, G., G. Hobom, and H. Kössel. 1976. DNA base sequence of the p_0 promoter region of phage λ. Nature 265:117–21.

Shimada, K., and A. Campbell. 1974. Int-constitutive mutants of bacteriophage lambda. Proc. Natl. Acad. Sci. USA 10:237–41.

Shine, J., and L. Dalgarno. 1974. The 3'-terminal sequence of *Escherichia coli* 16 S ribosomal RNA: Complementarity to nonsense triplets and ribosome binding sites. Proc. Nat. Acad. Sci. USA 71:1342–46.

Skalka, A. 1974. A replicator's view of recombination (and repair). *In* R. F. Grell, ed. Mechanisms in recombination. Pp. 421–32. Plenum Press, New York.

Sly, W. S., K. Rabideau, and A. Kolber. 1970. The mechanisms of lambda virulence. II. Regulatory mutations in classical lambda virulence. *In* A. D. Hershey, ed. The bacteriophage lambda. Pp. 575–88. Cold Spring Harbor Laboratory, Cold Spring Harbor, N.Y.

Smith, G. R., and J. Hedgpeth. 1975. Oligo(A) not coded by DNA generating 3'-terminal heterogeneity in λ phage RNA. J. Biol. Chem. 250:4818–21.

Stahl, F. W., and M. M. Stahl. 1974. Red-mediated recombination in bacteriophage lambda. *In* R. F. Grell, ed. Mechanisms in recombination. Pp 407–19. Plenum Press, New York.

Sussman, R., and H. Ben Zeev. 1975. Proposed mechanism of bacteriophage lambda induction: acquisition of binding sites for lambda repressor by DNA of the host. Proc. Natl. Acad. Sci. USA 72:1973–76.

Szybalski, W. 1969. Initiation and patterns of transcription during phage development. *In* Canadian Cancer Conference (Proceedings of the Eighth Canadian Cancer Research Conference, Honey Harbor, Ont., 1968). 8:183–215. Pergamon Press, New York.

Szybalski, W. 1970. Various controls of transcription in coliphage lambda. *In* L. Silvestri, ed. RNA polymerase and transcription. Lepetit Colloquia on Biology and Medicine 1. Pp. 209–17. North-Holland, Amsterdam.

Szybalski, W. 1971. Controls of transcription and replication in coliphage lambda. p. 1–45. *In* Karl-August-Forster Lectures: Informationsgesteuerte Synthese, Akad. Wiss. Literat. Mainz. Mathem. Naturwiss. Klasse. 6:1–45. F. Steiner Verlag, Wiesbaden, Germany.

Szybalski, W. 1972. Transcription and replication in *E. coli* bacteriophage lambda. *In* L. Ledoux (ed.). Uptake of informative molecules by living cells. North-Holland, Amsterdam.

Szybalski, W. 1974a. Initiation and regulation of transcription in coliphage lambda. *In* B. B. Biswas, R. K. Mondal, A. Stevens, and W. E. Cohn (eds.). Control of transcription. Pp. 201–12. Plenum Press, New York.

Szybalski, W. 1974b. Genetic and molecular map of *Escherichia coli* bacteriophage lambda (λ). *In* A. I. Laskin and H. A. Lechevalier (eds.). Handbook of microbiology. 4:611–18. CRC Press, Cleveland, Ohio.

Szybalski, 1974c. Bacteriophage lambda. *In* R. C. King (ed.). Handbook of genetics. 1:309–22. Plenum Press, New York.

Szybalski, W. 1976. Genetic and molecular map of *Escherichia coli* bacteriophage lambda (λ). *In* G. D. Fasman (ed.). Handbook of biochemistry and molecular biology. 3d ed. Vol. 2. Nucleic acids. Pp. 677–85. CRC Press, Cleveland, Ohio.

Szybalski, W., K. Bøvre, A. Guha, Z. Hradecna, S. Kumar, H. A. Lozeron, V. Maher, Sr., H. J. J. Nijkamp, W. C. Summers, and K. Taylor. 1969. Transcriptional controls in developing bacteriophages. J. Cell Physiol. 74 Suppl; 1:33–70.

Szybalski, W., K. Bøvre, S. Hayes, Z. Hradecna, S. Kumar, H. Z. Lozeron, H. J. J. Nijkamp, and W. F. Stevens. 1970. Transcriptional units and their controls in *Escherichia coli* phage λ: Operons and scriptions. Cold Spring Harbor Symp. Quant. Biol. 35:341–53.

Thomas, R. 1971. Control circuits. *In* A. D. Hershey (ed.). The bacteriophage lambda. Cold Spring Harbor Laboratory, Cold Spring Harbor, N.Y.

Thomas, R. 1973. Boolean formalization of genetic control circuits. J. Theor. Biol. 42:563–85.

Walz, A., and V. Pirrotta. 1975. Sequence of the P_R promoter of phage λ. Nature 254:118–21.

MICHAEL CASHEL

Pleiotropic Regulatory Effects of ppGpp in Bacteria

2

The ability of any cell to adapt and coordinate its biochemical activities is the source of endless fascination in regulatory biology. How does a cell regulate its components? How does a cell coordinate its constructive and destructive biochemical activities so as to take advantage of nutritional abundance but survive impoverishment?

There is little doubt that strong selective pressures have led to the evolution of cells possessing the enzymatic means of adaptively exploiting changes in nutritional.abundance. On the one hand, such mechanisms already known are often highly specific for particular substrates or biochemical pathways as in cases of induction, repression, and feedback effects. Even in the recently appreciated instances of autogenous regulation (Goldberger and Deeley, this volume), regulation is highly specific. On the other hand, it seems likely that during nutritional deprivation cellular survival could require mechanisms with more widespread effects that simultaneously serve to economize a variety of cellular activities. Many nonessential cellular enzymatic activities could be turned off in a cell on a metabolically tight budget. Alternatively such mechanisms can enhance the cellular efficiency of utilization of an excellent carbon source, such as glucose. A well-known regulatory signal in this case is $3'5'$ cyclic AMP. This nucleotide is known to exert its pleiotropic effects simultaneously at many genetic sites, operating through interactions with a cyclic AMP binding protein.

This review article concerns a second mode of pleiotropic regulation that seems to restrict a variety of cellular activities during nutritional impoverish-

Laboratory of Molecular Genetics, National Institute of Child Health and Human Development, National Institutes of Health, Bethesda, Maryland 20014.

ment. Evidence will be reviewed that seems to implicate guanosine 3'5' bispyrophosphate as the negative regulatory effector in this system. Guanosine 3'5' bispyrophosphate is now abbreviated as ppGpp, but is often called magic spot I, or MS I, a name given it before structure determination (Cashel and Gallant, 1969; Cashel and Kalbacher, 1970; Sy and Lipmann, 1973; Que et al., 1973). A natural analogue of ppGpp exists that is closely related both structurally and metabolically and often accompanies ppGpp accumulation. This also bears a 3' pyrophosphate residue but otherwise is identical to GTP and is abbreviated pppGpp, magic spot II or MS II. Evidence relating to the mechanism of formation of ppGpp and pppGpp as well as their interrelationships has been reviewed and will only be summarily considered here (Block and Haseltine, 1974; Cashel and Gallant, 1974; Cashel, 1975). The concern here is with regulatory effects exerted by ppGpp on gene expression and bacterial physiology.

THE REL A GENE-DEPENDENT REGULATION SYSTEM

The bacterial regulatory system that led to the identification of ppGpp is functionally defined by mutant behavior. Single gene mutants (Borek, Rockenbach, and Ryan, 1956) were originally termed "relaxed RNA control" mutants (Stent and Brenner, 1961; Alfoldi, Stent, and Clowes, 1962) and are now denoted as mutants in the *rel* A locus. These relaxed mutants grow nearly as well as parental wild-type strains in both rich and minimal media but show a variety of differences in physiological activities during restriction of aminoacyl tRNA availability for protein synthesis (Alfoldi et al., 1963; Neidhardt, 1966). Historically, the first difference noted between mutant and wild-type strains was in the dependence of continued stable RNA accumulation on amino acid availability (Stent and Brenner, 1961). In wild-type bacteria stable RNA accumulation is dependent upon a sufficient supply of all twenty amino acids for continued protein synthesis. If protein synthesis is limited for any amino acid, then stable RNA accumulation is abruptly restricted or said to be under "stringent amino acid control" (Stent and Brenner, 1961). In otherwise isogenic but *rel* A mutants, stable RNA accumulation continues for a time unabated despite amino acid starvation. As will be discussed later, subsequent comparisons of the amino acid dependence of many physiological activities displayed by stringent-relaxed strain pairs during amino acid starvation have not only revealed many differences in addition to RNA accumulation but also a general pattern. The starved stringent strain curtails activities that persist in the starved relaxed strain. Such differences collectively define the "stringent response" to amino acid starvation. This regulatory system is by definition pleiotropic; its operation is governed by the expression of a single gene, but the regulatory manifestations of the activity of this gene are biochemically diverse, as we shall see.

IS PPGPP AN EFFECTOR OR AN EFFECT?

Rather strong but nevertheless circumstantial evidence has been adduced to implicate ppGpp as an inhibitor mediating the pleiotropic response of stringent strains to amino acid starvation.

The accumulation of ppGpp in stringent bacteria is the first detectable consequence of the stringent response other than restricted formation of aminoacylated tRNA (Cashel, 1969; Gallant et al., 1970). Amino acid-starved relaxed bacterial mutants do not accumulate ppGpp. In a variety of independent *rel* A mutants in *Escherichia coli,* closely related *Salmonella typhimurium*, and in distantly related *Bacillus subtilis*, the relaxed RNA control phenotype occurs, and such mutants also fail to accumulate ppGpp during amino acid starvation (Cashel, 1971; De Boer et al., 1971; Fiil, von Meyenberg, and Friesen, 1972; Kaplan, Atherly, and Barrett, 1973; Swanton and Edlin, 1972). There is also a close correlation between conditions provoking ppGpp accumulation and those triggering the stringent responses (Cashel, 1970; Gallant et al., 1970; Lund and Kjeldgaard, 1972; Kaplan, Atherly, and Barrett, 1973). The accumulation of ppGpp and the stringent response are not amino acid specific but occur after removal of any one of several different amino acids. These effects occur whether amino acids are removed from auxotrophs or inhibitors of amino acid biosynthesis are employed. The notion of ppGpp functioning as a pleiotropic inhibitor to mediate the stringent response is also consistent with the observed dominance of the wild-type allele in merodiploids (Fiil, 1969).

Elegant *in vitro* studies point to a role of the *rel* A$^+$ gene product in ppGpp formation. A purified protein termed the stringent factor does catalyze the synthesis of ppGpp and pppGpp by a pyrophosphate transfer reaction from ATP to GDP or GTP (Haseltine et al., 1972; Cochran and Byrne, 1973; Sy and Lipmann, 1973; Block and Haseltine, 1975). The *in vitro* formation of ppGpp and pppGpp is both stimulated and stabilized by the interaction of ribosomes, stringency factor, mRNA and codon-specified uncharged tRNA bound to the ribosomal acceptor site (Pedersen, Lund, and Kjeldgaard, 1973; Haseltine and Block, 1973). Uncharged tRNA can be displaced from the ribosomal A site by enzymatic binding (EF Tu mediated) of the cognate aminoacylated tRNA, an event that occasions the shutdown of ppGpp formation (Haseltine and Block, 1973). Generally these studies provide a reasonable account of whole cell ppGpp accumulation behavior in response to amino acid starvation. The conclusions bear on the regulatory effects of ppGpp only insofar as it can be demonstrated that the *rel* A$^+$ gene product is, in fact, the stringent factor. Block and Haseltine (1973) have analyzed the *in vitro* ppGpp biosynthetic activities of a number of independent, missense mutations of the *rel* gene derived by Fiil and Friesen (1968). Such studies enabled correlation of *in vitro* ppGpp synthetic rates with the degree of amino acid dependence of uridine labeling of RNA accumulation. Thus the evidence linking the *rel* A$^+$ gene product with the stringent factor is fairly strong.

CRITERIA FOR ASSESSING PPGPP REGULATORY EFFECTS

Thus *rel* A gene-dependent regulation defines a pleiotropic regulatory system, and strong circumstantial evidence allows the working notion that regulation is accomplished as a consequence of ppGpp accumulation.

There is a possibility that other regulatory signals exist that are *rel* gene-dependent in addition to ppGpp. Specifically, pppGpp accumulation often accompanies that of ppGpp, and it is a very real possibility that there are regulatory effects associated with only the guanosine pentaphosphate. Analysis of the regulatory differences between those strains accumulating only ppGpp (called *spo* T by Laffler and Gallant, 1974) and those accumulating both ppGpp and pppGpp (*spo* T$^+$) would provide information on this point. However our general experience with *spo* T$^+$ and *spo* T strains does not suggest a regulatory role for pppGpp that cannot be satisfied by ppGpp. Instead attention is usually focused on ppGpp as the effective regulator; detailed studies are necessary before this focus is really justified.

For purposes of estimating whether a cellular function might be regulated by ppGpp, the first question is whether the activity is subject to stringent amino acid control in diverse genetic backgrounds, in other words, in different relaxed-stringent pairs of strains. Amino acid-specific consequences of starvation do occur, such as derepression of specific biosynthetic pathways. Therefore it is important to verify that the activity measured is not amino acid-specific. Another interesting but troublesome consequence of starving certain auxotrophs for single amino acids or starving prototrophs for all amino acids simultaneously is that the pools of all four ribonucleoside 5' triphosphates are decreased in stringent strains but not in relaxed strains (Cashel and Gallant, 1969; Irr and Gallant, 1969; Sokawa, Nakao-Sato, and Kaziro, 1970). Such effects are not crucial to the operation of the stringent response since the response can be triggered by mild starvation conditions that reduce only GTP pool values with relatively minor effects on ATP pool levels (Nierlich, 1968; Gallant and Harada, 1969; Gallant et al., 1970). Such situations entail the use of conditional aminoacyl synthetase mutants at restrictive temperatures or more simply by valine addition to *E. coli* K 12 strains (Blatt, Pledger, and Umbarger, 1972). The depletion of all ribonucleoside 5' triphosphate pools may reflect a very major energy drain, as pointed out by

Gallant et al. (1970). For example, histidine deprivation of a histidine auxotroph blocked prior to the AICAR branch point in histidine biosynthesis can result in accumulation of purine rings as an early intermediate in histidine biosynthesis and ATP consumption. However starvation of a histidine auxotroph blocked beyond the AICAR branch point allows recycling of the purine ring, and the ATP pools remain fairly stable. The simultaneous withdrawal of all amino acids might well provoke a high energy drain through an analogous mechanism operating through rather massive derepression of virtually all the amino acid biosynthetic pathways.

Thus if all nucleotide pools are depleted, a mild dependence of a given cellular activity may not indicate ppGpp regulation but merely that biological energy is necessary for the cellular activity in question.

Another possible way of estimating ppGpp regulation of a given cellular function is provided by *rel* gene-independent accumulation of ppGpp during energy source starvation (Lazzarini, Cashel, and Gallant, 1971; Harshman and Yamazaki, 1971). In this manner even relaxed mutants can be made to accumulate ppGpp. The proposed mechanism for *rel* A-independent ppGpp accumulation is that the rate of degradation of ppGpp is decreased but without increasing the ppGpp synthetic rate (Gallant, Margason, and Finch, 1972). The result is a slow accumulation of ppGpp that might be correlated with the onset of regulation, provided there are no complications due to catabolite repression or to generalized consequences of energy source starvation.

The above criteria for estimating whether a cellular function is regulated by ppGpp at best provide only strong correlations between ppGpp accumulation and the regulation of a particular cellular activity. In none of the instances in which correlations of this sort have been described have mutants been isolated that are resistant to the regulatory effects of ppGpp. Such a search might be worthwhile; the verification of ppGpp resistance of such activities *in vitro* would constitute the first compelling indication that regulation by ppGpp really occurs.

It is also worthwhile noting that no mutants are yet known that are absolutely deficient in ppGpp; thus there is no way of assessing whether ppGpp provides a cellular function other than regulation. Several laboratories, including our own, are attempting to isolate an amber mutation in the *rel* A locus to answer this question. If ppGpp does indeed provide an essential cellular function, it will be interesting to know the mechanism of magic spotless death under restrictive conditions. If not, ppGpp probably functions primarily as a regulatory signal.

We now turn to a survey of a fairly enormous and diverse literature describing cellular activities that have been proposed to be under stringent control and thus quite probably regulated by ppGpp. For any given activity, published disagreement is the rule rather than the exception,[1] and objective justice cannot be done to the arguments favoring one or another interpretation.

RIBOSOMAL AND TRANSFER RNA REGULATION

As alluded to earlier, RNA accumulation was historically the first cellular activity noted to be *rel* gene-dependent. A provocative review has been written on this topic (Gallant and Lazzarini, 1975).

Estimates of the rates of ribosomal RNA (rRNA) and tRNA transcription as a function of the stringent response are complicated by ppGpp inhibition of membrane transport of nucleobases and nucleosides. Thus early measurements of reduced RNA synthesis by nucleoside or base labeling made without appropriate corrections for stringent control of isotope equilibration were grossly overestimated. More recent measurements clearly indicate a moderate reduction (4- to 10-fold) of rRNA formation during the stringent response (Nierlich, 1968; Winslow and Lazzarini, 1969; Lazzarini and Dahlberg, 1971; Stomato and Pettijohn, 1971). This inhibition of rRNA synthesis is generally taken to be exerted at the level of initiation of transcription partly as a result of electron microscopic visualization of ribosomal cistron gene expression (Hamkalo and Miller, 1973) and also because of only mild degrees of inhibition of chain elongation rates. A recurring question arises concerning the possibility of increased rRNA degradation accounting for the inhibition of RNA accumulation rather than decreased rates of rRNA synthesis. Measurements by Lazzarini and Dahlberg (1971) indicate that if degradation of nascent RNA does occur, it is too fast to be measurable under their pulse conditions. Such a rapid time scale for degradation would be faster than occurs during purine or pyrimidine starvation of auxotrophs and therefore is unprecedented.

Clear evidence of stringent regulation of tRNA synthesis has been obtained. Primakoff and Berg (1970) have demonstrated that ϕ 80 phage bearing the suIII suppressor tRNA gene produces phage mRNA but not suppressor tRNA during the stringent response. More recently, Ikemura and Dahlberg (1973) have shown that most tRNA species, but not all, are subject to stringent control as judged from phosphate labeling of tRNA bands visualized after electrophoresis in acrylamide gels.

The verification of these putative regulatory effects of ppGpp with *in vitro* systems has been fitful. There were early indications that EF-Tu and EF-Ts comprised a factor (psi) capable of selectively stimulating rDNA cistron transcription and that this activity was selectively inhibited by ppGpp (Travers, Kamen, and Cashel, 1970). These early experiments, however, could not be confirmed (Haseltine 1972; Birnbaum and Kaplan, 1972). Alternative attempts to show ppGpp inhibition of rRNA transcription have since been made with gently lysed extracts showing high rates of rRNA synthesis; the results are conflicting (Murooka and Lazzarini, 1973; van Ooyen et al., 1975). Similarly, permeabilized cells support rRNA synthesis, but accompanying the acquisition of permeability is a loss of stringent control that cannot be restored by exogenous addition of ppGpp (Lazzarini and Johnson, 1973; Atherly, 1974). Very recently promising reports have been made showing ppGpp-induced inhibition of rRNA synthesis in crude extracts (Van Ooyen et al., 1975; Block, 1975; Reiness et al., 1975). The pendulum on the issue of *in vitro* ppGpp effects on rRNA transcription may finally be damped through an analysis of mutants defective in factors apparently specifying rRNA transcription (Chaney and Schlessinger, 1975). Once the way cells turn on expression of rRNA genes is understood, a better understanding of how. they are turned off might be achieved.

In vitro transcription of tRNA genes can be demonstrated (Yang et al., 1974; Reiness et al., 1975), but no inhibitory effects of ppGpp have been noted. This is all the more remarkable since the tRNA transcript generally studied is the same suIII species demonstrated by Primakoff and Berg (1970) to be under stringent control.

MESSENGER RNA REGULATION

Measurements of the proportion of stable RNA in transcripts isolated during the stringent response indicate at least a twofold reduction in mRNA transcription in *E. coli* (Lazzarini and Dahlberg, 1971). In *Bacillus subtilis,* where the normal portion of unstable RNA transcription is larger than in *E. coli,* higher estimates of inhibition of mRNA formation have been made during the stringent response (Gallant and Margason, 1972). On the other hand, since amino acid biosynthetic enzymes can be derepressed during amino acid starvation in stringent cells, the mRNA species encoding these enzymes must escape stringent control. Measurements of stringent control of individual mRNA species reported in the literature yield not only different conclusions about different species but also are in conflict for the same species.[2] There is a recent, clear indication that ribosomal proteins and the mRNA species encoding them are under stringent control (Dennis and Nomura, 1974; 1975), but so far there is no *in vitro* evidence for ppGpp inhibition of ribosomal protein synthesis (Kaltschmidt, Kahan, and Nomura, 1974).

In vitro systems sustaining transcription coupled to translation have, of course, been incubated in the presence and absence of ppGpp. Both stimulatory and inhibitory effects have been observed that seem to operate at the level of initiation of transcription (Varmus, Perlman, and Pastan, 1971; Zubay, Gielow, and Englesberg, 1971; deCrombruggie et al., 1972; Aboud and Pastan, 1973, 1975; Yang and Zubay, 1973; Yang et al., 1974). The effects are reproducible, nucleotide-specific, and promoter-dependent. They are also often inconsistent with what is known of the ability to form certain enzymes in growing cells. For example, synthesis *in vitro* of an enzyme in the arginine ECBH gene cluster is inhibited by ppGpp but derepressed in stringent strains by arginine starvation (Yang et al., 1974). Another is that beta galactosidase synthesis *in vitro* seems to be dependent upon ppGpp in a fashion additive with cAMP effects, yet the enzyme is massively inducible during exponential growth on glycerol when ppGpp levels are very low.

It is clear from rifampicin sensitivities of rRNA, tRNA, and mRNA transcription that the enzyme transcribing all these RNA species in *E. coli* shares at least a beta subunit. How a single enzyme can transcribe various genetic elements selectively during normal cellular growth as well as during the stringent response is a central problem. By analogy with the cAMP system one cannot but wonder whether there exists a ppGpp binding protein that functions at the transcription level.

In vitro studies with homogeneous RNA polymerase preparations and synthetic templates have led to the demonstration that ppGpp inhibits initiation of transcription with d(I-C) as a template whereas d(A-T) transcription is unaltered (Cashel et al., 1975). At the same time, both structural features of ppGpp that distinguish it from GTP serve to prevent nonspecific inhibition of RNA chain elongation by ppGpp (Cashel et al., 1975). However, the simple notion that ppGpp operates by selectively restricting initiations of RNA chains beginning with GTP (Cashel, 1970) is rather seriously quenched by Ikemura and Dahlberg's (1973) observation of RNA chains made very efficiently during the stringent response that have a GTP 5' terminus. Perhaps more significantly, Ginsberg and Steitz (1975) have demonstrated that the 5' terminus of the 30S precursor of rRNA bears an A start.

Thus although transcriptional control by ppGpp seems quite a palatable notion from cellular experiments, *in vitro* studies are sometimes promising but more often not.

REGULATION AT THE LEVEL OF PROTEIN FORMATION AND DEGRADATION

Resupplementing amino acid-starved stringent cells with the missing amino acid results in the disappearance of ppGpp with a half-life of about twenty seconds (Cashel, 1970; Fiil, von Meyenberg, and Friesen, 1972; Lund and Kjeldgaard, 1972), and thereafter protein synthesis and growth resume. Using *spo*T mutants having 10 to 20 times slower rates of ppGpp decay, Laffler and Gallant (1974) have noted that appreciable protein accumulation does not occur until after ppGpp disappears despite the presence of a full complement of amino acids. Similar correlations have been obtained for rRNA accumulation (Stamminger and Lazzarini, 1974). These observations have been taken to mean that ppGpp inhibits protein synthesis directly and severely. Numerous *in vitro* protein synthesis experiments have demonstrated that ppGpp can inhibit all phases of protein synthesis under certain conditions in a manner analogous to GDP (Arai et al., 1972; Legault, Jeantet, and Gros, 1972; Yoshida, Travers, and Clark, 1972). In all cases the inhibition is reversed by increasing the GTP concentration. Considerations of the pool sizes of ppGpp, GDP, and GTP lead to the prediction that only moderate inhibition of protein synthesis (Hamel and Cashel, 1973; 1974) could be exerted nonspecifically at ribosomal binding events. These studies raise a dilemma concerning the lack of specificity of ppGpp effects as well as the prediction that is not borne out by cellular behavior. If ppGpp inhibits protein synthesis nonspecifically, a stringent strain should not be as efficient as a relaxed strain in depressing its biosynthetic enzymes and growing when shifted from amino acid-rich media to amino acid-poor media. Quite the opposite is observed (Sokawa, Sokawa, and Kaziro, 1971; 1974). I suspect that nonspecific inhibitory effects of ppGpp on protein-synthetic components are physiologically reversible. For example, ppGpp binds to EF-Tu even more tightly than GDP, which binds about 100 times more tightly than GTP (Miller, Cashel, and Weissbach, 1973). Yet in the presence of EF-Ts and charged tRNA, ppGpp is readily displaced by GTP to form a functional complex. *In vitro* attempts to measure ppGpp inhibition of phage coat protein synthesis using phage RNA as messenger have been negative (Lang 1974).

Work from Kaziro's group (Sokawa, Sokawa, and Kaziro, 1974) has led to the suggestion that relaxed mutants might be defective in aminoacyl tRNA binding, a hypothesis not yet verified in the literature. An alternative explanation to the sluggish outgrowth behavior of relaxed strains (first noticed by Alfoldi et al., 1963) has been pursued by Hall and Gallant (1971a,b). They found lowered specific activities of proteins formed in relaxed strains in addition to lowered enzymatic activities; this suggested that a consequence of the *rel* A mutation could be an impairment of coding fidelity. This perturbation could well be an effect on ribosomal function quite independent of the presence or absence of ppGpp and reflecting another role for the *rel* A gene product in ribosomal function. *In vitro* verification of this notion using measurements of error frequencies in the presence and absence of ppGpp have also not yet been published. A functional difference in rates of polysome assembly has been noted in careful experiments by Cozzone and Donini (1973). However, although it has been suggested that ppGpp may be involved in protein synthesis initiation (Rapaport, Svihovec, and Zamecnik, 1975), this does not fit with what is known of *E. coli* ppGpp synthesis *in vitro*.

Relaxed and stringent strains do clearly differ in their ability to proteolytically degrade proteins (Sussman and Gilvarg, 1969). This phenomenon has been extensively studied by Goldberg (1971a, 1972) who found proteolysis exhanced under conditions where ppGpp accumulates. Although proteolysis behaves as if it might be dependent upon ppGpp, no *in vitro* evidence of such a dependence has yet appeared. Conversely, abolishing proteolytic activity by adding PMSF (Goldberg, 1971b) during the stringent response does not result in disappearance of ppGpp, suggesting at least that proteolysis is not the cause for ppGpp accumulation behavior (M. Cashel, unpublished).

REGULATION OF DE NOVO NUCLEOTIDE SYNTHESIS AND TRANSPORT

The GTP pool values are subject to stringent control in a fashion not simply accountable for by consumption of GTP for ppGpp synthesis. Instead ppGpp inhibition of IMP dehydrogenase is implicated as well as an analogous but weaker inhibition observed with adenylosuccinate synthetase (Gallant, Irr, and Cashel, 1971). There may well be further inhibition by ppGpp at early steps in purine and pyrimidine biosynthesis during the stringent response. This speculation comes from the fact that intermediates in purine and pyrimidine biosynthesis do not seem to accumulate during the stringent response despite the almost complete abolition of RNA accumulation.

The first clue to transport defects were noted as resistance to 5-fluorouracil during the stringent response, which led to demonstration of a stringent control of uracil permeation and conversion to UTP (Edlin and Neuhard, 1967). Uridine or uracil transport has been reported to be diminished as much as 200-fold in the presence of ppGpp (Winslow and Lazzarini, 1969). Guanine or guanosine transport and equilibration with GTP is reduced about 20-fold, and adenine or adenosine equilibration is reduced about 4-fold during the stringent response (Nierlich, 1968; Lazzarini and Dahlberg, 1971). Studies with membrane vesicles sustaining transport of 6-hydroxypurine, adenine, and uridine reveal ppGpp inhibition kinetics that can account for whole-cell behavior (Hochstadt-Ozer and Cashel, 1972). Two separate purine-specific enzymes catalyzing phosphoribosylpyrophosphate-dependent formation of GMP and AMP are inhibited by ppGpp when the enzymes are purified free of membrane vesicles. Transport of pyrimidines in vesicles is less well defined enzymatically than purines, but can be completely inhibited by ppGpp. Bacterial membranes isolated from growing cells uniformly labeled with ^{32}P are indeed rich in ppGpp; over 50% of the acid-extractible phosphate is ppGpp, whereas ATP and GTP are barely detectable (Konigs and Cashel, unpublished). Thus ppGpp binding to vesicles is not simply due to nonspecific binding of the hydrophobic guanine ring.

REGULATION OF LIPID AND PHOSPHOLIPID SYNTHESIS

Evidence has been published that leads to the proposal that both the formation of lipids (Sokawa, Nakao, and Kaziro, 1968) and phospholipids (Sokawa, Sokawa, and Kaziro, 1972; Merlie and Pizer, 1973) are subject to stringent control. Support for these observations comes from *in vitro* measurements of synthesis in the presence of ppGpp (Merlie and Pizer, 1973; Polakis, Guchhait, and Lane, 1973). However, not all of these studies are consistent with one another. For example, Sokawa, Sokawa, and Kaziro (1972) find the major block in amino acid-starved stringent cells to be exerted at the formation of phosphatidyl ethanolamine, whereas Merlie and Pizer find it at the other side of the CDP diglyceride branch point affecting phosphatidyl glycerol phosphate synthetase as well as an effect on glycerol phosphate acyltransferase. More recently, Lueking and Goldfine (1975) have shown that glycerol phosphate acyl transferase inhibition by ppGpp is substrate specific. Use of palmityl CoA as a substrate is inhibited, but palmityl acyl carrier protein is not. This report is consistent with the observations of Polakis, Guchhait, and Lane (1973); in addition both laboratories found that chelation of divalent metal ions by ppGpp could account for its inhibitory effects. This property might well account for some effects of ppGpp on other systems. The physiological role of the effects on acetyl CoA carboxylase have been challenged (Nunn and Cronan, 1974). In addition to these effects on the formation of phospholipids, stringent control of phospholipid turnover may occur (Golden and Powell, 1972).

REGULATION OF GLYCOLYSIS AND RESPIRATION

Irr and Gallant (1969) noted that phosphate labeling of glycolytic intermediates was subject to stringent control while phosphate uptake was not. Labeling of all four ribonucleoside 5' triphosphates was also under stringent control; the deficiency of glucose-6-phosphate labeling could be cured by ATP addition. These observations can thus be accounted for by the high-energy-drain mechanisms mentioned earlier. The question arises whether glycolytic intermediates are subject to stringent control when energetically mild starvations provoke the stringent response. Sokawa, Nakao-Sato, and Kaziro (1970) have shown that respiration on glucose is under stringent control along with virtually all cellular components, but again energy-drain mechanisms are sufficient explanation. Although lowering of ATP pool levels is not an obligate aspect of the stringent response, why do relaxed strains behave differently? A possible clue to this answer seems to come from experiments with ^{32}P uniformly labeled cells chased with a 20-fold excess of cold phosphate at the time the stringent response is gently provoked by valine addition. Figure 1 shows that in a stringent prototroph, the pattern of chase of the four ribonucleoside 5' triphosphates is very different from that of growing cells. Normalizing the chased nucleotide activities to those at the time of valine addition reveals that even though GTP pool levels drop typically during

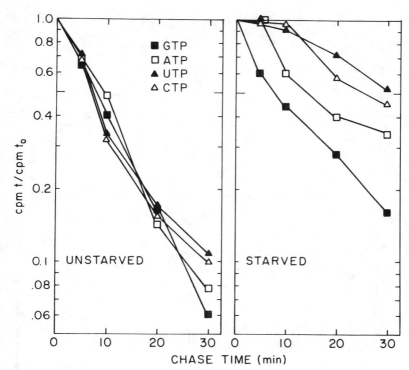

Fig. 1.   The effects of a phosphate chase on GTP, ATP, CTP, and UTP activities during cell growth and during the stringent response. Prototrophic *E. coli* K-12 cells were labeled in 0.4 mM ^{32}Pi for two generations, and an 8 mM phosphate chase was imposed at the time of valine addition (starved, right panel) at a cell density of 1.2×10^8 cells per ml. For comparison, nucleotides were also determined in a parallel culture that was not chased (unstarved, left panel). In each case the radioactivities of GTP, ATP, CTP, and UTP were measured (indicated by the symbol key on the figure) by thin-layer chromatography. The individual activities are normalized to the activities observed at time zero (t_0) when the phosphate chase was imposed alone or together with valine.

the first few minutes (Gallant and Harada, 1969; Gallant et al., 1970), the rate of chase is similar to that found in growing cells. During starvation other nucleotides chase differently; the ATP pool remains constant in size and is not chased as fast as GTP. UTP and CTP pools also remain constant in size, but are chased even slower than ATP and perhaps by phosphate flowing through ATP. Figure 2 shows that this curious pattern of chase is not observed in a similarly starved relaxed strain; thus it is under stringent control. Analysis of the rates of chase of individual phosphate residues of guanine nucleotides reveals a preferential chase of the gamma phosphate of GTP and pppGpp, while both ppGpp and ATP remain stably labeled (Cashel, unpublished). This puzzling anomaly in chase kinetics has been shown to be independent of

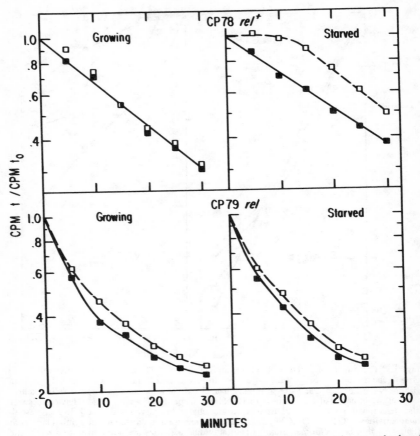

Fig. 2.   The effects of a phosphate chase on ATP and GTP activities in stringent and relaxed strains during growth and amino acid starvation. Strain CP 78 (*rel*A+) and CP 79 (*rel*A) were labeled with ^{32}Pi and treated as in figure 1. The activities of GTP (—) and ATP (—) are shown. The UTP and CTP chase kinetics generally parallel that of ATP in all cases.

phosphate permeability regulation and is affected by the *rel* allele in several relaxed-stringent strain pairs. It seems reasonable that this transient stability of ATP to phosphate chase in stringent strains, which is so far inseparable from the operation of the stringent response, may relate to different responses of stringent and relaxed strains to severe energy challenges.

CONCLUSIONS AND PROJECTIONS

Cellular activities that can be subject to regulation by the *rel* gene-dependent system range from transcription to intermediary metabolism. Some interesting aspects not discussed here are covered in a review by Edlin and

Broda (1968). The polyamine problem (Holffa, Janne, and Pispa, 1974) and leucine sensitivity (Alfoldi et al., 1963) are particularly interesting. How generalized is the pleiotropic stringent response?

Recently, Dr. Patrick O' Farrell has developed an elegant technique for two-dimensional gel analysis of proteins that permits the visualization of most, if not all, of the proteins synthesized in *E. coli*. Dr. O'Farrell (unpublished) has performed such analyses on isogenic stringent and relaxed strains to determine whether there are differences in the proteins formed during the course of residual protein synthesis under conditions that cause the stringent response. The results indeed indicate numerous differences in the radioactive spots resolved, comprising at least 30 percent of the proteins visualized. Dr. Anthony Furano has performed similar analyses but with stringent and relaxed strains bearing a conditional valyl synthetase. He compared the proteins formed at only partially restrictive temperatures while growth is slower but still logarithmic and the pools of ppGpp are elevated in the stringent strain. Again, the gel analysis shows surprising massive qualitative and quantitative differences in the proteins produced in the two strains. Although there are many temperature-sensitive and temperature-dependent changes in the relaxed strain, the over-all relaxed pattern at restrictive temperatures resembles that of the stringent strain grown at 30° or the normal valyl synthetase parent grown at either temperature.

The range of proteins possibly under stringent control from both sorts of experiments leads to a heightened appreciation of how many differences in protein production the cell can sustain. At the same time possibilities of simple intracellular signals provoking coordination of large sets of cellular enzymes must be more seriously entertained. Although the massive differences in proteins made can be qualitatively correlated with ppGpp levels, one again questions whether effects on this scale are simply due to direct or even indirect consequences of ppGpp accumulation.

It is intriguing in this respect that cyclic 3'5' AMP would appear to stimulate the synthesis of about 5 percent of *E. coli* proteins and that, with a few exceptions, the synthesis of this same set of proteins is inhibited by cyclic 3'5' GMP (O'Farrell, unpublished). These three likely pleiotropic effectors (cAMP, cGMP, ppGpp) share several structural features: they all are purine derivatives; they all are nucleotides; they all bear diestertified phosphates on both the 3' and 5' hydroxyls of ribose. One cannot help but wonder whether there are other analogous pleiotropic inhibitors and whether they can interact.

ACKNOWLEDGMENTS

I am grateful to Dr. Patrick O'Farrell of the Department of Biochemistry and Biophysics, University of California at San Francisco, and to Dr. Anthony Furano of the Laboratory of Biochemical Pharmacology, National Institute of Arthritis, Metabolism, and Digestive Diseases, National Institutes of Health, Bethesda, Maryland, for permission to discuss some salient features of data not yet published.

1. Several years ago Dr. R. A. Lazzarini made a table with about eight columns listing various cellular activities possibly regulated during the stringent response. Under each column there were three boxes labeled either "increased, decreased, or unchanged." Every box but a few contained at least one reference.

2. For example, see J. Mol. Biol. 37, no. 2, which contains four articles on this subject sustaining different conclusions.

LITERATURE CITED

Aboud, M., and I. Pastan. 1973. Stimulation of *lac* transcription by guanosine 5'-diphosphate 2' (or 3')-diphosphate and transfer ribonucleic acid. J. Biol. Chem. 248:3356–58.

Aboud, M., and I. Pastan. 1975. Activation of transcription by guanosine 5'-diphosphate, 3'-diphosphate, transfer ribonucleic acid, and a novel protein from *Escherichia coli*. J. Biol. Chem. 250:2189–95.

Alfoldi, L., G. S. Stent, and R. C. Clowes. 1962. The chromosome site for the RNA control (R.C.) locus in *Escherichia coli*. J. Mol. Biol. 5:348–55.

Alfoldi, L., G. S. Stent, M. Hoogs, and R. Hill. 1963. Physiological effects of the RNA control (R.C.) gene in *E. coli*. Z. Vererbungs. 94:285–302.

Arai, K., N. Arai, M. Kawakita, and Y. Kaziro. 1972. Interaction of guanosine 5'diphosphate, 2'-(or 3'-) diphosphate (ppGpp) with elongation factors from *E. coli*. Biochem. Biophys. Res. Commun. 48:190–96.

Atherly, A. G. 1974. Ribonucleic acid regulation in permeabilized cells of *Escherichia coli* capable of ribonucleic acid and protein synthesis. J. Bacteriol. 118:1186–89.

Birnbaum, L. S. and S. Kaplan. 1973. *In vitro* synthesis of *Escherichia coli* ribosomal RNA. J. Mol. Biol. 75:73–81.

Blatt, J. M., W. J. Pledger, and H. E. Umbarger. 1972. Isoleucine and valine metabolism in *Escherichia coli*. XX. Multiple forms of acetohydroxy acid synthetase. Biochem. Biophys. Res. Commun. 48:444–50.

Block, R. 1975. Synthesis of ribosomal RNA in a partially purified extract from *Escherichia coli*. A. Benzon Symp. 9:226–38.

Block, R., and W. A. Haseltine. 1975. Purification and properties of stringent factor. J. Biol. Chem. 250:1212–17.

Block, R., and W. A. Haseltine. 1973. Thermolability of the stringent factor in rel mutants of *Escherichia coli*. J. Mol. Biol. 77:625–29.

Block, R., and W. A. Haseltine. 1974. *In vitro* synthesis of ppGpp and pppGpp. *In* M. Nomura, A. Tissieres, and P. Lengyel (eds.). Ribosomes. Pp. 746–61. Cold Spring Harbor Press, Cold Spring, N.Y.

Borek, E., J. Rockenbach, and A. Ryan. 1956. Studies on a mutant of *Escherichia coli* with unbalanced ribonucleic acid synthesis. J. Bacteriol. 71:318–23.

Cashel, M. 1969. The control of ribonucleic acid synthesis in *Escherichia coli*. IV. Relevance of unusual phosphorylated compounds from amino acid starved stringent strains. J. Biol. Chem. 244:3133–41.

Cashel, M. 1970. Inhibition of RNA polymerase by ppGpp, a nucleotide accumulated during the stringent response to amino acid starvation in *E. coli*. Cold Spring Harbor Symp. Quant. Biol. 35:407–13.

Cashel, M. 1975. Regulation of bacterial ppGpp and pppGpp. Ann Rev. Microbiol. 29:301–18.

Cashel, M., E. Hamel, P. Shapshak, and M. Bouquet. 1975. Interactions of ppGpp structural analogs with RNA polymerase. A. Benzon Symp. 9.

Cashel, M., and J. Gallant. 1968. Control of RNA synthesis in *Escherichia coli*. I. Amino acid dependence of the synthesis of the substrates of RNA polymerase. J. Mol. Biol. 34:317–30.

Cashel, M., and J. Gallant. 1969. Two compounds implicated in the function of the RC gene of *Escherichia coli*. Nature 221:838–41.

Cashel, M., and J. Gallant. 1974. Cellular regulation of guanosine tetraphosphate and guanosine pentaphosphate. *In* M. Nomura, A. Tissieres, and P. Lengyel (eds.). Ribosomes. Pp. 733–45. Cold Spring Harbor Press, Cold Spring Harbor, N.Y.

Cashel, M., and B. Kalbacher. 1970. The control of ribonucleic acid synthesis in *Escherichia coli*. V. Characterization of a nucleotide associated with the stringent response. J. Biol. Chem. 245:2309–18.

Chaney, S. G., and D. Schlessinger. 1975. *Escherichia coli* mutants deficient in RNA accumulation at high temperature. Biochim. Biophys. Acta 378:80–91.

Cochran J. W., and R. W. Byrne. 1974. Isolation and properties of a ribosome-bound factor required for ppGpp and pppGpp synthesis in *Escherichia coli*. J. Biol. Chem. 249:353–60.

Cozzone, A., and P. Donini. 1973. Turnover of polysomes in amino acid starved *Escherichia coli*. J. Mol. Biol. 76:149–62.

De Boer, H. A., H. A. Raue, G. Ab, and M. Gruber. 1971. Role of the ribosome in stringent control of bacterial RNA synthesis. Biochim. Biophys. Acta 246:157–60.

deCrombruggie, B., I. Pastan, W. V. Shaw, and J. L. Rosner. 1972. Stimulation by cyclic AMP and ppGpp of chloramphenicol acetyl transferase synthesis. Nature New Biol. 241:237–39.

Dennis, P. P., and M. Nomura. 1974. Stringent control of ribosomal protein gene expression in *Escherichia coli*. Proc. Nat. Acad. Sci. USA 71:3819–23.

Dennis, P. P., and M. Nomura. 1975. Stringent control of the transcriptional activities of ribosomal protein genes in *E. coli*. Nature 255:460–65.

Edlin, G., and P. Broda. 1968. Physiology and genetics of the "Ribonucleic Acid Control" locus in *Escherichia coli*. Bacteriol. Rev. 32:206–26.

Edlin, G., and J. Neuhard. 1967. Regulation of nucleoside triphosphate pools in *Escherichia coli*. J. Mol. Biol. 24:225–32.

Fiil, N. 1969. A functional analysis of the *rel* gene in *Escherichia coli*. J. Mol. Biol. 45:195–203.

Fiil, N., and J. D. Friesen. 1968. Isolation of "relaxed" mutants of *Escherichia coli*. J. Bacteriol. 95:729–31.

Fiil, N. P., K. von Meyenberg, and J. D. Friesen. 1972. Accumulation and turnover of guanosine tetraphosphate in *Escherichia coli*. J. Mol. Biol. 71:769–83.

Gallant, J., H. Erlich, B. Hall, and T. Laffler. 1970. Analysis of the RC function. Cold Spring Harbor Symp. Quant. Biol. 35:397–405.

Gallant, J., and B. Harada. 1969. The control of RNA synthesis in *Escherichia coli*. III. The functional relationship between purine ribonucleoside triphosphate pool sizes and the rate of ribonucleic acid accumulation. J. Biol. Chem. 244:3125–32.

Gallant, J., J. Irr, and M. Cashel. 1971. The mechanism of amino acid control of guanylate and adenylate biosynthesis. J. Biol. Chem. 246:5812–16.

Gallant, J., and R. A. Lazzarini. Regulation of ribosomal RNA synthesis and degradation in bacteria. *In* E. H. McConkey, ed., Protein Synthesis: A Series of Advances. Marcel-Dekker, New York, in press.

Gallant, J., and G. Margason. 1972. Amino acid control of messenger ribonucleic acid synthesis in *Bacillus subtilis*. J. Biol. Chem. 247:2289–94.

Gallant, J., G. Margason, and B. Finch. 1972. On the turnover of ppGpp in *Escherichia coli*. J. Biol. Chem. 247:6055–58.

Ginsburg, D., and J. A. Steitz. 1975. The 30S ribosomal precursor RNA from *E. coli*: A primary transcript containing 23S, 16S and 5S sequences. J. Biol. Chem. 250:5647–54.

Golden, N. G., and G. L. Powell. 1972. Stringent and relaxed control of phospholipid metabolism in *Escherichia coli*. J. Biol. Chem. 247:6651–58.

Goldberg, A. L. 1971a. A role of aminoacyl-tRNA in the regulation of protein breakdown in *Escherichia coli*. Proc. Nat. Acad. Sci. USA 68:362–66.

Goldberg, A. L. 1971b. Effects of protease inhibitors on protein breakdown and enzyme induction in starving *Escherichia coli*. Nature New Biol. 234:51–53.

Goldberg, A. L. 1972. Degradation of abnormal proteins in *Escherichia coli*. Proc. Nat. Acad. Sci. USA 69:422–26.

Hall, B., and J. Gallant. 1972. Defective translation in RC⁻ cells. Nature New Biol. 237:131–35.

Hall, B., and J. Gallant. 1971. Effect of the RC gene product on constitutive enzyme synthesis. J. Mol. Biol. 61:271–73.

Hamel, E., and M. Cashel. 1973. Role of guanine nucleotides in protein synthesis, elongation factor G and guanosine 5′-triphosphate, 3′-diphosphate. Proc. Nat. Acad. Sci. USA 70:3250–54.

Hamel, E., and M. Cashel. 1974. Guanine nucleotides in protein synthesis. Utilization of pppGpp and dGTP by initiation factor 2 and elongation factor Tu. Arch. Biochem. Biophys. 162:293–300.

Hamkalo, B. A., and O. L. Miller, Jr. 1973. Electronmicroscopy of genetic activity. Ann. Rev. Biochem. 42:379–96.

Harshman, R. B., and H. Yamazaki. 1971. Formation of ppGpp in a relaxed and stringent strain of *Escherichia coli* during diauxic lag. Biochem. 10:3980–82.

Haseltine, W. A. 1972. *In vitro* transcription of *Escherichia coli* ribosomal RNA genes. Nature 235:329–33.

Haseltine, W. A., and R. Block. 1973. Synthesis of guanosine tetra- and pentaphosphate requires the presence of a codon-specific, uncharged transfer ribonucleic acid in the acceptor site of ribosomes. Proc. Nat. Acad. Sci. USA 70:1564–68.

Haseltine, W. A., R. Block, W. Gilbert, and K. Weber. 1972. MSI and MSII made on ribosome in idling step of protein synthesis. Nature 238:381–84.

Hochstadt-Ozer, J., and M. Cashel. 1972. The regulation of purine utilization in bacteria. V. Inhibition of purine phosphoribosyl-transferase activities and purine uptake in isolated membrane vesicles by guanosine tetraphosphate. J. Biol. Chem. 247:7067–72.

Holffa, E., J. Janne, and J. Pispa. 1974. The regulation of polyamine synthesis during the stringent control in *Escherichia coli*. Biochem. Biophys. Res. Commun. 57:1104–11.

Ikemura, T., and J. E. Dahlberg. 1973. Small ribonucleic acids of *Escherichia coli*. II. Noncoordinate accumulation during stringent control. J. Biol. Chem. 248:5033–41.

Irr, J., and J. Gallant. 1969. The control of RNA synthesis in *Escherichia coli*. II. Stringent control of energy metabolism. J. Biol. Chem. 244:2233–39.

Kaltschmidt, E., L. Kahan, and M. Nomura. 1974. *In vitro* synthesis of ribosomal proteins directed by *Escherichia coli* DNA. Proc. Nat. Acad. Sci. USA 71:446–50.

Kaplan, S., A. G. Atherly, and A. Barrett. 1973. Synthesis of stable RNA in stringent *Escherichia coli* cells in the absence of charged transfer RNA. Proc. Nat. Acad. Sci. USA 70:689–92.

Laffler, T., and J. Gallant. 1974a. Spo T, a new genetic locus involved in the stringent response in *E. coli*. Cell 1:27–30.

Laffler, T., and J. Gallant. 1974b. Stringent control of protein synthesis in *E. coli*. Cell 3:47–49.

Legault, L., C. Jeantet, and F. Gros. 1972. Inhibition of *in vitro* protein synthesis by ppGpp. FEBS Lett. 27:71–75.

Lazzarini, R. A., M. Cashel, and J. Gallant. 1971. On the regulation of guanosine tetraphosphate levels in stringent and relaxed strains of *Escherichia coli*. J. Biol. Chem. 246:4381–85.

Lazzarini, R. A., and A. E. Dahlberg. 1971. The control of ribonucleic acid synthesis during amino acid deprivation in *Escherichia coli*. J. Biol. Chem. 246:420–29.

Lazzarini, R. A., and L. D. Johnson. 1973. Regulation of ribosomal RNA synthesis in cold-shocked *E. coli*. Nature New Biol. 243:17–19.

Lueking, D. R., and H. Goldfine. 1975. The involvement of ppGpp in the regulation of phospholipid biosynthesis in *Escherichia coli:* Lack of ppGpp inhibition of acyl transfer from acyl-ACP to sn-glycerol-3-phosphate. J. Biol. Chem. 250:4911–17.

Lund, E., and N. O. Kjeldgaard. 1972. Metabolism of guanosine tetraphosphate in *Escherichia coli*. Eur. J. Biochem. 28:316–26.

Merlie, J. P., and L. I. Pizer. 1973. Regulation of phospholipid synthesis in *Escherichia coli* by guanosine tetraphosphate. J. Bacteriol. 116:355–66.

Miller, D. L., M. Cashel, and H. Weissbach. 1973. The interaction of guanosine 5'-diphosphate, 2'(3')-diphosphate with bacterial elongation factor Tu. Arch. Biochem. Biophys. 154:675–82.

Murooka, Y., and R. A. Lazzarini. 1973. *In vitro* synthesis of ribosomal ribonucleic acid by a deoxyribonucleic acid-protein complex isolated from *Escherichia coli*. J. Biol. Chem. 248:6248–50.

Neidhardt, F. C. 1966. Role of amino acid activating enzymes in cellular physiology. Bacteriol. Rev. 30:701–19.

Nierlich, D. P. 1968. Amino acid control over RNA synthesis, a re-evaluation. Proc. Nat. Acad. Sci. USA 60:1345–52.

Nunn, W., and J. Cronan. 1974. rel gene control of lipid synthesis in *Escherichia coli*. Evidence for eliminating fatty acid synthesis as the sole regulatory site. J. Biol. Chem. 249:3994–96.

Pederson, F. S., E. Lund, and N. O. Kjeldgaard. 1973. Codon specific, tRNA-dependent *in vitro* synthesis of ppGpp and pppGpp. Nature New Biol. 243:13–15.

Polakis, S. E., R. B. Guchhait, and M. D. Lane. 1973. Stringent control of fatty acid synthesis in *Escherichia coli:* Possible regulation of acetyl CoA carboxylase by ppGpp. J. Biol. Chem. 248:7957–66.

Primakoff, P., and P. Berg. 1970. Stringent control of transcription of phage ϕ 80psu$_3$. Cold Spring Harbor Symp. Quant. Biol. 35:391–96.

Que, L., G. R. Willie, M. Cashel, J. W. Bodley, and G. R. Gray. 1973. Guanosine 5'diphosphate, 3'diphosphate; assignment of structure by ^{13}C nuclear magnetic resonance spectroscopy. Proc. Nat. Acad. Sci. USA 70:2563–66.

Rapaport, E., S. K. Svihovec, and P. C. Zamecnik. 1975. Relationship of the first step in protein synthesis to ppGpp: Formation of A(5')ppp5'Gpp. Proc. Nat. Acad. Sci. USA 72:2653–57.

Reiness, G., H. L. Yang, G. Zubay, and M. Cashel. 1975. Effects of guanosine tetraphosphate on cell-free synthesis of *Escherichia coli* ribosomal RNA and other gene products. Proc. Nat. Acad. Sci. USA 72:2881–85.

Sokawa, J., Y. Sokawa, and Y. Kaziro. 1972. Stringent control in *Escherichia coli*. Nature New Biol. 240:242–45.

Sokawa, Y., J. Sokawa, and Y. Kaziro. 1971. Function of the *rel* gene in *Escherichia coli*. Nature New Biol. 234:7–10.

Sokawa, Y., J. Sokawa, and Y. Kaziro. 1974. Role of *rel* gene in translation during amino acid starvation in *Escherichia coli*. Nature 249:59–62.

Sokawa, Y., E. Nakao, and Y. Kaziro. 1968. On the nature of the control by RC gene in *Escherichia coli;* amino acid dependent control of lipid synthesis. Biochem. Biophys. Res. Commun. 33:108–12.

Sokawa, Y., E. Nakao-Sato, and Y. Kaziro. 1970. RC gene control in *Escherichia coli* is not restricted to RNA synthesis. Biochim. Biophys. Acta 199:256–64.

Stamminger, G., and R. A. Lazzarini. 1974. Altered metabolism of the guanosine tetraphosphate, ppGpp, in mutants. Cell 1:85–90.

Stent, G. S., and S. Brenner. 1961. A genetic locus for the regulation of ribonucleic acid synthesis. Proc. Nat. Acad. Sci. USA 47:2005–14.

Sussman, A. J., and C. Gilvarg. 1969. Protein turnover in amino acid-starved strains of *Escherichia coli* K-12 differing in their ribonucleic acid control. J. Biol. Chem. 244:6304–6.

Sy, J., and F. Lipmann. 1973. Identification of the synthesis of guanosine tetraphosphate (MS I) as insertion of a pyrophosphoryl group into the 3'-position in guanosine 5'-diphosphate. Proc. Nat. Acad. Sci. USA 70:306–9.

Swanton, M., and G. Edlin. 1972. Isolation and characterization of an RNA relaxed mutation of *B. subtilis*. Biochem. Biophys. Res. Commun. 46:583–88.

Travers, A., R. Kamen, and M. Cashel. 1970. The *in vitro* synthesis of ribosomal RNA. Cold Spring Harbor Symp. Quant. Biol. 35:415–18.

Van Ooyen, A. J. J., D. A. de Boer, G. Ab, and M. Gruber. 1975. Specific inhibition of ribosomal RNA synthesis *in vitro* by guanosine 3'diphosphate 5'diphosphate. Nature 254:530–31.

Varmus, H. E., R. L. Perlman, and I. Pastan. 1971. Regulation of lac transcription in *E. coli*. Nature New Biol. 230:41–43.

Winslow, R. M., and R. A. Lazzarini. 1969. The rates of synthesis and chain elongation of ribonucleic acid in *Escherichia coli*. J. Biol. Chem. 244:1128–37.

Yang, H-L., and G. Zubay. 1973. Synthesis of the arabinose operon regulator protein in a cell-free system. Molec. gen. Genet. 122:131–36.

Yang, H. L., G. Zubay, E. Urm, G. Reiness, and M. Cashel. 1974. Effects of guanosine tetraphosphate, guanosine pentaphosphate, and β-γ methylenyl-guanosine pentaphosphate on gene expression of *Escherichia coli in vitro*. Proc. Nat. Acad. Sci. USA 71:63–67.

Yoshida, M., A. Travers, and B. F. C. Clark. 1972. Inhibition of translation initiation complex formation by MS 1. FEBS Lett. 23:163–66.

Zubay, G., L. Gielow, and E. Englesberg. 1971. Cell-free studies on the regulation of the arabinose operon. Nature New Biol. 233:164–65.

MARY D. BARKLEY AND SUZANNE BOURGEOIS

The *Lac* Operon

3

INTRODUCTION

The ability of *E. coli* to ferment lactose is an adaptive process of the organism. The two enzymes that permit the bacterium to utilize lactose, 4-O-β-D-galactopyranosyl-D-glucose, as a carbon source are a membrane permease, which directs the transport and accumulation of lactose inside the cell, and β-galactosidase, which cleaves lactose into galactose and glucose. These two enzymes, plus a third, a transacetylase having no known function in lactose metabolism, are coded for by the structural genes of the lactose operon. Very low amounts of these enzymes are found in cells growing on glucose. In the presence of lactose or other galactosides, about 5% of the cell protein is *lac* enzymes. The regulation of their synthesis occurs in a coordinate fashion. (For a comprehensive account, see Beckwith and Zipser, 1970.)

The genetic map of the *lac* operon is shown in figure 1. The *z* gene is the structural gene for β-galactosidase, a tetrameric protein composed of identical 135,000 molecular weight subunits. The enzyme catalyzes hydrolytic as well as transfer reactions of sugars at a β-galactoside linkage; the glycone residue of the substrate may be transferred to water or to some other hydroxylic acceptor. (For a review, see Wallenfels and Malhotra, 1961.) The *y* gene is the structural gene for lactose permease, a system that functions via a protein of molecular weight 30,000 when isolated from the bacterial membrane. The *a* gene is the structural gene for thiogalactoside transacetylase, a dimeric protein composed of identical 32,000 molecular weight subunits; it is not an

Department of Chemistry, University of California, San Diego, La Jolla, California 92093; Salk Institute for Biological Studies, San Diego, California 92112

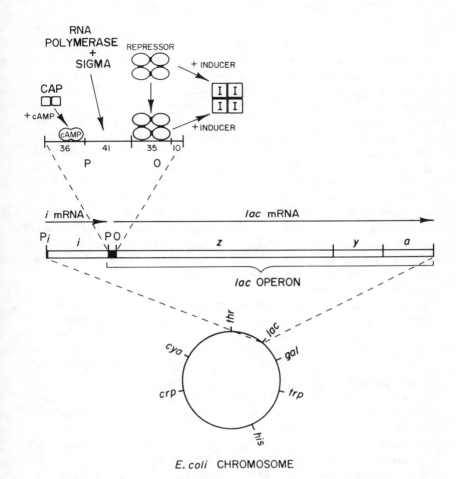

Fig. 1. Genetic map of the *lac* operon. The expanded *lac* region is inverted relative to its orientation on the chromosome; the structural genes are drawn roughly to scale. The upper part of the figure shows a schematic drawing of the negative and positive control systems. See text for details. Abbreviations: *crp,* gene for CAP protein; *cya,* gene for adenyl cyclase; *gal,* genes essential for galactose metabolism; *thr, trp, his,* genes essential for biosynthesis of threonine, tryptophan, and histidine, respectively.

essential gene. Thiogalactoside transacetylase catalyzes the transfer of the acetyl moiety from acetyl coenzyme A to the 6-OH group of thiogalactoside acceptors. Transcription of the operon into a single polycistronic messenger RNA (mRNA) begins in the *lac* promoter region P, which includes the binding site for RNA polymerase. Adjacent to the promoter, but not part of the *lac* operon, is the *i* gene, which codes for the regulatory protein of the operon, the *lac* repressor. Presumably, transcription of the *i* gene into a separate mRNA begins at the promoter P_i (see fig. 1).

In 1961 Jacob and Monod formulated the model of negative control that predicted the mechanism of regulation of the *lac* operon. In the absence of galactosides, the repressor protein binds to the DNA at the operator site O and inhibits transcription of the operon by RNA polymerase. Under conditions of repression, only a very low rate of synthesis of *lac* enzymes occurs, amounting to about 10 molecules of each enzyme per cell; the repressed level of synthesis is called the basal level. In the presence of an inducing galactoside, the repressor protein comes off the operator and transcription proceeds. Within a few minutes the rate of synthesis of *lac* enzymes increases 1,000-fold. This phenomenon is called induction. Inducer molecules interact with the *lac* repressor, presumably causing a conformational transition in the protein, and thus reduce its affinity for the operator. Isolation and purification of the *lac* repressor protein (Gilbert and Müller-Hill, 1966; Riggs and Bourgeois, 1968) and subsequent studies of its interaction with *lac* operator DNA *in vitro* (Riggs et al., 1968) confirmed the essential features of the model of negative control.

In addition to the negative control by the *lac* repressor protein, the *lac* operon is subject to catabolite repression, a general regulatory process affecting all inducible operons for sugar catabolism in *E. coli*. Catabolite repression insures that when the bacterium is confronted with a mixture of glucose and other sugars, the utilization of which requires inducible enzyme synthesis, the cell will preferentially use glucose as carbon source. In the case of the *lac* operon, the rate of synthesis of *lac* enzymes in a fully induced culture growing on glucose is weakly repressed to about half that of cells growing on glycerol. Glucose lowers the intracellular level of cyclic 3',5'-adenosine monophosphate (cAMP) in *E. coli;* catabolite repression is relieved by exogenous cAMP (Perlman and Pastan, 1968; Ullmann and Monod, 1968). A protein that mediates the effects of cAMP, called the catabolite activator protein (CAP), as well as cAMP are essential for maximal expression of the *lac* operon. This positive control acts at the *lac* promoter region P.

Before presenting details of the regulation of the *lac* operon, we will describe briefly some experimental techniques standard in investigations of the *lac* system and some pertinent facts about the components of the negative and positive control.

Methodology

Genetic tools have proved invaluable throughout the history of the *lac* operon, by providing both insight into the mechanism of regulation through genetic analysis of mutants and reagents for biochemical investigations. Because of the finesse developed in the genetic manipulation of the *lac* region, a wide variety of mutant strains are available, bearing mutations either in the *i* gene for the repressor protein or in the promoter or operator sites on the DNA. We will postpone discussion of the various classes of regulatory mutants to later sections. Two feats of genetic engineering have been crucial for the recent progress in the biochemical characterization of the *lac* system: the introduction of the *lac* region on the chromosome of temperate bacteriophage and the isolation of mutants that overproduce *lac* repressor protein.

The isolation of lambdoid-transducing phages carrying the *lac* region yielded a source of DNA enriched about 70-fold in the *lac* genes over the *E. coli* chromosome (Beckwith and Signer, 1966). Several advantages accrue from having the *lac* region on the phage genome. A homogenous *lac* DNA molecule is readily purified in quantity from the bacteriophage. That the phage DNA has one *lac* operator site per 3×10^7 molecular weight genome, instead of one operator site per 2×10^9 molecular weight *E. coli* chromosome, was critical to the development of the membrane filter assay, as we shall see shortly. Recently, a restriction enzyme map of DNA in the vicinity of the *lac* control region has been established (Gilbert, Gralla, and Maxam, in preparation, cited by Gilbert et al., 1975). It is now possible to isolate DNA fragments, about 100–200 base pairs long, containing the promoter and operator.

Several mutants have been isolated that overproduce *lac* repressor protein to varying degrees. A wild-type strain of *E. coli* synthesizes about 10 repressor molecules per cell per generation. The first i^q quantity mutant made 10 times more repressor protein than normal (Müller-Hill, Crapo, and Gilbert, 1968). Now, there is a mutant, i^{q1}, that produces 100 times the normal amount of repressor protein (Müller-Hill et al., 1975). These quantity mutants are believed to arise from mutations in the *i* gene promoter P_i, since they map at the extreme left end of the *i* gene and since the repressor proteins from wild-type and i^q strains show no differences in sequence of the first five amino acids (Platt et al., 1972). Increasing the *i* gene dosage by placing the i^q mutation on a *lac* phage yields an additional 10-fold increase in the amount of repressor protein synthesized after induction of the prophage. Under optimal conditions as much as 7% of the cell protein can be *lac* repressor.

Several biochemical procedures have been developed in order to study the *lac* system. Here we will outline the *in vitro* binding assays for the *lac* repressor protein (for reviews, see Bourgeois, 1971a, 1971b). Other techniques will be discussed in context. The *lac* repressor protein is defined by its two biological activities, the ability to bind inducer and to recognize the *lac* operator. The inducer commonly used is isopropyl-1-thio-β-D-galactoside

(IPTG), a so-called gratuitous inducer because it induces the *lac* operon *in vivo* without itself being a substrate of β-galactosidase. The operator DNA is a *lac* phage DNA.

The membrane filter technique has been especially fruitful for quantitating the binding of repressor protein and operator DNA (Riggs, Suzuki, and Bourgeois, 1970a; Riggs, Newby, and Bourgeois, 1970b; Riggs, Bourgeois, and Cohn, 1970c). This assay depends on the fact that under appropriate conditions of ionic strength (I), *lac* repressor protein, as do many other proteins (Kihara and Kuno, 1968), adheres to nitrocellulose filters. Moreover, radioactively labeled ligands that bind to repressor, such as sugars and DNAs, do not stick to nitrocellulose when free, but remain bound to the protein on the filter. The operator-binding assay can be adapted for use with crude preparations of repressor. Also, the repressor-operator complex immobilized on membrane filters dissociates upon washing of the filter with buffer-containing inducer. The operator DNA thus released can be reclaimed. This property of the repressor protein has been exploited for purifying fragments of DNA containing the *lac* operator (Bourgeois and Riggs, 1970) and the *lac* operator itself (Gilbert, 1972) away from non-operator DNA.

The binding of repressor protein and inducer IPTG can also be determined by membrane filtration. The filter assay is most useful for rapid estimates of repressor concentrations, for example, for monitoring IPTG-binding activity during column chromatography. For quantitative measurement of IPTG binding to *lac* repressor protein, whether purified or in crude extracts, equilibrium dialysis is still the most reliable method. Another type of technique, which is more sensitive than equilibrium dialysis for detecting low levels of IPTG binding, is precipitation by ammonium sulfate (Bourgeois and Jobe, 1970) or antibody (Riggs and Bourgeois, 1968). However, binding constants determined by the ammonium sulfate method must be viewed with caution, since they differ significantly from the values determined by equilibrium dialysis. The antibody precipitation technique has been employed as the basis of a small-scale purification scheme for mutated *lac* repressors for the purpose of sequence analysis (Platt et al., 1972).

Components of the Regulatory System

The dual control system of the *lac* operon is schematized in figure 1. Negative control of transcription is accomplished by the *lac* repressor protein, the operator site on the DNA, and small effecting ligands. The *lac* repressor is a tetrameric protein of 150,000 molecular weight, composed of identical subunits of 38,000 molecular weight each. The tetramer has one binding site for *lac* operator, and four binding sites for inducer, one per monomer. The repressor tetramer is a globular protein, whose amino-acid sequence is known (Beyreuther et al., 1973, 1975); its properties will be enumerated in the "*Lac* Repressor Protein" section. The *lac* operator is a region of double-stranded DNA from 21 to 35 base pairs long, whose nucleotide sequence is known (Gilbert and Maxam, 1973; Dickson et al., 1975). The most striking feature of the operator sequence is the existence of a quasi-dyad symmetry between adjacent anti-polar repeats on the complementary DNA strands. There are actually two classes of effecting ligands, low molecular weight sugars that alter the interaction of repressor protein and operator DNA: inducers (mentioned already) and anti-inducers. *In vivo,* anti-inducers are identified by their ability to prevent induction in competition with inducers. Inducing and anti-inducing ligands interact directly with repressor protein bound to the operator, forming a ternary complex and decreasing or increasing, respectively, the affinity of repressor for operator. The multiple interactions of repressor, operator, and inducer will be discussed in some detail under two headings: "Interaction of Repressor and DNA" and "Interaction of Repressor and Effecting Ligands."

The *lac* promoter region of the DNA comprises two functional sites that regulate transcription: the RNA polymerase binding site and the site of action of CAP protein. Its nucleotide sequence is also known (Dickson et al., 1975). The site recognized by RNA polymerase holoenzyme (core enzyme plus σ factor) adjoins the operator. In fact, the polymerase binding site penetrates the left side of the operator. Evidence for this partial overlap, as well as descriptions, of the promoter and operator regions will be presented in the section entitled "Regulatory Sites on DNA." The site for binding of CAP protein in the presenc of cAMP lies in the *i*-gene proximal half of the promoter. The properties of the CAP protein and its interactions with DNA and cAMP will be described in the "CAP Protein" section. The mechanism by which CAP protein plus cAMP stimulate transcription of the *lac* operon is not known; however, both are required, in addition to RNA polymerase holoenzyme, for initiation of mRNA synthesis at catabolite-sensitive promoters, as discussed under "Transcription of the Operon."

INTERACTION OF REPRESSOR AND DNA

The *lac* repressor protein binds not only at the *lac* operator site but also at non-operator nucleotide sequences on DNA. We will discuss the interaction of repressor and DNA in terms of a nonspecific binding to any DNA and a specific binding to operator, the latter by definition being sensitive to inducer IPTG. Since the binding of repressor to operator is a unique property of the protein, it has been the subject of intensive investigation. We shall summarize these results first.

A. Specific Recognition of Operator

The binding of *lac* repressor protein to operator DNA has been studied by the membrane filtration technique. It should become apparent in this and later sections that, at present, this is the only method available for characterizing the physical properties of this interaction. So far, all the data are consistent with the following bimolecular reaction for the binding of *lac* repressor R to the operator site O:

$$R + O \underset{k_b}{\overset{k_a}{\rightleftharpoons}} RO$$

where k_a is the specific rate constant of association of repressor and operator, and k_b is the specific rate constant of dissociation of repressor-operator complex. The equilibrium association constant K_O for the binding of repressor protein and operator DNA

$$K_O = \frac{[RO]}{[R][O]} = \frac{k_a}{k_b}$$

is extremely large, about 1×10^{13} M^{-1} under standard conditions (I = 0.05M, pH 7.4, 24°C; Riggs et al., 1970a). Because of the very high affinity of repressor for operator, binding reactions are carried out at low concentrations, of the order of 10^{-12} M in both reagents. Figure 2 shows an equilibrium binding curve. The value of the association constant K_O measured in equilibrium binding experiments, agrees with the value k_a/k_b calculated from the ratio of the rate constants from kinetic experiments. However, it is easier to detect small changes in the association constant from the more accurate kinetics measurements.

The kinetic data for the rate of formation of repressor-operator complex are plotted according to the integrated rate equation for a second-order reaction in figure 3a. The rate constant of association k_a of repressor and operator (the slope of the line) is very large, about 7×10^9 M^{-1} sec^{-1} (Riggs et al., 1970c). It is only possible to determine a rate constant of this magnitude in a conventional kinetics experiment because of the high affinity of repressor for operator; the time scale for the association reaction at 10^{-12} M is several minutes. A point to be noted, and to which we shall return in later discussion, is that the bimolecular rate constant k_a is at least an order of magnitude greater than the value normally expected for diffusion-limited reactions of molecules of this size.

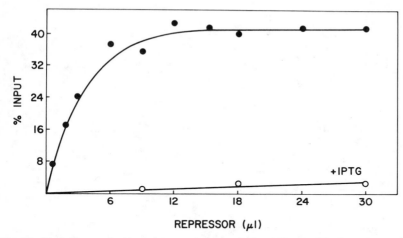

Fig. 2. Binding curve for *lac* repressor and operator DNA. Aliquots of purified *lac* repressor protein and radioactively labeled λh80d*lac* DNA (1.7×10^{-11} M operator) are equilibrated in standard binding buffer (I = 0.05M) at room temperature. λh80d*lac* is a λ phage that carries the bacterial *lac* genes. Samples of the reaction mixture are filtered on membrane filters; the filters are washed with buffer and counted for radioactivity. The background (4%) of DNA retained by the filters in the absence of repressor has been subtracted from each point. Solid circle = no IPTG; open circle = 10^{-3} M IPTG. Standard binding buffer is 0.01M Tris, pH 7.4, 0.01 M KCl, 0.01M Mg(CH_3CO_2)$_2$, 10^{-4} M EDTA, 10^{-4} M dithiothreitol, 5% dimethyl sulfoxide, 50 μg/ml bovine serum albumin. Data from Riggs et al. (1970a).

The kinetics data for the rate of disappearance of labeled repressor-operator complex are plotted on a semi-log scale in figure 3*b*. The rate constant of dissociation k_b of repressor-operator complex (the slope of the line) is about 6×10^{-4} sec^{-1} corresponding to a half life $t_{1/2}$ of about 30 min for the unimolecular decay process (Riggs et al., 1970c). For induction to occur as it does in the cell, without detectable lag after the addition of inducer, it is clear that the inducer molecule must accelerate the removal of repressor protein from the operator site on DNA. This fact is illustrated in figure 3*b*, where it is seen that inducer IPTG speeds up the rate of decomposition of repressor-operator complex, and conversely, anti-inducer o-nitrophenyl-β-D-fucoside (ONPF) retards it (Riggs et al., 1970b). Since inducing and anti-inducing ligands do not alter significantly the rate of association of repressor and operator (Jobe and Bourgeois, 1972b; Lin and Riggs, 1972b), their effect on the rate of dissociation can be ascribed directly to a decrease or increase in the affinity of repressor for operator in the presence of IPTG or ONPF, respectively. Further, these experiments establish the existence of a ternary ligand-repressor-operator complex by showing that effecting ligands interact with repressor-operator complex.

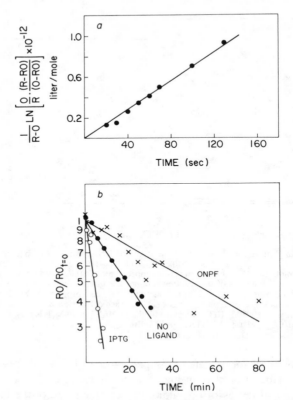

Fig. 3.   Kinetics of binding of *lac* repressor and operator DNA. *a*. Rate of association of repressor and operator. At time $t = 0$, active repressor protein (2.4×10^{-12} M) and labeled λh80d*lac* DNA (1.1×10^{-12} M) are mixed; at various times t, samples are removed and filtered. The specific rate constant of association k_a of repressor and operator is the slope of the straight line. Data from Riggs et al. (1970c). *b*. Rate of dissociation of repressor-operator complex. Repressor protein and labeled λh80d*lac* DNA are equilibrated to form labeled repressor-operator complex (8.6×10^{-12} M). At time $t = 0$, the reaction mixture is diluted 10-fold into buffer containing a 50-fold excess of cold λh80d*lac* DNA, in the absence or presence of various concentrations of effecting ligand, and the rate of exchange of repressor off the labeled operator DNA onto the unlabeled operator DNA is monitored; at various times t, samples are removed and filtered. The specific rate constant of dissociation k_b of repressor-operator complex is the slope of the straight line. Data from Riggs et al. (1970b). Solid circle = no ligand; open circle = 3×10^{-6} M IPTG: X = 1.8×10^{-3} M ONPF, o-nitrophenyl-β-D-fucoside. Standard conditions (see legend, fig. 2).

The effects of a variety of physical and chemical parameters on the interaction of *lac* repressor and operator DNA have also been investigated (Riggs et al., 1970c). The *lac* repressor binds to a thermodynamically stable, double-stranded structure of the operator DNA. Denaturation of the DNA destroys operator-binding; the binding to operator is restored upon renaturation of the

DNA. Actinomycin D inhibits the binding of repressor to operator DNA, presumably by competing with the protein for the operator site. This antibiotic, a cyclic polypeptide containing intercalative dye, binds preferentially to DNA between the base-paired sequences dG-dC, the peptide chains lying along the narrow groove of the DNA helix (Sobell, 1973). The sequence of the *lac* operator contains one putative actinomycin site (see fig. 9a). Substitution of 5-bromodeoxyuridine (BudR) for thymidine in *lac* operator DNA strengthens the interaction with repressor about a factor of ten, as evidenced by a 10-fold decrease in the rate constant of dissociation k_b (Lin and Riggs, 1972a). The affinity of repressor for operator is quite sensitive to ionic strength. A 10-fold increase in the ionic strength of the binding buffer (from I = 0.02M to I = 0.2M) decreases the rate constant of association k_a about 60-fold and increases the rate constant of dissociation k_b about 5-fold, corresponding to a 250-fold reduction in the equilibrium association constant K_O. At constant ionic strength, the stability of repressor-operator complex is the same in the presence or absence of Mg^{+2} ion (Barkley et al., 1975). Increasing the negative charge on the repressor protein (isoelectric point pH 5.6) by raising the pH of the binding buffer (from pH 7.0 to pH 9.0) causes a slight reduction in the affinity of repressor for operator; the rate constant of association k_a decreases about 3-fold, whereas the rate constant of dissociation k_b is essentially unchanged, over this range of pH. The effect of temperature on the repressor-operator interaction, although not pronounced, is noteworthy. In going from 1°C to 24°C, the rate constant of association k_a increases about 4-fold and the rate constant of dissociation k_b remains constant. Thus the activation energy for the association reaction is + 8.5 kcal/mole, about four times the value due to viscosity in a diffusion-controlled reaction; and for the dissociation reaction, close to zero. The equilibrium constant K_O increases 4-fold over this temperature range, so for the binding reaction $\Delta H = 8.5$ kcal/mole. At 24°C, $K_O = 1 \times 10^{13}$ M^{-1} and $\Delta G = -18$ kcal/mole. The entropy change, $\Delta S = 90$ cal/deg. mole, is the main driving force for the reaction.

These experimental results highlight two remarkable features of the *lac* repressor-operator interaction, namely, the very tight binding of repressor and operator and the rapidity with which the repressor protein finds the operator site on DNA. The question naturally arises whether the interaction achieves its extraordinary specificity through a mechanism in which the repressor protein binds to an unusual DNA structure. Several models for the recognition process have been discussed. One type includes models in which DNA base pairs in the operator region are disrupted, the repressor reading the sequence of the exposed bases. Gierer (1966) has proposed a cruciform model for specific repressor-operator interactions, for which the 2-fold symmetry of the operator sequence is a prerequisite. Alternate models are those in which the operator region is fully base-paired, the repressor reading the base sequence in the grooves of the helix. Along these lines are the general models suggested for the interaction of polypeptides with double-stranded RNA (Carter and Kraut, 1974) or DNA (Church, Sussman, and Kim, 1975) and of proteins with kinked DNA helices (Crick and Klug, 1975).

The question of whether the binding of *lac* repressor protein to operator DNA unwinds the DNA helix was resolved by experiments measuring the affinity of repressor for operator DNA having various degrees of negative superhelical twist (Wang, Barkley, and Bourgeois, 1974). Since the release of superhelical turns in DNA is favored thermodynamically, as documented by studies of the binding of intercalative dyes (Bauer and Vinograd, 1970), a protein that unwinds the duplex helix will bind with greater affinity to covalently closed circular DNA with negative superhelical twist than it will to the identical, untwisted DNA. The angle of unwinding can be computed from the ratio of the affinities of the ligand for these two DNAs (Davidson, 1972). The binding of *lac* repressor to superhelical λp*lac* DNA was determined in kinetic experiments by membrane filtration. As the number of negative superhelical turns in the DNA progressed from -10 to -350, the rate constant of association k_a increased about 4-fold, and the rate constant of dissociation k_b decreased about 3-fold; the increase in the equilibrium association constant K_o was at most 14-fold. The angle of unwinding for *lac* repressor, calculated on the basis of a 26° unwinding angle for ethidium (Wang, 1974), is about 90° per operator, corresponding to about 3° per base pair. The small amount of unwinding measured indicates a structural change in the operator duplex, which is probably important in recognition. Moreover, it is inconsistent with any mechanism of recognition involving substantial unwinding of the Watson-Crick helix by the repressor, either to form a Gierer-type structure (see fig. 9*b*) or to expose a number of bases.

The unwinding experiments preclude the possibility that the repressor protein promotes the formation of looped-out structures in the operator DNA. However, they do not address the question of whether the operator exists in a hairpin or other partially single-stranded structure in a stable state in the absence of repressor. It is highly unlikely that such a structure would be more stable than the fully paired duplex. The facts that the operator sequence does not contain any unpaired or modified bases and that purified operator, a 27 base-pair piece of DNA, has a T_m of 67°C in 0.15 M NaCl $-$ 0.015 M Na citrate suggest that the DNA is double-stranded (Gilbert and Maxam, 1973). However, the operator site on DNA is vulnerable to single-strand specific endonucleases (Chan and Wells, 1974). As few as 2-5 cuts by S_1 and mung bean nucleases, and about 300 cuts by nonspecific nicking agents, such as pancreatic DNase, micrococcal nuclease, and sonication, destroy the same fraction of operator sites in λp*lac* DNA. Also, binding of repressor protein to the operator prevents its degradation by the single-strand specific nucleases. Despite these facts it appears unlikely that the operator itself is the site of attack of S_1 nuclease, since nicking the λp*lac* DNA only reduces by a factor of two the half-life $t_{1/2}$ of the complex formed with repressor.

Recently Crick and Klug (1975) have postulated another type of unusual DNA structure, in which the double-stranded helix executes right-angle turns. These "kinks" in the DNA helix can be constructed by unstacking one base pair and unwinding the duplex helix by about 25°. The base sequences near a kink would be more exposed than they would be in a linear stretch of DNA. The authors speculate that when *lac* repressor binds to the operator site on DNA, the double helix becomes kinked in four places, thus accounting for the 90° unwinding measured. Although so far there is no experimental evidence attesting to the existence of kinks in DNA, and no reason on theoretical grounds to recommend kinking over smooth bending of the double helix (Kuhn and Thürkauf, 1961), the idea is tantalizing. Preliminary electron microscopy results do not lend much support to this hypothesis in the case of the repressor-operator interaction (J. Hirsh and R. Schleif, private communication). In positively stained electron micrographs of 200 base-pair restriction fragments of DNA containing the *lac* promoter-operator region, the DNA does not appear kinked in either the presence or absence of bound *lac* repressor protein. The mean length of the fragments with repressor bound to the operator is about 2% less than that of the naked DNA fragments. Although a model with two kinks in the operator site would not be inconsistent with the electron microscopy data (F. H. C. Crick, private communication), it would be premature to draw any conclusions from these findings.

The intriguing problem of explaining the very fast rate of association of *lac* repressor and operator DNA has elicited several mechanisms for facilitated diffusion. The enhancement of the rate constant k_a over the value for a diffusion-limited reaction calculated from the von Smoluchowski equation has been ascribed to a variety of processes: long-range electrostatic attraction, a reduction in dimensionality of diffusion, and direct transfer of repressor protein between DNA binding sites. In the latter two cases the binding of repressor to the operator site is visualized as a two-step process: the protein first binds nonspecifically to DNA, and then searches the DNA molecule for the operator. Adam and Delbrück (1968) have pointed out that diffusion reaction rates can be accelerated by reduction of dimensionality. The model for the association of repressor and operator consists of three-dimensional diffusion of the repressor to a DNA molecule, followed by one-dimensional diffusion along the DNA chain. Richter and Eigen (1974) have performed a theoretical treatment for the diffusion of a sphere toward a rod under the influence of an electric field. On the basis of their equations they reach two conclusions. First, electrostatic attraction between the repressor protein and the operator site on DNA is not the essential rate-enhancing mechanism. They show that dissociation rates are much more sensitive to ionic strength than are association rates, the reverse of what is observed in the case of the repressor-operator interaction. There is no doubt that electrostatic forces play an important role, because of the unusual sensitivity of the rate constant of association k_a to ionic strength. However, the electrostatic effects are probably exerted indirectly through the dissociation rate of the nonspecific DNA binding. Second, they estimate the size of the DNA target required to account for the observed rate of association k_a to be about 1,000 Å or 300 base pairs. An alternative mechanism for the searching process by direct transfer of the *lac* repressor from site to site on the DNA has been proposed (von Hippel et al., 1975; Bresloff and Crothers, 1975). This model would imply transitional binding of two DNA sites by the repressor protein. A direct transfer process has been invoked to explain the binding kinetics of the intercalative dye ethidium (Bresloff and Crothers, 1975). The advantage of this mechanism is that it allows a faster path for the ligand to seek a preferred binding site than mechanisms requiring dissociation to free ligand. In order for a direct transfer process to function as a rate-enhancing mechanism at dilute concentrations (10^{-12} M operator or 30 ng/ml *lac* phage DNA), one must postulate intramolecular transfer events within the domain of a single DNA molecule. Thus the rate constant of association k_a should be a function of the effective DNA concentration, that is, of the length of the DNA (von Hippel et al., 1975).

There is no experimental evidence bearing directly on either of these hypothetical mechanisms for facilitated diffusion. It is not known whether *lac* repressor has a second potential binding site for DNA, as required by the direct transfer model. The prediction of both models, that the rate constant k_a should decrease for small operator DNA fragments below a certain size, has not been tested experimentally. However, there are some data that are suggestive. For sonicated operator DNA fragments about 1,000–2,000 base pairs long, the equilibrium constant K_O (Riggs et al., 1970c) and rate constant of dissociation k_b (Gilbert, 1972) are the same as for the whole phage DNA, indicating that the rate constant of association k_a is not lowered for DNA pieces of that size. Also, the rate constant of dissociation k_b of repressor from the 200 base-pair restriction fragment carrying an intact *lac* control region is the same as for λp*lac* DNA (A. Maxam, private communication). Assuming that the affinity of the repressor for the operator site is independent of the size of the DNA piece in which it is embedded and that the principle of microscopic reversibility holds, if the rate constant of association k_a were to decrease for binding to a 200 base-pair fragment of DNA, then the rate constant of dissociation k_b should decrease. But it does not. It may be that facilitated diffusion is not the basis for the anomalously large value of the bimolecular rate constant, and that one should look elsewhere for an explanation of this phenomenon.

Nonspecific Recognition of DNA

Besides binding very tightly to the operator site on DNA, the *lac* repressor binds with lower affinity to other base sequences in natural and synthetic DNAs. On a given DNA molecule there are many nonspecific binding sites for repressor protein. The interaction of repressor and a single such site on DNA, according to the equation

$$R + DNA \rightleftharpoons R-DNA$$

is governed by the equilibrium association constant K_{DNA}

$$K_{DNA} = \frac{[R-DNA]}{[R][DNA]}$$

Here K_{DNA} is the average affinity per site; $[DNA]$ is the concentration of potential sites. Because of the low affinity of repressor for non-operator DNAs and because of the multisite binding, the nonspecific binding of repressor to DNA cannot be quantitated by the procedures developed to study the repressor-operator interaction. However, the association constant K_{DNA} can be measured in competition experiments on membrane filters, since the ability of unlabeled DNA to compete with labeled operator DNA for the repressor is a function of the affinity of repressor for the binding sites on the unlabeled DNA molecule. Because of the conditions prevailing in membrane filtration experiments, where the competing DNA is present in enormous excess of repressor protein, the association constant K_{DNA} measured is biased in the direction of the higher affinity sites on non-operator DNA. The nonspecific binding of repressor to DNA has been investigated by several physical chemical techniques, in addition to membrane filtration.

Two types of competition experiments have been employed to determine the affinity of repressor for non-operator DNA: equilibrium competition and a somewhat unconventional rate competition (Lin and Riggs, 1972b). For equilibrium competition experiments a constant concentration of repressor protein and labeled operator DNA is equilibrated with increasing concentrations of unlabeled non-operator DNA. Equilibrium competition curves are depicted in

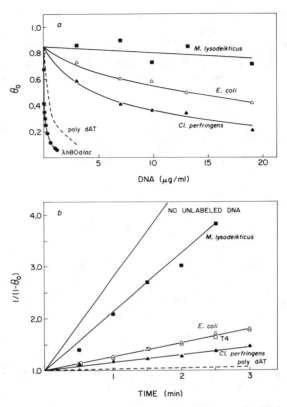

Fig. 4. Competition for *lac* repressor by non-operator DNAs. *a*. Equilibrium competition. Aliquots of unlabeled DNA and labeled λh80d*lac* DNA (2.2×10^{-12} M) are mixed, and then active repressor protein (2.2×10^{-12} M) is added. After equilibration, samples of the reaction mixture are filtered. θ_0 is the fraction saturation of labeled operator by repressor. *b*. Rate competition. At time $t = 0$, active repressor protein (2.2×10^{-12} M) is added to a mixture of labeled λh80d*lac* DNA (2.2×10^{-12} M) and cold non-operator DNA (0.65 μg/ml); at various times *t*, samples are removed and filtered. The apparent rate constant of association k_a (app) of repressor and labeled operator DNA is proportional to the slope of the straight line. Unlabeled DNAs: solid circle = λh80d*lac*; solid square = *M. lysodeikticus*; open square = T4; solid triangle = *Cl. perfringens*; open triangle = *E. coli*; dashed line = poly dAT. unbroken line = no unlabeled DNA. Standard conditions (see legend, fig. 2) except binding buffer has 3×10^{-3} M Mg(CH$_3$CO$_2$)$_2$. Data from Lin and Riggs (1972b).

figure 4*a*. The affinity K_{DNA} of repressor for the competing DNA relative to the affinity K_O for operator is computed from the concentration of unlabeled DNA required to reduce the amount of labeled repressor-operator complex by one-half. The equilibrium competition method requires relatively high concentrations of unlabeled DNA. The rate competition method is ten times more sensitive to the concentration of competing DNA. In these experiments the rate of association of repressor protein and labeled operator DNA is measured in the presence of a given concentration of unlabeled non-operator DNA. The apparent rate constant of association k_a(app) is smaller, since the concentration of free repressor protein is reduced due to binding to the competing DNA. Figure 4b shows the kinetics data from rate competition experiments; the apparent rate constant k_a(app) is proportional to the slope of the line. The equilibrium constant K_{DNA} can be calculated from the ratio of the rate constants in the presence and absence of competing DNA, assuming that repressor is in equilibrium with non-operator DNA during the reaction. Values for K_{DNA} obtained by the two techniques are in good agreement; for example, for poly dAT, K_{DNA} is $3\text{-}9 \times 10^7$ M^{-1} by equilibrium competition and $2\text{-}6 \times 10^7$ M^{-1} by rate competition.

The binding of *lac* repressor protein to a wide variety of non-operator DNAs has been characterized in competition experiments (Lin and Riggs, 1972b; Riggs, Lin, and Wells, 1972; Lin and Riggs, 1976; Richmond and Steitz, 1976; P. Lu, private communication). The outstanding result of these studies is that the repressor discriminates between DNAs having different sequences, even in its nonspecific binding to DNA. This is suggestive in the binding to natural DNAs where the affinity of repressor for non-operator DNAs correlates roughly with the (A + T) content of the DNA (Lin and Riggs, 1972b). Natural DNAs having a higher (A + T) content compete more effectively with operator, as evident in figure 4. On a weight basis DNA from *Cl. perfringens* (70 mole % (A + T)) competes at least ten times better than DNA from *M. lysodeikticus* (30 mole % (A + T)). Further, *lac* repressor binds to glucosylated DNAs from T2 and T4 phages with about the affinity expected on the basis of their (A + T) content. The extent of glucosylation of hydroxymethyl-cytosine residues is high: 75 % for T2 DNA and 100% for T4 DNA (Georgopoulos and Revel, 1971). The fact that the repressor has equal, as well as the expected, affinity for these two DNAs suggests that the nonspecific interaction is not affected by the presence of sugar groups in the major groove of DNA. Nevertheless, the interpretation that the repressor binds only to preferred, non-glucosylated sites cannot be completely rejected. No binding to ribonucleic acids could be detected. The effects of differences in the DNA bases and the base sequence on the nonspecific binding are more dramatically displayed in the binding to synthetic DNAs. The values of the association constant K_{DNA} for various DNA copolymers are collected in table 1. These synthetic polynucleotides exhibit a wide spectrum of affinities for *lac* repressor, ranging from 10^5 M^{-1} for poly(dG-dC): poly(dG-dC) to 10^{10} M^{-1} for poly(dA-dIU):poly(dA-dIU). The basis for the recognition process in the nonspecific binding to DNA is not known. Clearly, simple base composition, (A + T) content, is not the determining factor, since poly(dA-dT):poly(dA-dT) binds 30 times tighter than poly dA:poly dT. In the alternating copolymers the possibility that the repressor binds to branched structures existing because of intrastrand complementarity is effectively excluded by two facts: poly(dI-dC):poly(dI-dC) and poly(dG-dC): poly(dG-dC) bind poorly and crosslinked poly(dA-dU-HgX):poly(dA-dU-HgX) binds well. There is only minor correlation of the affinity K_{DNA} with the stability of the duplex structure (T_m) in the case of halogen-substituted analogues of poly(dA-dT):poly(dA-dT). Moreover, the notion that *lac* repressor makes extensive contacts with DNA bases in the major groove of the helix is jeopardized by the finding that the affinity K_{DNA} is not perturbed when the major groove is filled with sugar residues or bulky mercury mercaptans. Still, the fact remains that the binding is strengthened considerably by substitutions in positions 4 (S for O) and 5 (halogens for methyl) of thymine.

The effects of various parameters on this nonspecific binding have also been determined by membrane filtration. The dependence of the equilibrium

TABLE 1

BINDING OF REPRESSOR TO SYNTHETIC POLYNUCLEOTIDES

Polymer	K_{DNA} M^{-1a}	T_m°C	Reference
lac operator	2-5 × 10^{13}		
d(A-T):d(A-T)	3-10 × 10^7	60	1,2
	9-22 × 10^{6b}		3
d(A-4-thioT):d(A-4-thioT)	5 × 10^9		4
d(A-U):d(A-U)	1-1.4 × 10^6	57	2
	3-7 × 10^{6b}		3
d(A-FU):d(A-FU)	3-10 × 10^8	59	2
d(A-ClU):d(A-ClU)	1.7-5 × 10^9	67	2
d(A-BrU):d(A-BrU)	2.5-5 × 10^9	66	2
d(A-IU):d(A-IU)	5-14 × 10^9	66	2
d(A-U-Hg-X):d(A-U-Hg-X)			
X: dithiothreitol	1-2 × 10^{9b}	—^{c}	3
X: β-mercaptoethanol	2-5 × 10^{8b}	54	3
X: mercaptopropanediol	4-9 × 10^{7b}	56	3
d(G-C):d(G-C)	1.4 × 10^5		5
d(I-C):d(I-C)	3 × 10^5		5
dA:dT	1-1.3 × 10^6		1
dG:dC	1-3 × 10^6		1
dI:dC	3 × 10^5		1
d(T-T-G):d(C-A-A)	1-3 × 10^{8d}		5

a. K_{DNA} is the equilibrium association constant for the reaction

$$R + DNA \rightleftharpoons R\text{-}DNA$$

It is calculated relative to the association constant for operator $K_0 = 2\text{-}5 \times 10^{13}$ M^{-1}, assuming each base pair begins a potential binding site. Standard conditions (see legend of fig. 2) except binding buffer has 3×10^{-3} M Mg(CH$_3$CO$_2$)$_2$.

b. 0.01 M Tris, pH 7.4, 0.01 M KCl, 3×10^{-3} M Mg(CH$_3$Co$_2$)$_2$; 25°C.

c. This DNA probably has intrastrand crosslinks.

d. K_{DNA} calculated assuming every third base pair begins a potential binding site.

KEY TO REFERENCES: 1. Lin and Riggs (1972b). 2. Lin and Riggs (1976). 3. Richmond and Steitz (1976). 4. P. Lu (private communication). 5. Riggs et al. (1972).

association constant K_{DNA} upon ionic strength, pH, and temperature was measured in competition experiments (Lin and Riggs, 1972b, 1975b). The affinity K_{DNA} of repressor for non-operator DNA exhibits about the same dependence on ionic strength and pH as does the affinity K_O for operator, but appears to be independent of temperature. For conditions abolishing the binding of repressor to operator DNA, the effects on the nonspecific binding obviously could not be studied by the usual competition methods. Accordingly, an ingenious technique was developed for measuring the binding of repressor to labeled non-operator DNA directly on membrane filters (Lin and Riggs, 1975a). The procedure exploits the fact that at low ionic strength $(I = 0.05 M)$ *lac* repressor protein can be photochemically attached to BrdU-substituted λh80 DNA (Lin and Riggs, 1974). In this type of experiment, actinomycin D inhibits the binding of *lac* repressor to nonoperator DNA. On the other hand, the inducer IPTG does not alter the affinity K_{DNA} of repressor for three non-operator DNAs (BrdU-λh80, poly(dA-dT):poly(dA-dT), and poly(dT-dT-dG): poly(dC-dA-dA).

Physical methods have also been employed to study the nonspecific binding of *lac* repressor to the bulk of the sites on DNA. Two notable results have come out of these experiments: namely, the size of the binding site on non-operator DNA and the detection of a change in conformation of DNA upon binding of repressor. The number of base pairs comprising the non-operator DNA site was measured in titration experiments by three techniques: light scattering with poly dAT (Maurizot, Charlier, and Hélène, 1974), glycerol gradient sedimentation and circular dichroism (CD) with both λ DNA and poly dAT (von Hippel et al., 1975; Butler, Revzin, and von Hippel, 1975). In all cases one *lac* repressor tetramer binds per 11-13 base pairs; this non-operator DNA site is roughly half the length of the 27 base-pair operator piece. At low ionic strength the CD spectra of poly dAT and λ DNA is enhanced in the 260–280 nm region by repressor (Maurizot et al., 1974; Butler et al., 1975). The increased ellipticity of the strong DNA circular dichroism band when repressor protein is bound is evidence for a conformational change in the secondary structure of the DNA. The CD effect was not observed at high ionic strength, perhaps because the binding of repressor to poly dAT is greatly reduced (Maurizot et al., 1974). Moreover, *lac* repressor is a helix-stabilizing protein; at very low ionic strength it increases the melting temperature of poly dAT appreciably (von Hippel et al., 1975). Inducer IPTG affects neither the conformational change (Maurizot et al., 1974) nor the glycerol gradient sedimentation results (von Hippel et al., 1975), further testifying that the nonspecific binding is not sensitive to inducer. The interaction of repressor and non-operator DNAs has also been studied by observing changes in the tryptophan fluorescence of the protein that occur upon binding to DNA (Sommer, Lu, and Miller, 1975). Results from these binding experiments are in qualitative agreement with those obtained by the membrane filter technique.

After all this, what, if anything can we conclude about the factors important in the repressor-DNA recognition process? First, compare the properties of the interaction of repressor with operator and non-operator DNAs. The specific and nonspecific binding share these traits:

1. Sensitivity to electrostatic conditions. Increased shielding (ionic strength) and negative charge on the protein (pH) weaken the interaction.
2. Inhibition by actinomycin D. The antibiotic intercalates at dG-dC sequences and blocks the narrow groove of the DNA helix.
3. Effect of Br substitution in DNA. Replacement of methyl by Br at the 5 position of thymine in the major groove of the DNA helix strengthens the interaction.
4. Conformational change in DNA.

The specific and nonspecific binding differ in the following respects:

1. Effect of inducer IPTG. Inducer lowers the affinity K_O for operator DNA, but does not change the affinity K_{DNA} for non-operator DNA. The binding of repressor to non-operator DNA is insensitive to effecting ligands, even in the case of poly(dT-dT-dG):poly(dC-dA-dA), which provides, in order, the sequences TTGT of four of the six bases of the symmetrical region of the *lac* operator (see fig. 9a).
2. Temperature dependence. The affinity K_O for operator DNA increases slightly with temperature. The affinity K_{DNA} for non-operator DNA apparently does not depend on temperature.
3. Size of the DNA site. The length of the operator site is about 27 base pairs; the length of non-operator sites is about 12 base pairs. A rationalization of this discrepancy will be presented later.

Detailed models for protein-nucleic acid interactions, where the protein lies in one of the grooves of double helical nucleic acids, have been proposed. Sung and Dixon (1970) constructed a model for histone binding to DNA, in which they demonstrate that the major groove of DNA in the B conformation readily accommodates an α-helical structure of the amino-terminal region of the protein. An analogous model has been suggested for the case of *lac* repressor (Adler et al., 1972). Carter and Kraut (1974) have constructed a highly plausible model for the complementary binding of helical antiparallel β-polypeptide chain segments in the minor groove of double-stranded RNA.

The RNA helix assumes a hybrid form between the A and A′ conformations; hydrogen bonds form between the ribose 2′-hydroxyls and the peptide carbonyl oxygens. The 2′-hydroxyl group, present in RNA but absent in DNA, plays an important role in the precise complementarity between the RNA and polypeptide double helices. Mimicking this model is one for binding to DNA in the B conformation (Church et al., 1975). Here, unusual hydrogen bonds form between alternate deoxyribose 3′-hydroxyls and peptide nitrogens; most amino acid side groups could interact with DNA bases in the minor groove without distortion of the backbone conformation. The possible involvement of the major and minor grooves in the binding of repressor to DNA, operator or otherwise, is difficult to pinpoint. The minor groove is mentioned by the fact that actinomycin D inhibits the interaction with both operator and non-operator DNAs. However, it is conceivable that intercalation of the dye abolishes the binding by distorting the DNA structure. And the stereochemistry of the actinomycin-DNA complex is itself based on model studies. As for the major groove, the experimental results are frankly confusing. The affinity of repressor for halogen-substituted operator and non-operator DNAs is decidedly enhanced. On the other hand, blocking the major groove has no profound effect on the nonspecific binding; and the effect of such a perturbation on the specific binding is not known. Perhaps, as numerous authors suggest, the key to the major groove mystery lies in some structural subtlety of the DNA helix. The fact that the length of the DNA sites differs by a factor of two, in the cases of operator and non-operator DNA binding, raises additional questions about the geometry of the repressor, which we will take up later. It is tempting to imagine that the *lac* repressor makes some common contacts with both operator and non-operator DNAs, and additional contacts with the operator, which are disrupted upon binding of inducer. But it is by no means necessary to seek a uniform recognition process for the specific and nonspecific interactions with DNA.

INTERACTION OF REPRESSOR AND EFFECTING LIGANDS

The other important activity of the *lac* repressor is the binding of effecting ligands, inducers or anti-inducers. These low-molecular-weight sugar molecules, primarily β-galactosides, can bind to repressor protein whether it is free in solution or bound to DNA. The binding sites on the protein for DNA and for effecting ligands are distinct and non-overlapping; this is amply documented both genetically and biochemically. However, these sites are mutually interacting; binding of effecting ligand alters the affinity of repressor for operator, and vice versa. The interplay between the DNA and ligand binding sites is mediated by a conformational change in repressor protein, and is the substance of the regulatory mechanism. We shall discuss separately the interaction of effecting ligands with repressor protein and with repressor-operator complex.

Binding to Free Repressor

The interaction of *lac* repressor protein and effecting ligands has been studied with two intents: to quantitate the binding and to investigate the conformational change. The equation for the stoichiometry of the binding of repressor and an effecting ligand L is

$$R + 4L \rightleftharpoons RL_4$$

In general, this reaction is characterized by a single equilibrium association constant K_L for the binding of ligand to a site on the protein

$$K_L = \frac{[R'L]}{[R'][L]}$$

where now $[R']$ is the concentration of sites for ligand, theoretically four times the concentration of tetrameric repressor.

The binding of a wide variety of effecting ligands to repressor has been measured by equilibrium dialysis, either directly using labeled ligand or by competition with labeled IPTG (Barkley et al., 1975). The binding constants K_L, which range from $3 M^{-1}$ to about $2 \times 10^6 \ M^{-1}$, for a few compounds are presented in Table 2. The sugars are classified as inducers or anti-inducers by their effect on the stability of repressor-operator complex; most ligands which bind to *lac* repressor turn out to be inducers. The common inducer IPTG has a high affinity for repressor, $K_L = 1 \times 10^6 \ M^{-1}$. The value of K_L depends slightly on pH, but not on Mg^{+2}; it decreases about 6-fold as the temperature increases from 4°C to 40°C (Ohshima, Mizokoshi, and Horiuchi, 1974; Butler et al., 1975). At 25°C, $\Delta G = -7.7$ kcal/mole, $\Delta H = -6.2$ kcal/mole, and $\Delta S = 5$ cal/deg. mole; the enthalpy change is the main driving force for the reaction. Allolactose, the natural inducer of the *lac* operon *in vivo*, binds slightly tighter than IPTG (Jobe and Bourgeois, 1972a). Melibiose, the α-galactoside isomer of allolactose, binds with moderate affinity. One neutral ligand, o-nitrophenyl-β-D-galactoside (ONPG) was found that binds with moderate affinity to *lac* repressor, but exerts no effect on the repressor-operator interaction. Anti-inducers are competitive inhibitors of inducer binding; presumably, they bind at the same site. The evidence that inducers and anti-inducers share a common, or partly overlapping, binding site is purely circumstantial; the arguments are three. First, the two types of effecting ligands are chemically

TABLE 2

BINDING OF REPRESSOR AND REPRESSOR-OPERATOR COMPLEX TO EFFECTING LIGANDS

	K_L, M^{-1a}	Reference	^0K_L [b]	$K_0/^LK_0$ [c]	Reference
Inducers					
methyl-1-thio-β-D-galactoside	1.1×10^5	1	$(3.3\pm1.1)\times10^2$	6.5×10^2	1
isopropyl-β-D-galactoside	$(9.9\pm1.5)\times10^3$	1			
isopropyl-1-thio-β-D-galactoside	$(1.2\pm0.2)\times10^6$	1	$(5.0\pm1.3)\times10^3$	1×10^3	1
	1.4×10^{6d}	2			
	5.5×10^{5e}	2			
	1.04×10^{6f}	3			
p-aminophenyl-1-thio-β-D-galactoside	$(7.2\pm0.5)\times10^{5g}$	3			
galactose	$(7.6\pm1.7)\times10^2$	1			
melibiose (6-0-α-D-galactopyranosyl-D-glucose)	$(9.9\pm1.0)\times10^2$	1			
allolactose (6-0-β-D-galactopyranosyl-D-glucose)	$(1.7\pm0.2)\times10^6$	1	$(7.7\pm2.4)\times10$	6×10^2	1
Neutral					
o-nitrophenyl-β-D-galactoside	$(9.2\pm1.5)\times10^3$	1			
Anti-inducers					
phenyl-β-D-galactoside	$(1.1\pm0.3)\times10^3$	1	$(6.7\pm4.5)\times10^{h}$	5.6×10^{-1h}	1
o-nitrophenyl-β-D-fucoside	$(7.1\pm2.7)\times10^3$	1	$(4.0\pm0.2)\times10^{3h}$	3.3×10^{-1h}	1,4
glucose	$(1.4\pm0.2)\times10$	1	$(5.3\pm3.0)\times10^{h}$	4.9×10^{-1h}	1,4
lactose (4-0-β-D-galactopyranosyl-D-glucose)	3.0 ± 1.2	1	$(2.2\pm0.3)\times10^{h}$	1.8×10^{-1h}	1,4

a. K_L is the equilibrium association constant for the reaction

$$R' + L \rightleftharpoons R'L$$

where R' is a ligand-binding site. 0.1 M potassium phosphate buffer, pH 7.8, 10^{-3} M dithioerythritol, 10^{-3} M sodium azide, 4°C.

b. ^0K_L is the equilibrium association constant for the reaction

$$RO + L \rightleftharpoons ORL$$

calculated assuming one site for ligand on repressor bound to operator DNA. Standard conditions (see legend of fig. 2).

c. $K_0/^LK_0$ is the ratio of the affinity of repressor for operator DNA in the absence of ligand to the affinity at saturation with ligand. Standard conditions (see legend of fig. 2).

d. 0.01 M Tris, pH 8.2, 0.2 M KCl, 0.02 M Mg(CH₃CO₂)₂, 10^{-4} M EDTA, 5×10^{-4} M dithiothreitol, 4°C.

e. 0.047 M KH₂PO₄, 0.027 M Na₃BO₄, 0.1 M KCl, 0.02 M Mg(CH₃CO₂)₂, 10^{-4} M EDTA, 5×10^{-4} M dithiothreitol, pH 8.2 at 4°C.

f. 0.01 M Tris, pH 7.6, 0.2 M KCl, 10^{-4} M EDTA, 4°C.

g. Same as f, except pH 8.2

h. Standard conditions (see legend of fig. 2) except binding buffer (I = 0.1 M) has 0.06 M KCl. As noted in the text, ^0K_L and $K_0/^LK_0$ are independent of ionic strength.

KEY TO REFERENCES: 1. Barkley et al. (1975). 2. Ohshima et al. (1974). 3. Butler et al. (1975). 4. Jobe and Bourgeois (1972c).

and structurally related compounds. Second, as just stated, their binding to *lac* repressor protein is competitive. And lastly, their effects on the repressor-operator interaction are simultaneously altered by mutation in the case of the i^sY18 mutated repressor to be described later (Jobe, Riggs, and Bourgeois, 1972). Anti-inducers generally bind to repressor with low affinity. The common anti-inducer ONPF has a moderate affinity for repressor, $K_L = 7 \times 10^3$ M^{-1}. Lactose, the substrate for β-galactosidase *in vivo* and itself an anti-inducer of the operon, binds with low affinity (Jobe and Bourgeois, 1972c). Glucose also binds with low affinity; perhaps it acts to repress the operon by stabilizing repressor-operator complex as well as by catabolite repression. At low temperatures the binding of all effecting ligands is non-cooperative, indicating that the multiple ligand binding sites on repressor are identical and independent. At temperatures above 30°C slight positive cooperativity in the binding of IPTG appears (Butler et al., 1975); under somewhat different conditions, both negative and positive cooperativity have been observed (Ohshima et al., 1974).

The problem of the number of sites N for effecting ligand actually measured in equilibrium binding experiments has been tacitly ignored in the literature; it is assumed to be four per repressor tetramer. In fact, it is some number between two and four (Ohshima et al., 1974; Butler et al., 1975; M. D. Barkley, unpublished result; C. Hélène, private communication). The reason for this evasion is simple; it is not clear how to account for the observations. Some investigators report a reversible change in the value of N with temperature (Ohshima et al., 1974), whereas others find no significant change (Butler et al., 1975). Substantial variation in the value of N between preparations of purified repressor protein is also encountered (Butler et al., 1975; M. D. Barkley, unpublished result); we will take up the implications of this later.

Evidence for a conformational change in *lac* repressor protein upon binding of inducer IPTG, but not anti-inducers, derives from several sources. A shift in the fluorescence maximum of the protein, from 338 nm to 330 nm, with essentially no change in peak shape or intensity, occurs in the presence of saturating concentrations of IPTG (Laiken, Gross, and von Hippel, 1972). Glucose has no effect on the fluorescence. The spectrum is characteristic of tryptophan residues, of which there are two per repressor subunit (see table 4). Through the use of suppressed nonsense mutations in each of the two tryptophan positions, amino acids 190 and 209, (see fig. 8 and table 5), the fluorescence change resulting from IPTG binding has been imputed to tryptophan 209 (Sommer, Lu, and Miller, 1976); both tryptophans contribute to the changes mentioned earlier for non-operator DNA binding (Sommer et al., 1975). Titration experiments, monitoring the quenching of the protein fluorescence at 360 nm with inducer concentration, confirm the results obtained by equilibrium dialysis, with regard to the affinity (Laiken et al., 1972) and the noncooperative aspect of the binding (Butler et al., 1975). However, the observed fluorescence quenching (28%) at saturation with IPTG is independent of N, the number of ligand binding sites per tetramer. This result implies that those subunits that do not bind IPTG nevertheless undergo the conformational change detected by fluorescence, confounding in view of the absence of cooperativity in ligand binding. The kinetics of the IPTG binding reaction have also been studied by monitoring the fluorescence quenching in stopped-flow experiments (Laiken et al., 1972). The rate process has two steps: a bimolecular step characterized by a rate constant smaller than expected for a diffusion-limited reaction and a slow unimolecular step equated with a change in conformation of repressor protein upon binding of IPTG. Recently, by monitoring intensity changes in the fluorescence at 360 nm in temperature-jump experiments, a very fast, unimolecular relaxation process has been discovered to occur in *lac* repressor independently of inducer binding (Wu, Bandyopadhyay, and Wu, 1976). This result suggests a rapid conformational transition between two states of repressor protein, which takes place in the absence of bound IPTG and could account for the low apparent value of the bimolecular rate constant. The relative significance of these two conformational changes for the induction mechanism is not known. Ultraviolet difference spectroscopy provides additional documentation of a conformational change (Ohshima, Matsuura, and Horiuchi, 1972; Matthews et al., 1973). Here, changes in the environment of multiple aromatic residues of *lac* repressor were detected in the presence of IPTG, but not in the presence of anti-inducers, glucose and ONPF. Besides the optical techniques, a conformational change has been detected by a differential sedimentation method. The sedimentation coefficient of *lac* repressor protein increases about 3% in the presence of saturating concentrations of IPTG (Ohshima et al., 1972; M. D. Barkley, unpublished result). Nanosecond depolarization studies of repressor protein tagged with a fluorescent probe reveal no gross structural changes in the protein in the presence of IPTG (Bandyopadhyay and Wu, 1975).

Binding to Repressor-DNA Complex

Effecting ligands interact with *lac* repressor protein when it is bound to DNA, either specifically at the operator site or nonspecifically. As mentioned previously, the complex formed between repressor and operator is sensitive to effecting ligand; those formed between repressor and non-operator DNAs are not. The ligand-repressor-operator interaction has been investigated by membrane filtration. The data are most easily reconciled by the following simple reaction scheme.

$$R + O \underset{k_b}{\overset{k_a}{\rightleftharpoons}} RO$$

$$+ \qquad +$$

$$L \qquad L$$

$$K_L \updownarrow \;\; {}^L k_a \;\; \updownarrow \;\; {}^O K_L$$

$$RL + O \rightleftharpoons ORL$$

$${}^L k_b$$

As before, k_a and k_b are the specific rate constants of association and dissociation, respectively, of repressor and operator, where $K_O = k_a/k_b$. And now ${}^L k_a$ and ${}^L k_b$ are the effected rate constants, the specific rate constants of association and dissociation of repressor-ligand complex and operator. The equilibrium constants for the reactions leading to induction are ${}^O K_L$, for the binding of ligand and repressor-operator complex, and ${}^L K_O = {}^L k_a/{}^L k_b$, for the binding of repressor-ligand complex and operator.

In vivo the differential rate of β-galactosidase synthesis displays a sigmoidal dependence on inducer concentration. Figure 5a shows the characteristic induction curve. Half the maximal differential rate is achieved at about 2×10^{-4}M IPTG (Clark and Marr, 1964). The sigmoidicity of the induction curve *in vivo*, expressed by an index analogous to a Hill coefficient of 3, is indicative of a positively cooperative process (Bourgeois, 1966). Presumably, the first event in the sequence is the removal of the repressor from the operator by inducer. This is demonstrated *in vitro* by an equilibrium release curve in figure 5b. Here, the solid lines show the effects of various ligands on the repressor-operator binding equilibrium. The order of effectiveness of the inducers, IPTG > methyl-l-thio-β-D-galactoside (TMG) > melibiose, as inhibitors of the formation of repressor-operator complex parallels that of their capacities to induce the *lac* operon *in vivo* (Riggs et al., 1970b) and to bind to free repressor protein. In this assay anti-inducers have no visible effect. Although these experiments are a reliable measure of the relative potency of inducing ligands, the data are not suitable for quantitative treatment because the proportion of labeled complexes in the reaction mixture actually retained by the filters varies with inducer concentration.

Kinetics experiments provide a sound basis for quantitating the interaction of inducers and anti-inducers with repressor-operator complex; in particular, the measurement of the rate of dissociation as a function of concentration of effecting ligand. The effect of IPTG on the kinetics of the repressor-operator binding reaction has been investigated in detail (Barkley et al., 1975). Figure 6 shows a plot of the apparent specific rate constant of dissociation k_{bapp} of repressor and operator versus IPTG concentration; the data points (o) are the

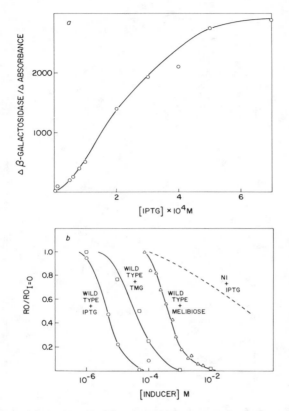

Fig. 5. Degree of induction as a function of inducer concentration. *a*. Induction of β-galactosidase synthesis *in vivo*. Cultures of *E. coli* strain ML3 ($i^+o^+z^+y^-$) growing exponentially on glycerol are induced with various concentrations of IPTG. Δ β-galactosidase/Δ absorbancy is the final differential rate of synthesis of β-galactosidase. Data from Clark and Marr (1964). *b*. Effect of inducers on the repressor-operator binding equilibrium *in vitro*. Constant concentrations of repressor protein and operator DNA are equilibrated in the presence of various concentrations of inducing ligand, as described in the legend of figure 2. Solid line = wild-type repressor protein; circle = IPTG; square = TMG; triangle = melibiose. Data from Riggs et al. (1970b) and M. D. Barkley (unpublished result). Broken line = i^sNI (see table 3) mutated repressor protein: IPTG. Data from Jobe et al. (1972).

results of individual experiments as in Figure 3*b*. The value of the rate constant at saturation with IPTG is the effected rate constant $^Lk_b = 2 \times 10^{-1}$ sec^{-1} under standard conditions, about 1,000-fold greater than in the absence of inducer. The rate constant of association of repressor protein and operator DNA is essentially the same in the presence or absence of effecting ligand: $k_a = {}^Lk_a$. Thus the equilibrium association constant ^LK_O for the binding of repressor-IPTG complex to operator DNA is about 3×10^{10} M^{-1}. Two simple

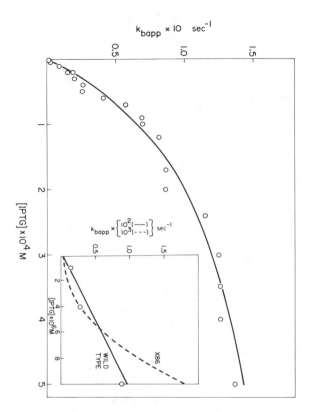

Fig. 6.   Dependence of apparent rate constant of dissociation k_{bapp} of *lac* repressor-operator complex upon IPTG concentration. Circle = data from individual kinetics experiments with wild-type repressor protein, similar to those described in the legend of figure 3*b*. Because of the very short half-lives measured at high IPTG concentrations, the dissociation reaction is stopped precisely 30 sec prior to filtration by addition of anti-inducers (0.3M glucose and 3×10^{-3}M ONPF). Solid line = theoretical curve fit to data for wild-type repressor protein assuming one site for IPTG. Data from Barkley et al. (1975). *Insert*. Expansion of scale at low concentrations of IPTG. Broken line = experimental curve for i^rX86 mutated repressor protein (see table 3). The procedure for the individual kinetics experiments is modified slightly. Purified active i^rX86 repressor protein and labeled $\lambda plac$ DNA are equilibrated to form labeled i^rX86 repressor-operator complex (6×10^{-12}M). To reduce nonspecific binding of i^rX86 repressor to labeled DNA, the reaction mixture contains 2-6 μg/ml chicken blood DNA. At time $t = 0$, a 30-fold excess of cold $\lambda plac$ DNA and various concentrations of IPTG are added; at various times t, samples are removed and filtered. Binding buffer (I = 0.2M) has 0.16M KCl. Data from Pfahl (1976).

mechanisms for induction were treated mathematically: an extreme cooperative model, in which the binding of inducer causes a concerted allosteric
transformation in repressor tetramer; and a noncooperative model, in which
the conformational transition occurs independently in each subunit. The ex-

treme cooperative model predicts a sigmoid curve of k_{bapp} vs. [IPTG], whereas the noncooperative model predicts a hyperbolic curve. Since the observed plot of k_{bapp} vs. [IPTG] is hyperbolic, mechanisms of induction involving highly cooperative interactions between inducer sites on repressor bound to operator DNA are excluded; this result is surprising in view of the *in vivo* results. Also, the value of the equilibrium association constant $^{O}K_L$ for the binding of IPTG to repressor-operator complex is extracted from the plot of k_{bapp} vs. [IPTG] by fitting the theoretical curves to the data. Assuming one site for IPTG on repressor bound to operator DNA (solid line in figure 6), the affinity $^{O}K_L$ is about 5×10^3 M^{-1}.

The effects of various reaction conditions on the ternary interaction of repressor protein, operator DNA, and inducer IPTG have also been investigated. The affinity $^{L}K_O$ of repressor-IPTG complex for operator is altered by changes in ionic strength, pH, and temperature to the same degree as is the affinity K_O of repressor for operator. The affinity $^{O}K_L$ of IPTG for repressor-operator complex is independent of ionic strength and temperature, and slightly dependent on pH. On the other hand, Mg^{+2} has profound effects on both affinities. A 100-fold increase in Mg^{+2} concentration (from zero to 0.01 M) results in a 200-fold decrease in the affinity $^{L}K_O$ of repressor-IPTG complex for operator and a 50-fold decrease in the affinity $^{O}K_L$ of IPTG for repressor-operator complex. The ternary complex is maximally stable in the absence of Mg^{+2}, the affinity of repressor for operator being reduced only 5-fold by saturation with inducer.

The interaction of other effecting ligands with repressor-operator complex has been similarly characterized in kinetic experiments. Table 2 contains a summary of the results. For all the inducers the value of the effected rate constant $^{L}k_b$ at saturation is the same within experimental error (Barkley et al., 1975). Thus all inducers destabilize repressor-operator complex about 1,000-fold, presumably by triggering the identical conformational change in repressor protein. Anti-inducers, on the other hand, have small stabilizing effects on repressor-operator complex, about 5-fold in the case of lactose (Jobe and Bourgeois, 1972c). As expected from simple thermodynamic arguments, inducers bind with greater affinity to free repressor (K_L) than to repressor-operator complex ($^{O}K_L$), and conversely for the natural anti-inducers, glucose and lactose. Phenyl-β-D- galactoside and ONPF behave anomalously, apparently binding with greater affinity to free repressor than to repressor-operator complex and at the same time stabilizing repressor-operator complex 2- to 3-fold.

In the case of *lac* repressor bound to non-operator DNAs, IPTG binding has been studied by fluorescence. The changes in the fluorescence of repressor protein upon binding of IPTG are the same in the presence or absence of DNA (von Hippel et al., 1975). This fact implies that *lac* repressor undergoes equivalent conformational transitions whether free in solution or bound nonspecifically to DNA; however, there is no concomitant change in the affinity of repressor for non-operator DNA. Titration experiments with IPTG show that inducer binds to repressor-DNA complexes of poly dAT (Maurizot et al., 1974) and of calf thymus DNA (von Hippel et al., 1975; Butler et al., 1975) identically as it does to free repressor protein.

LAC REPRESSOR PROTEIN

So far we have been describing the behavior of wild-type *lac* repressor protein. Many mutations exist in the *i* gene, the structural gene for the *lac* repressor, that alter the properties of the protein. In this section we shall discuss the genetic qualities of these mutants, as well as the biochemical characteristics of the wild-type and mutated repressor proteins. Since these subjects have been reviewed recently (Bourgeois and Pfahl, 1976; Müller-Hill, 1975), our presentation will be brief.

The i Gene

The *i* gene adjoins the *lac* promoter region P, without itself being part of the operon. As shown in figure 1, transcription of the *i* gene initiates at the *i* gene promoter P_i and proceeds in the same direction as that of the operon, but results in a separate piece of messenger RNA (Miller, Beckwith, and Müller-Hill, 1968). Little is known about the factors governing synthesis of the *lac* repressor. The amount of repressor protein present in cells is proportional to the number of copies in the *i* gene (Edelmann and Edlin, 1974). The only regulatory element in evidence to date is the promoter P_i, based on the existence and mapping data of i^q mutants that overproduce wild-type repressor (Müller-Hill et al., 1968; Miller et al., 1968). The assumption is that *lac* repressor protein is synthesized constitutively by the cell. An alternative suggestion is that synthesis of repressor protein occurs in a burst during replication of the *i* gene DNA (Edelmann and Edlin, 1974), but the experimental data in this regard are not decisive.

Hundreds of *i* gene mutants have been isolated, analyzed genetically, and mapped, by a number of investigators. The mutants can be categorized on the basis of their behavior *in vivo*. Additionally, several dozen mutated repressor proteins have been characterized *in vitro*. The phenotypes of the major classes of *i* gene mutants along with the biochemical activities of the corresponding mutated repressors are summarized in table 3. We will describe the properties of these mutants below.

TABLE 3

Properties of *Lac* Regulatory Mutants

Locus	Phenotype — Lactose Fermentation[a]	Phenotype — Inducibility	Phenotype — Dominance	Predictable Characteristics[b] — DNA Binding	Predictable Characteristics[b] — IPTG Binding	Predictable Characteristics[b] — Tetramer Formation
i Gene Allele						
i^+	lac$^+$	inducible	*trans* dominant to i^-, recessive to i^s, i^{-d}	+	+	+
i^-	lac$^+$	constitutive	recessive to i^+	−	−	−
i^-	lac$^+$	constitutive	recessive to i^+	−	+	+
i^{-d}	lac$^+$	constitutive	*trans* dominant to i^+, recessive to i^q	−	+	+
i^s	lac$^-$, (lac$^+$)	non-inducible or inducible at high inducer concentration	*trans* dominant to i^+, recessive to i^q	+	−	+
i^r	(lac$^+$)	constitutive, repressible at low inducer concentration, inducible at high inducer concentration	*trans* dominant to i^+ in the presence of inducer	(+)	+	+
i^{rc}	(lac$^+$)	constitutive, repressible by inducer	*trans* dominant to i^+ in the presence of inducer, recessive to i^+	(+)	+	(+)
i^{TL}	lac$^+$	constitutive after incubation at high temperature	recessive to i^+	(−)	(−)	(−)
i^{TSS}	lac$^+$	constitutive after growth at high temperature	recessive to i^+	(−)	(−)	(−)
				Repressor Binding	RNAp+σ Binding	CAP Binding
Operator						
o^+	lac$^+$	inducible	recessive to o^c	+	+	+
o^c	lac$^+$	constitutive	*cis* dominant to $i^+ o^+$, i^q	−	+	+
o^s	lac$^-$	non-inducible	recessive to $i^+ o^+$, $i^+ o^c$	++	+	+
Promoter						
p^+	lac$^+$	inducible		++	+	+
p class I	lac$^-$	non-inducible		++	−	−
p class II	lac$^-$	non-inducible		++	−	+
p class III	lac$^+$	inducible		++	+	++

a. Strains indicated as (lac$^+$) have a reduced growth rate in lactose minimal medium.

b. (−) means negative only at non-permissive temperature; (+) means positive only in the presence of inducer.

The *trans* dominant i^{-d} mutants have a constitutive *lac* positive phenotype. There are two types of such mutants: strong i^{-d}'s, which are fully constitutive and produce a high level of *lac* enzymes in the absence of inducer, and weak i^{-d}'s, which are partially constitutive and can be induced several-fold by IPTG (Pfahl, 1972; Pfahl, Stockter, and Gronenborn, 1974). The dominance of the i^{-d} allele over the i^{+} allele occurs by negative complementation, or the formation of inactive mixed tetramers containing i^{-d} and i^{+} repressor subunits. Three different repressor species have been found in extracts of these merodiploids (Miwa, Sadler, and Smith, 1974). *In vitro*, i^{-d} mutated repressor proteins do not bind operator DNA detectably (Pfahl et al., 1974); some i^{-d} repressors bind non-operator DNA, and others do not (Müller-Hill, 1975). They bind IPTG with affinities close to that of wild-type repressor, and they form stable tetramers.

The superrepressed i^{s} mutation confers a *lac* negative phenotype; it is dominant over the wild-type. The i^{s} mutant strains are of two kinds: strong i^{s}'s, which are not inducible, and weak i^{s}'s, which are inducible at high concentrations of IPTG (Bourgeois and Jobe, 1970; Pfahl, 1972; Pfahl et al., 1974). *In vitro*, i^{s} mutated repressors exhibit normal ($i^{s}44$, $i^{s}2A$, $i^{s}16Z$, $i^{s}14A$, $i^{s}N2$, $i^{s}43$, $i^{s}Y18$, $i^{s}45$) or slightly increased ($i^{s}277$, $i^{s}N1$, $i^{s}272$) affinity for operator DNA, but impaired IPTG binding (Jobe et al., 1972). For most i^{s} mutated repressors the complex formed with operator DNA shows the same response to inducer as that of wild-type repressor, only shifted to higher concentrations of IPTG. Three strong i^{s} mutated repressors, $i^{s}N1$, $i^{s}272$, and $i^{s}45$, have altered allosteric properties, as evidenced by a qualitatively different shape of the equilibrium release curve (broken line in figure 5b).

An intriguing class of mutants are the repressible i^{r} mutants; *in vivo* the action of IPTG is reversed. These mutants have a *lac* positive phenotype. They are constitutive, and repressible by low concentrations of inducer. The $i^{r}X86$ mutant is inducible by high concentrations of inducer (Chamness and Willson, 1970); the i^{rc} mutant is not (Myers and Sadler, 1971). *In vitro,* the $i^{r}X86$ mutated repressor has a 50-fold increased affinity for operator DNA, and binds IPTG normally (Jobe and Bourgeois, 1972b). It also has increased affinity for *E. coli* DNA (Pfahl, 1976). The $i^{r}X86$ repressor differs somewhat from the wild-type repressor in its allosteric properties. As depicted by the broken line in figure 6, the curve of $k_{b app}$ vs. [IPTG] is slightly sigmoidal, indicating that more than one inducer molecule is required to release $i^{r}X86$ repressor from the operator (Pfahl, 1976). Pfahl (1976) proposed the following explanation of the *in vivo* behavior of this mutant, which might apply for other i^{r} mutants as well. In the absence of inducer the $i^{r}X86$ repressor is bound to other high-affinity pseudo-operator sites, of the type which will be described later, on the *E. coli* chromosome. At low concentrations of inducer it is released preferentially from these sites and binds the operator site, for which it retains considerable affinity. At high concentrations of inducer the i^rX86 repressor dissociates from the operator.

The *trans* dominant i^{-d}'s and the superrepressed i^s's are the two major classes of *i* gene mutants that have been examined. The mutational defect in the repressor protein affects operator binding for i^{-d}'s and IPTG binding for i^s's. In both cases the ability of the protein to form a stable tetramer is intact. Recently, a few recessive i^- constitutive mutants have been obtained that are assembly mutants. *In vitro* the i^- mutated repressor proteins bind IPTG and appear to be mixtures of monomers and dimers of repressor subunits (Schmitz et al., 1976). And lastly, there are a few temperature-sensitive *i* gene mutants. These mutants have the wild-type *lac* positive inducible phenotype at the permissive temperature. At elevated temperatures they are recessive i^- constitutives after incubation of the thermolabile i^{TL} mutant (Horiuchi and Novich, 1961) or after growth of the temperature-sensitive synthesis i^{TSS} mutant (Sadler and Novick, 1965).

Figure 7 is a map of the *i* gene showing the locations of the above-mentioned mutations (Pfahl 1972, 1976; Pfahl et al., 1974; Müller-Hill et al., 1975). These sites on the genetic map have not yet been correlated with the physical map past the first 81 amino acids, although this will be greatly facilitated by the recent development of a fine structure mapping system (Miller et al., 1975; Schmeissner, Ganem, and Miller, in preparation cited by Miller et al., 1975). At present this mapping system consists of a set of over 100 ordered deletions, all but one of which enter the *i* gene from the left. The end points of these deletions effectively divide the *i* gene into intervals corresponding to an average length of three amino acids on the repressor polypeptide chain. The colinearity of the genetic map with the amino acid sequence of the *lac* repressor, established first for the amino-terminal portion of the protein (Weber et al., 1972; Müller-Hill et al., 1975), is now complete (J. H. Miller, private communication). Based on the mapping data of *i* gene mutants, it is possible to link the biological activities of the repressor protein and specific regions on the polypeptide chain. As seen in figure 7, the i^{-d} mutations map at the extreme left of the *i* gene, which codes for the amino-terminal region of the repressor. The genetic evidence implicating the amino-terminal portion of the protein in the DNA-binding site is overwhelming; all the strong i^{-d} variants map at the left end of the *i* gene. Adjacent to this region, there is an interval of the *i* gene that may determine the allosteric or conformational properties of the protein. The weak i^{-d} mutants, some strong i^s mutants, including two (i^sN1 and i^s272) with allosteric defects, the i^r mutants i^rX86 and i^{rc}, and the thermolabile mutant i^{TL} all map in this area. In the middle of the *i* gene, there is a cluster of i^s mutations. Since all the weak i^s variants map in

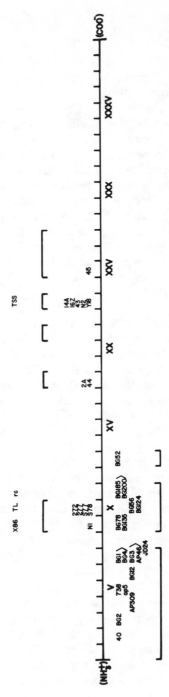

Fig. 7. Functional map of the i gene. The figure shows the relative locations of i^{-d} and i^s mutations, as well as certain i gene mutations mentioned in the text and in table 5. Brackets, and names enclosed, below the line represent i^{-d} mutations. Brackets, and names enclosed, above the line represent i^s mutations. Roman numerals denote deletion groups, arbitrarily spaced at equal distances along the gene. Data and description of mapping system from Pfahl (1972) and Pfahl et al. (1974), except the i^s mutations originally assigned to deletion group VIII have been reassigned to deletion group X (Pfahl, unpublished result). Correlation of the first X deletion groups with the first 81 amino acids is from Müller-Hill et al. (1975).

this region, it probably codes for amino acids in the inducer binding site of the repressor.

In addition to the usual procedures for isolating the missence mutants described above, Miller and coworkers (1975) have generated a spectrum of *i* gene variants by suppression of nonsense mutations. This genetical technique offers unique advantages. It allows substitution of several different amino acids for a given residue in the polypeptide chain, some of which could not be achieved by a single base change. And it permits the isolation of neutral variants, which make repressor protein with wild-type activity but having an amino acid substitution. The effects of some of the changes achieved by nonsense suppression will be described in the next section.

Protein Chemistry

The physical properties of the *lac* repressor protein are listed in table 4. This protein has no peculiar features that obviously explain its biological activities. It has an acidic isolectric point; at neutral pH the net charge on the protein is negative. In order for the repressor to neutralize the negative charges on the phosphate groups of DNA, the DNA-binding site of the protein must be a positively charged domain, however.

The shape of the repressor molecule, as well as the arrangement of subunits within the tetramer, are very much unsettled questions. Individual *lac* repressor molecules have been examined by electron microscopy in several laboratories (Ohshima, Horiuchi, Yanagida, 1975; Humphreys, 1975; C. Brack, private communication). Negatively stained repressor tetramer is visualized as a cubical molecule of dimensions 91 ± 3 Å by 102 ± 9 Å by 90 ± 5 Å (Humphreys, 1975). The four identical subunits are arranged in a U, with their long axes perpendicular to the plane of the U. The cleft is 15 ± 4 Å wide, and the subunits appear as rods of dimensions 90 Å × 45 Å. There is a plane of rotational symmetry passing through the base of the U. Neither IPTG nor ONPF discernibly alter the size or configuration of the repressor tetramer. With heavier staining procedures the tetramer appears as a somewhat smaller, squarish molecule of dimensions 80 ± 5 Å by 70 ± 5 Å (Ohshima et al., 1975). The tetramer has an inter-subunit space of about 15–20 Å filled with stain. The subunits are visible under these conditions as rods of dimensions 70 Å by 35 Å, but without sufficient resolution to decipher their arrangement. Although these authors find different absolute values for the dimensions of the *lac* repressor, their results are qualitatively consistent. The larger tetramer dimensions probably provide the better estimate of size, since less of the molecule is covered with stain when the coat of stain is thin. Microcrystals of *lac* repressor protein have been examined by a combination of electron microscopic and powder x-ray diffraction techniques (Steitz et al., 1974). The

TABLE 4

PHYSICAL AND CHEMICAL PROPERTIES OF Lac REGULATORY PROTEINS

Property	Lac Repressor	Reference	CAP Protein	Reference
Molecular weight[a]	148,800	1	45,000	10
M_w of native protein[b]	140,000	2	44,600	10
Oligomeric structure[c]	4 identical subunits	1	2 identical subunits	10
Subunit amino acid composition	347 residues[d] $Lys_{11}, His_7, Arg_{19}$, $Asp_{15}, Asn_{11}, Thr_{18}$, $Ser_{30}, Glu_{13}, Gln_{28}$, $Pro_{13}, Gly_{22}, Ala_{44}$, Cys_3, Val_{33}, Met_9, $Ile_{17}, Leu_{40}, Tyr_8$, Phe_4, Trp_2	1	200 residues[a] $Lys_{13}, His_5, Arg_{10}$, Asp_{14}, Thr_{13}, Ser_9, Glu_{31}, Pro_7, Gly_{16}, Ala_{12}, Cys_2, Val_{14}, Met_5, $Ile_{16}, Leu_{21}, Tyr_5$, Phe_5, Trp_2	10
Amino terminus	methionine		valine[c]	11
Carboxy terminus	glutamine			
Subunit molecular weight[a]	37,200	1	22,500	10
M_w of reduced-alkylated subunits in 6 M GuHCl[b]			22,300	10
Partial specific volume[a]	0.741 ml/g	2	0.752 ml/g	10
Sedimentation coefficient of native protein[e]	7S	3	3.53 S	10
Isoelectric point[f]	pH 5.6	4	pH 9.12	10
$E_{280}^{1\%}$, 1cm	5.9[a,g]	2,5	6.9[h]	10
A_{280}/A_{260}	1.9	5	1.8	10
% a-helix[i]	38%, 40%	6,7	31%	10
% β-sheet[i]	27%, 42%	6,7		
Molecular dimensions of native protein	90Å × 100Å × 90Å[j]; 140Å × 60Å × 45Å[k]	8,9		

a. Amino acid analysis.

b. Equilibrium sedimentation.

c. End group determination.

d. Sequence analysis.

e. Velocity sedimentation.

f. Isoelectric focusing.

g. Dry weight.

h. Lowry, estimated from data in reference 10.

i. Circular dichroism.

j. Electron microscopy of dilute solution.

k. Electron microscopy and powder X-ray diffraction of microcrystals.

KEY TO REFERENCES: 1. Beyreuther et al. (1973). 2. Butler et al. (1975). 3. Riggs and Bourgeois (1968). 4. K. Weber (unpublished result cited by Müller-Hill, 1971). 5. M. D. Barkley (unpublished result). 6. Matsuura, Ohshima, and Horiuchi (1972). 7. Chou et al. (1975). 8. Humphreys (1975). 9. Steitz et al. (1974). 10. Anderson et al. (1971). 11. H. Niall (unpublished result cited by Anderson et al., 1971).

results are at odds with the studies on individual molecules. The proposed shape of the repressor molecule in the crystals is asymmetric, with dimensions of 140 Å by 60 Å by 45 Å.

At this point, there is no evidence pertaining to the geometry of the *lac* repressor-operator interaction. It is not even known how many subunits of the protein make contact with DNA. Comparing the size of the operator site, about 60–90 Å, with the size of the tetramer, about 90 Å, it seems likely that the operator accommodates one repressor molecule. In this situation at least two subunits could, and quite likely do, interact with the operator.

The amino acid composition per subunit of *lac* repressor protein is also given in table 4. The repressor has a normal amino acid content, somewhat low in aromatic amino acids. There are eight tyrosines, four phenylalanines, and two tryptophans per 347 residues, accounting for the low value of the extinction coefficient of the protein at 280 nm, $E_{1cm}^{1\%} = 5.9$. The primary structure of the *lac* repressor polypeptide chain is shown in figure 8 (Beyreuther et al., 1973, 1975). Again, there is nothing inherently revealing in the amino acid sequence. The 60-residue sequence at the amino terminus contains four of the eight tyrosine residues at positions 7, 12, 17, and 47, eight positively charged residues, and four negatively charged residues. Both the amino and carboxy terminal portions of the polypeptide chain have a higher proportion of positively charged residues relative to the intervening region. The remaining four tyrosine residues are located at positions 126, 193, 260, and 269, and the two tryptophans at positions 190 and 209. The three cysteine residues are at positions 107, 140, and 268; there are no disulfide bridges in the repressor molecule. From the amino acid sequence Chou, Adler, and Fasman (1975) made a detailed prediction of the secondary structure of *lac* repressor protein. The predictive value of 37% α-helix content is in reasonable accord with the estimates from circular dichroism experiments on the native protein.

A number of investigators have determined the amino acid substitutions of *i* gene variants (Weber et al., 1972; Files, Weber, and Miller, 1974; Miller et al., 1975; Beyreuther et al., in preparation cited by Müller-Hill, 1975; J. G. Files, private communication). The results of their efforts are compiled in table 5. As anticipated from the mapping data, all strong i^{-d} mutants specify amino acid substitutions in the first 58 residues of the polypeptide chain. The i^rX86 mutated repressor, which has increased affinity for both operator and non-operator DNAs, has an exchange at residue 61, very close to the amino terminal region. The i^- assembly mutants, which make repressor proteins of subunit molecular weight that bind IPTG, specify amino acid substitutions in the regions of residues 210–216 and 257–277 (Schmitz et al., 1976). The effects of multiple amino acid substitutions at given residues, created by

MET LYS PRO VAL THR   LEU TYR ASP VAL ALA   10   GLU TYR ALA GLY VAL   SER TYR GLN THR VAL   20
SER ARG VAL VAL ASN   GLN ALA SER HIS VAL   30   SER ALA LYS THR ARG   GLU LYS VAL GLU ALA   40
ALA MET ALA GLU LEU   ASN TYR ILE PRO ASN   50   ARG VAL ALA GLN GLN   LEU ALA GLY LYS GLN   60
SER LEU LEU ILE GLY   VAL ALA THR SER SER   70   LEU ALA LEU HIS ALA   PRO SER GLN ILE VAL   80
ALA ALA ILE LYS SER   ARG ALA ASP GLN LEU   90   GLY ALA SER VAL VAL   VAL SER MET VAL GLU   100
ARG SER GLY VAL GLU   ALA CYS LYS ALA ALA   110   VAL HIS ASN LEU LEU   ALA GLN ARG VAL SER   120
GLY LEU ILE ILE ASN   TYR PRO LEU ASP ASP   130   GLN ASP ALA ILE ALA   VAL GLU ALA ALA CYS   140
THR ASN VAL PRO ALA   LEU PHE ILE ILE PHE   150   SER HIS GLN ASP GLY   THR ARG LEU GLY VAL   160
GLU HIS LEU VAL ALA   LEU GLY HIS GLN GLN   170   ILE ALA LEU LEU ALA   GLY PRO LEU SER SER   180
VAL SER ALA ARG LEU   ARG LEU ALA GLY TRP   190   HIS LYS TYR LEU THR   ARG ASN GLN ILE GLN   200
PRO ILE ALA GLU ARG   GLU GLY ASP TRP SER   210   ALA MET SER GLY PHE   GLN GLN THR MET LEU   220
ASN GLU GLY ILE VAL   PRO THR ALA MET LEU   230   VAL ALA ASN ASP GLN   MET ALA LEU GLY ALA   240
MET ARG ALA ILE THR   GLU SER GLY LEU ARG   250   VAL GLY ALA ASP ILE   SER VAL VAL GLY TYR   260
ASP ASP THR GLU ASP   SER SER CYS TYR ILE   270   PRO PRO LEU THR THR   ILE LYS GLN ASP PHE   280
ARG LEU LEU GLY GLN   THR SER VAL ASP ARG   290   LEU LEU GLN LEU SER   GLN GLY GLN ALA VAL   300
LYS GLY ASN GLN LEU   LEU PRO VAL SER LEU   310   VAL LYS ARG LYS THR   THR LEU ALA PRO ASN   320
THR GLN THR ALA SER   PRO ARG ALA LEU ALA   330   ASP SER LEU MET GLN   LEU ALA ARG GLN VAL   340
SER ARG LEU GLU SER   GLY GLN   347

Fig. 8. Amino acid sequence of the *lac* repressor. Data from Beyreuther *et al.* (1973, 1975).

TABLE 5

Amino Acid Substitutions in the *Lac* Repressor

Amino Acid Number	Wild-type Amino Acid	Mutant Name or Type	Amino Acid Substitution	Phenotype after Substitution		Reference
5	Thr	40	Met	i^{-d}	strong	1
7	Tyr	amber	Lys	i^-		2
			Gln, Ser, Leu	i^-	weak	2
9	Val	BG2	Ile	i^{-d}	strong	3
12	Tyr	amber	Gln,Ser,Leu	i^+		2
16	Ser	AP309	Pro	i^{-d}	strong	4
17	Tyr	amber	Gln,Ser,Leu,Lys	i^-		2
18	Gln	amber	Ser,Leu,Tyr,Lys	i^-		2
19	Thr	op5,738	Ala	i^{-d}	strong	4
26	Gln	amber	Ser,Leu,Tyr	i^+		4
29	His	BG12	Tyr	i^{-d}	strong	3
53	Ala	BG4,BG1	Thr	i^{-d}	strong	5
		BG3,AP46	Val	i^{-d}	strong	4,5
54 or 55	Gln	ochre	Tyr,Lys	i^-		2
54 55 56		JD24	deletion	i^{-d}	strong	5
58	Gly	BG78	Asp	i^{-d}	strong	5
		BG135	Ser	i^{-d}	strong	5
61	Ser	X86,amber	Leu	i^s,i^r		2,3,6
		amber	Tyr	i^s		2
		amber	Gln	i^+		2
74	His	S77	Tyr	i^s		3
75	Ala	S78	Val	i^s		3
76	Pro	BG56	Leu	i^{-d}	weak	3
77	Ser	BG124	Leu	i^{-d}	weak	5
		amber	Lys	i^-		2
		amber	Gln,Leu,Tyr	i^-	weak	2
78	Gln	ochre	Tyr	i^+		2
		ochre	Lys	i^s		2
81	Ala	BG200,BG185	Val	i^{-d}	weak	5
118	Arg	BG52	His	i^{-d}	weak	3
126	Tyr	amber	Gln,Ser,Leu	i^+		2
		amber	Lys	i^-		2
190	Trp	amber	Gln,Ser,Leu,Lys	i^-		2
		amber	Tyr	i^-	t.s.	2
193	Tyr	amber	Gln,Ser,Leu	i^+		2
		amber	Lys	i^-	weak	2
209	Trp	amber	Lys	i^-		2
		amber	Gln,Ser,Leu	i^s		2
		amber	Tyr	i^s	weak	2
235	Gln	amber	Ser,Leu,Tyr,Lys	i^s		2
246	Glu	amber	Leu	i^+		2
		amber	Lys	i^-		2
		amber	Tyr	i^-	weak	2
		amber	Gln,Ser	i^-	t.s.	2
256	Ser	amber	Leu,Tyr,Lys	i^-		2
		amber	Gln	i^-	t.s.	2
260	Tyr	ochre	Lys	i^-		2
		ochre	Gln	i^r		2
269	Tyr	amber	Gln,Ser,Lys	i^-		2
		amber	Leu	i^+		2

KEY TO REFERENCES: 1. Files et al. (1971). 2. Miller et al. (1975). 3. Beyreuther et al. (in preparation, cited by Müller-Hill, 1975). 4. Weber et al. (1972). 5. Müller-Hill et al. (1975). 6. J. G. Files (private communication).

suppression of amber and ochre mutations with characterized nonsense suppressors, are diverse. In some cases a particular exchange results in a mutant phenotype, whereas in others an exchange conserves the wild-type phenotype. In the amino-terminal portion of the protein, the tyrosine at position 12 and the glutamine at position 26 are replaceable by amino acids other than the wild-type residue with no change in activity of the repressor; these residues appear to be dispensable for operator binding. All substitutions of the wild-type residue for tyrosines 7 and 17 and glutamines 18, 54, and 55 in available suppressor strains destroy operator-binding in the altered repressor protein. This finding is circumstantial evidence that the latter residues make contacts with the DNA.

Further evidence for the essential role of the amino-terminal portion of the *lac* repressor protein in operator binding comes from studies of repressor molecules missing this region. Truncated repressor proteins, which no longer bind DNA but which bind IPTG and form tetramers, are derivable by genetic or enzymatic means. A few *i*⁻ amber mutants are *trans* dominant in nonsuppressing strains; these translational reinitiation mutants map at the extreme left of the *i* gene (Platt et al., 1972; Ganem et al., 1973; Files et al., 1974). Depending on the particular amber codon, translation of the *i* gene mRNA reinitiates at sites corresponding to the valine 23, methionine 42, and leucine 62 residues. *In vitro* the restart repressors bind IPTG normally and have a tetrameric structure; they are missing 23, 42, and 61 residues, respectively, from the amino-terminal region of the wild-type polypeptide chain.

Mild proteolytic digestion of native *lac* repressor protein produces a resistant "core" protein with similar properties (Platt, Files, and Weber, 1973). The core protein obtained after treatment with trypsin lacks 59 amino acids from the amino-terminal region (Platt et al., 1973) and 20–35 amino acids from the carboxy-terminal region (Beyreuther et al., 1973). Very gentle conditions yield a more homogeneous tryptic core protein missing 50 or 59 amino terminal residues with only moderate cleavage at the carboxy terminus (Huston et al., 1974). Circular dichroism measurements indicate a drop in helical content of tryptic core protein compared with native *lac* repressor (Huston et al., 1974), in line with the predictions of secondary structure (Chou et al., 1975). Loss of the capacity to bind operator and non-operator DNAs happens simultaneously in repressor protein exposed to trypsin (Lin and Riggs, 1975a). The tryptic core protein binds IPTG with the same affinity as the intact protein (Platt et al., 1973). Changes in the ultraviolet spectra identical to those observed for native repressor occur upon binding of IPTG to tryptic core protein, despite the absence of four of the eight tyrosine residues per subunit (Matthews, 1974). The molecular weight of the tryptic core tetramer is roughly 120,000, of the subunit species 28,000–35,000 (Platt et al., 1973;

Huston et al., 1974). The IPTG-binding activity and tetrameric structure can be recovered after treatment with denaturing solvent, implying that the tryptic core protein retains the ability to fold correctly (Platt et al., 1973). A variety of core proteins can be generated by the action of other proteases (Platt et al., 1973; Beyreuther, Bohmer, and Raufuss, in preparation, cited by Müller-Hill, 1975).

Investigations of modified wild-type *lac* repressor also elucidate the roles played by particular amino acid residues in the activities of the protein. So far, only tyrosine and cysteine residues have been studied quantitatively. Iodination of repressor protein at low molar iodine excess is a rapid reaction essentially confined to three tyrosine residues, 7, 12, and 17, with concomitant loss of operator binding (Fanning, 1975). This result indicates that these tyrosine residues in the amino-terminal region are exposed and probably not involved in interactions with other amino acid side chains. Operator and non-operator DNAs provide some protection against inactivation, whereas IPTG and ONPF do not. In contrast, iodination by lactoperoxidase selectively modifies one tyrosine residue per subunit (Bandyopadhyay and Wu, 1975). This iodotyrosine displays a fluorescence change when iodinated *lac* repressor binds either IPTG or operator DNA fragments, but not non-operator DNA. The sulfhydryl reagent 2-chloromercuri-4-nitrophenol reacts at two cysteine residues, 107 and 268, without effect on the activities of the protein (Yang and Matthews, 1975). A change in the ultraviolet spectrum of the chromophore is detected upon binding of inducers, but not anti-inducers, to the labeled *lac* repressor. This latter finding supports the implication from the spectral changes in the tryptic core protein that the conformational change in the repressor upon binding of inducer is transmitted through the protein core.

The tetrameric structure of *lac* repressor protein is very stable, presumably maintained by strong subunit interactions. Some dissociation of the tetramer into IPTG-binding subunits occurs in aged repressor preparations (Riggs et al., 1970a). In 0.1% SDS the *lac* repressor protein is a monomeric species without detectable activity (Hamada, Ohshima, and Horiuchi, 1973). Attempts to dissociate the tetramer into subunits that bind IPTG have been largely unsuccessful, although at lower concentrations of SDS, IPTG binding was detected in a mixture of monomers and dimers. In contrast, operator binding and possibly IPTG binding are not stable functions of *lac* repressor tetramer. Purification of repressor protein is usually accompanied by differential loss of operator-binding activity; in the best preparations, only about 50% of the theoretical number of sites for operator DNA are assayable by membrane filtration. Further deactivation of the capacity to bind operator often occurs with storage. Although the IPTG-binding activity of repressor protein appears relatively constant throughout purification and storage, there is commonly a 2-fold discrepancy in the number of sites for IPTG, as discussed previously. Whether the underlying causes of this apparent inactivation are significant or trivial is not clear. However, it seems safe to say that purified, homogeneous *lac* repressor protein is heterogeneous with respect to its biological activities. Despite attempts in a number of laboratories, to this date no single crystals of *lac* repressor protein have been obtained that are suitable for X-ray analysis; they are badly needed.

In sum, the *lac* repressor protein remains an enigma. It is a typical globular protein that performs some exceptional functions, defying instant analyses. We outline below the various attributes of the repressor that contribute to its biological activity. Genetic and biochemical data concur that:

1. The amino-terminal region is responsible for DNA binding, and probably comprises at least part of the actual site itself.
2. The protein core contains the IPTG binding site; it also plays some role in the allosteric transition.
3. An area near the carboxy-terminal region is involved in subunit interactions.
4. Both amino- and carboxy-terminal regions are near the surface of the protein; they appear to have some α-helical structure.

CAP PROTEIN

As is the case for other inducible operons, the *lac* operon is also under positive control by CAP protein plus cAMP. The CAP protein has two biological activities: it binds cAMP, and the resulting CAP protein-cAMP complex binds to DNA at specific promoters. Presumably, the binding of cAMP to CAP protein causes a conformational transition in the protein, enabling it to recognize the promoter. We will describe the properties of the CAP protein and its interactions with small ligands and DNA.

Genetics and Protein Chemistry

Two genetic loci, *cya* and *crp*, contribute to the regulatory system mediated by cAMP in *E. coli* (see fig. 1). Mutations in either gene result in a pleiotropically negative phenotype for utilization of several sugars. The *cya* gene codes for adenyl cyclase. It is not an essential gene, since deletions of *cya* are not lethal to the cell (Brickman, Soll, and Beckwith, 1973). The *crp* gene codes for CAP protein (Zubay, Schwartz, and Beckwith, 1970; Emmer et al., 1970). Addition of cAMP restores the wild phenotype in *cya* mutants, but not in *crp* mutants. *In vivo* and *in vitro* CAP protein plus cAMP are required for proper initiation of transcription by RNA polymerase at the promoters of inducible operons.

The CAP protein has been purified (Riggs, Reiness, and Zubay, 1971; Anderson et al., 1971) and characterized (Anderson et al., 1971). The physical properties are listed in table 4. The CAP protein is a dimer of 45,000 molecular weight, composed of seemingly identical subunits of 22,500 molecular weight. The dimer dissociates into subunits in 6 M guanidine-HCl. The CAP protein has a basic isoelectric point. On the basis of hydrodynamic measurements, it is a roughly spherical molecule (Anderson et al., 1971; Wu, Nath, and Wu, 1974). The α-helical content is 31%, estimated from circular dichroism measurements. The amino acid composition per subunit of CAP protein is also given in table 4. Although there are two cysteine residues per subunit, there are no disulfide bridges in the protein.

Interactions of CAP Protein

The interaction of CAP protein with cyclic nucleotides has been studied by several techniques. The equilibrium association constant of CAP protein and cAMP is 1.1×10^5 M^{-1}, measured by equilibrium dialysis; the dimer has only one apparent site for cAMP (Anderson et al., 1971). Cyclic 3',5'-guanosine monophosphate (cGMP) is a competitive inhibitor of cAMP binding. In competition experiments using the ammonium sulfate precipitation technique, a number of cyclic nucleotides were found to have considerable affinity for the CAP protein (Anderson, Perlman, and Pastan, 1972). The ability of the various cyclic nucleotides to stimulate *in vitro* transcription of the *gal* operon was also determined. Cyclic 3',5'-tubercidine monophosphate (cTuMP), which has a carbon substituted for nitrogen at position 7 of cAMP, was the only compound found to have the biological activity of cAMP. It has about the same affinity as cAMP for the CAP protein, and is equally effective in promoting *gal* transcription. All the other analogues inhibited the stimulation of *gal* transcription by cAMP, in rough proportion to their ability to bind CAP protein.

There is strong biochemical and physical evidence for a conformational change in the CAP protein upon binding of cAMP. In the presence of cAMP, proteolytic enzymes cleave native CAP protein, reducing the subunit molecular weight from 22,500 to 12,500 and altering its DNA-binding properties (Krakow and Pastan, 1973). In the absence of cAMP, the CAP protein is resistant to proteolysis. Moreover, cGMP does not convert the protein to a trypsin-sensitive form. In CAP protein tagged with fluorescent probes, an increase in fluorescence occurs upon binding of cAMP and cTuMP, but not upon binding of competitive inhibitors (Wu et al., 1974). A third biologically active analogue, $N^6,O^{2'}$-dibutyryl cAMP, was identified by this criterion, and found to stimulate *gal* transcription. Nanosecond fluorescence depolarization studies reveal no gross structural change in CAP protein in the presence of cAMP. By monitoring the fluorescence change of the probe in temperature-jump experiments, Wu and Wu (1974) detected a single, concentration-independent relaxation process, indicating a conformational transition between two states of CAP protein. In similar experiments in the presence of cAMP, two well-defined relaxation processes occur, the slower one being associated with the conformational change seen in the absence of cAMP. The kinetic data are consistent with reaction mechanisms in which the CAP protein exists in two states, to one of which cAMP binds preferentially.

The CAP protein does not bind to RNA polymerase in the presence or absence of cAMP (Nissley et al., 1972). The negative result in this experiment does not exclude interactions between CAP protein-cAMP complex and RNA polymerase bound to DNA at promoter sites. It is evident from *in vitro* transcription studies, which will be described later, that CAP protein-cAMP complex binds to a specific site in the *lac* promoter. However, for a long time, only nonspecific binding of CAP protein and DNA could be demonstrated in membrane filtration experiments. The nonspecific DNA binding is of two types: a cAMP-independent binding and a cAMP-dependent binding, both being eliminated by cGMP (Riggs et al., 1971). The cAMP-independent binding is a strong function of pH (Krakow and Pastan, 1973). At pH 6.0, CAP protein binds to DNA to a comparable extent in the presence or absence of cAMP, whereas at pH 8.0, it binds to DNA essentially only in the presence of cAMP. The CAP protein-cAMP complex binds about equally well to native and denatured DNAs from a variety of natural sources, including double and single strands of *lac* phage DNAs (Nissley et al., 1972). It also binds with roughly the same affinity to polydeoxynucleotides (Krakow and Pastan, 1973), exhibiting the same order of preference for halogen-substituted analogues of poly dAT as the *lac* repressor (Lin and Riggs, 1976).

Recently, Majors (1975) showed specific binding of CAP protein-cAMP complex to the *lac* promoter by membrane filtration. The CAP protein binds to labeled DNA restriction fragments containing the *lac* promoter-operator region in the presence of cAMP, but not to other labeled *lac* DNA fragments. The binding is abolished by cGMP. Fragments having promoters mutated in the CAP site, the point mutation L8 and the deletion L1, do not bind CAP protein-cAMP complex, establishing that the protein is interacting with its putative site in the *lac* promoter, to be described later. Previously, the only evidence of a specific interaction of CAP protein-cAMP complex with the *lac* promoter came from spectral studies of fluorescent-labeled CAP protein (Wu et al., 1974). A decrease in fluorescence of the probe occurs in CAP protein bound to λh80d*lac* DNA, but not to λh80 DNA, in the presence of cAMP; no change occurs in the absence of cAMP. So far, it has not been possible to determine the affinity of CAP protein for DNA, because of uncertainties in stoichiometry and the activity of the protein preparations. The recent detection of a specific interaction between CAP protein-cAMP complex and *lac* promoter DNA should permit quantitation of the DNA binding.

REGULATORY SITES ON DNA

We turn now to the control region of the *lac* operon, the interval on the chromosome between the end of the i gene and the beginning of the z gene. Within this small segment of DNA, there are three sites at which control functions are exerted: the operator, the RNA polymerase site, and the CAP protein site. Mutations in these loci alter *in vivo* the expression of the operon, *in vitro* the protein-DNA interactions. Again, for a more detailed discussion, we refer to a recent review (Bourgeois and Pfahl, 1976).

Lac Operator

The *lac* operator is defined genetically by the o^c operator constitutive mutation (see Table 3). The o^c mutants are partially constitutive, and have a lactose positive phenotype. The o^c mutation is *cis* dominant over i^+ and o^+; it only increases the level of expression of an adjacent z gene. Besides having higher basal levels, many o^c mutants exhibit small promoter-like effects: increases or decreases, compared to wild type, in the fully induced levels of *lac* enzyme synthesis. Smith and Sadler (1971) isolated and characterized hundreds of mutants carrying o^c point mutations. They assigned the o^c mutants to six different classes on the basis of the P value, the ratio of the basal to the maximal β-galactosidase level. Because of promoter effects, the functional P value, instead of the constitutive (basal) level itself, is the best *in vivo* measure of the relative affinity of *lac* repressor protein for o^c mutated operators. The origin of the promoter effects is not known. One can imagine that an o^c mutation might also affect transcription or translation, since there is evidence, to be mentioned later, for the overlap of the pertinent nucleic acid sequences. However, the less-interesting explanation that these effects result from secondary mutations in the z gene or in the positive control system cannot be excluded. Sadler and Smith (1971) later mapped the o^c mutants. The close linkage of the loci in the operator prohibits unambiguous ordering of the o^c mutations by genetic means. To date, o^c mutants, whose operator DNA has reduced affinity for *lac* repressor, represent the only known class of operator mutants. In theory, as we shall see shortly, there should exist at least one other type of operator mutant, containing a "superoperator," having increased affinity for repressor.

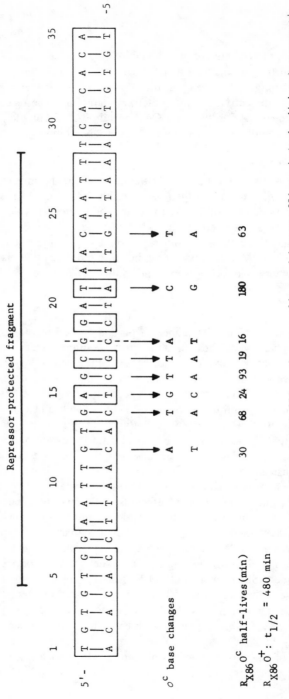

Fig. 9a. Nucleotide sequence of the *lac* operator. Figure shows the 35 base-pair sequence of the extended operator; 28 base pairs (enclosed in boxes) are symmetric about a 2-fold axis (broken line). The DNA fragment protected from nuclease digestion by *lac* repressor is indicated above the sequence. Data from Gilbert and Maxam (1973) and Dickson et al. (1975). Base-pair substitutions of o^c mutations and the corresponding half-lives of i^rX86 repressor-o^c operator complex are given below the o^+ sequence. Sequence data from Gilbert et al. (1975); binding data from Jobe et al. (1974).

Gilbert and Maxam (1973) isolated the *lac* operator as a double-stranded DNA fragment protected from nuclease digestion by *lac* repressor protein. The protected fragment is about 27 base pairs long; as already mentioned, its T_m of 67°C indicates a duplex structure. The nucleotide sequence of 24 base pairs, derived from the sequences of RNA transcripts of the two DNA strands, is indicated in figure 9a. The protected fragment has a normal base composition: 60%(A + T). However, the sequence reveals a high degree of symmetry; 16 out of 21 bases are symmetric about a 2-fold axis. In the process of determining the sequence of the entire promoter-operator region, Dickson and coworkers (1975) confirmed the operator sequence and discovered an addi-

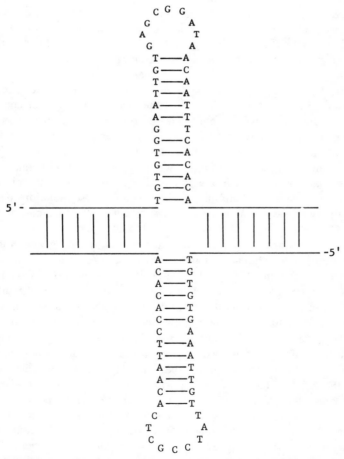

Fig. 9b. Possible cruciform structure of the *lac* operator. Formation of this structure requires unwinding of the linear duplex by 3.5 helical turns.

tional symmetric sequence, which extends the operator by 14 bases (see fig. 9a). Recently, Gilbert and Maxam (private communication) verified the extended operator sequence by DNA sequencing techniques.

The symmetrical aspect of the operator has prompted much speculation as to its function. Previously, we presented evidence against cruciform structures in the operator (see fig. 9b). The competing hypothesis is that the symmetry in the operator site fits a corresponding symmetry in the repressor tetramer. However, the available experimental data do not lend much support to the notion of a symmetric interaction of repressor protein and operator DNA. The first indications of asymmetry came from the analysis of o^c mutated operators. Jobe, Sadler, and Bourgeois (1974) measured the affinity of *lac* repressor protein for 11 o^c operators. For the tight-binding i^rX86 repressor, the stability of the complex formed with o^c operator DNA *in vitro* is proportional to the P value of the mutant *in vivo*: the more highly constitutive the o^c mutant, the shorter the half-life of the complex. Gilbert and Maxam (in preparation; cited by Gilbert et al., 1975) determined the sequence of 13 o^c operators, including the 11 just mentioned, and found 8 mutated loci. The positions of the o^c mutations did not fit the map order of Sadler and Smith (1971). Figure 9a shows the base-pair substitutions, as well as the corresponding half-lives of the i^rX86 repressor-o^c operator complexes, for the various o^c operators. All the o^c mutations are within the protected fragment; most of them are in the left half and toward the center of the operator. No o^c mutations have been found in the extended operator. Five of the eight substitutions are in symmetrically disposed base pairs; these mutations decrease the symmetry of the operator. However, substitutions that increase the symmetry (G-C→T-A at positions 14 and 16) also damage the operator. Moreover, repressor protein apparently interacts more strongly with the left side of the operator. Equivalent mutations (G-C→A-T at position 12 and C-G→T-A at position 24; A-T→G-C at position 15, and T-A→C-G at position 21) have a greater effect on the affinity for repressor when the substitution occurs in the left (promoter proximal) half of the operator than when it occurs in the right half. Also, no highly constitutive o^c mutant loci lie on the right side of the operator. If symmetry is an important factor in the repressor-operator interaction, then one would predict that a mutation which increased the symmetry of the operator so that the right half is made to resemble more closely the left half (A-T→C-G at positions 20 and 22) would result in a superoperator, with higher affinity for repressor than wild-type operator.

Recent results from chemical modifications of the operator are consistent with the o^c story (W. Gilbert and A. Maxam, private communication). Methylation by dimethyl sulfate of purine bases in the operator, but not in the extended operator, weakens the repressor-operator interaction. In the presence of repressor protein the reaction is blocked at some sites, enhanced at others, with no obvious symmetry in the pattern. The repressor protects the operator, but not the extended operator, against attacks by bleomycin. This antibiotic, a complex glycopeptide, breaks DNA at pyrimidine bases (Müller et al., 1972) preceded by a purine, predominantly of sequence dG-dT. Ultraviolet irradiation of *lac* repressor bound to BrdU-λh80d*lac* DNA results in photochemical attachment of the protein to the operator (Lin and Riggs, 1974). Gilbert and Maxam (private communication) found that some uracil bases in the operator, but not the extended operator, form cross-links with repressor protein. They infer from these data that the repressor makes contacts with thymine bases in the major groove of the DNA, at least in the case of the two large symmetry regions.

In addition to the *lac* operator site there are secondary binding sites for the *lac* repressor protein on the *E. coli* chromosome. The repressor has relatively high affinity for these pseudo-operators, so called because the binding is abolished by IPTG (W. S. Reznikoff, private communication), in contrast to the nonspecific interaction with DNA described previously. One such site has been located in the operator-proximal third of the *z* gene (Reznikoff, Winter, and Hurley, 1974) and its nucleotide sequence determined (Gilbert and Maxam, private communication). This pseudo-operator has 16 out of 21 bases homologous with the operator, but only two out of 14 with the extended operator. The symmetry of the pseudo-operator is substantially reduced; only eight base pairs in the operator region are symmetrically related, and two in the extended operator region. The pseudo-operator site lies about 400 base pairs (10%) into the *z* gene in an orientation opposite to that of the *lac* operator site. Its affinity for *lac* repressor is 10- to 30-fold lower than that of wild-type operator (Reznikoff et al., 1974; Gilbert et al., 1975). Genetic and biochemical evidence exists for a second pseudo-operator site, created by a mutation at the end of the *i* gene (M. Pfahl, unpublished result). The biological meaning of these pseudo-operators is not known.

The over-all picture emerging from the genetical and biochemical investigations of the *lac* operator is one in which the repressor binds primarily to the central 15 base-pair portion of the operator. This length is not inconsistent with the size of the binding site for non-operator DNA, 11-13 base pairs. Resolution of the symmetry question will probably require three-dimensional visualization of the repressor-operator complex by X-ray crystallography. Several investigators are pursuing chemical synthesis of the *lac* operator DNA necessary for these experiments (Itakura, Katagiri, and Narang, 1974; Caruthers, Goeddel, and Yansura, 1975).

Lac Promoter

The *lac* promoter is defined by mutations that alter the level of transcription of the operon, without affecting induction (Ippen et al., 1968). Genetic analysis has revealed two distinct sites in the *lac* promoter region (see fig. 10): the *i* gene proximal half being the site for CAP protein plus cAMP stimulation of transcription, and the operator proximal half being the site for recognition and initiation of transcription by RNA polymerase (Beckwith, Grodzicker, and Arditti, 1972). The various promoter mutants fall into three classes (see Hopkins, 1974). In the absence of CAP protein and cAMP, the wild-type promoter functions at 2% of its maximum level. Class I mutations only affect the stimulation of *lac* operon expression by CAP protein plus cAMP. Class I mutants map in the left half of the promoter, defined by the deletion mutant L1. The class II and class III mutations alter the RNA polymerase interaction. Class II and class III mutants map in the right half of the promoter. Compared with the wild-type, class II mutants have defective promoters, whereas class III mutants have more efficient promoters.

Dickson and coworkers (1975) determined the nucleotide sequence of the *lac* promoter-operator region. The promoter-operator region is the 122 base pair sequence, between the stop codon (UGA) at the end of the *i* gene and the formylmethionine initiation codon (AUG) at the beginning of the *z* gene, shown in figure 10. Gilbert and Maxam (private communication) confirmed this sequence, and extended it about 40 base pairs to the left of the sequence presented in figure 10.

The CAP site comprises the left half of the promoter, from the end of the *i* gene to the end point of the class I L1 deletion (Dickson et al., 1975). In the right half of the CAP site there is a symmetry region: 14 out of 16 base pairs are symmetric about a 2-fold axis. Dickson and coworkers (1974) proposed that this symmetric sequence is the binding site for the CAP protein dimer plus cAMP. Recent evidence for this putative binding site derives from two sources. First, the base-pair substitutions of two class I point mutations, L8 and L614, are in the symmetry region (Dickson et al., 1977; A. Maxam and V. Sundaresan, private communication). *In vitro* the CAP protein-cAMP complex does not bind to labeled promoter-operator DNA restriction fragments carrying the L8 mutation (Majors, 1975). And second, *alu* restriction enzyme of *Arthrobacter luteus* has a cleavage site in the center of the symmetric sequence. The *alu* scission diminishes the binding of CAP protein-cAMP complex to wild-type promoter-operator DNA fragments relative to fragments containing an intact CAP region (J. Majors, private communication).

The RNA polymerase site occupies the right half of the promoter, and overlaps the operator site. Transcription of *lac* mRNA from both the class III

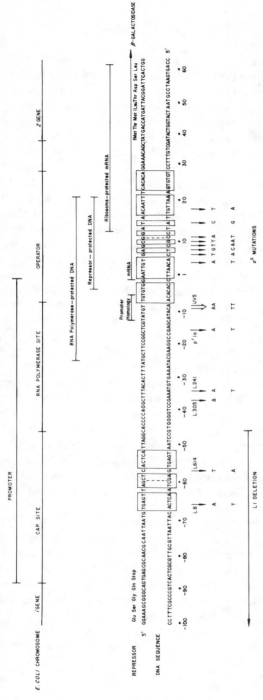

Fig. 10. Nucleotide sequence of the *lac* promoter-operator region. The symmetric regions of the operator and CAP sites are enclosed in boxes. Data for residues −100 to +47 from Dickson et al. (1975), for residues −100 to +63 from W. Gilbert and A. Maxam (private communication). The upper part of the figure indicates various sequences mentioned in the text. *Lac* mRNA, residues 1 to 63, transcribed from: UV5 promoter, data from Maizels (1973); wild-type promoter, data from J. Majors (private communication). Promoter homology, data from Pribnow (1975). RNA polymerase-protected DNA fragment: UV5 promoter, data from J. Gralla (private communication); wild-type promoter, data from J. Majors (private communication). *Lac* repressor-protected DNA fragment, data from Gilbert and Maxam (1973). Largest ribosome-protected RNA fragment, data from Maizels (1974). The lower part of the figure shows the base-pair substitutions or deletions of various promoter and operator mutations. Class I promoter mutations: L1 deletion, data from Dickson et al. (1975) and W. Gilbert and A. Maxam (private communication); L8, data from R. C. Dickson et al. (1977) and A. Maxam and V. Sundaresan (private communication); L614, data from R. C. Dickson et al. (1977). Class II promoter mutations: L305 and L241, data from Dickson et al. (1975). Class III promoter mutations: p⁺la, data from Dickson et al. (1975); UV5, data from J. Gralla (private communication). The *o^c* mutations, data from Gilbert et al. (1975).

UV5 mutated promoter (Maizels, 1973) and wild-type promoter (J. Majors, in preparation, cited by Gilbert et al., 1975) commences at the first base of the operator. Moreover, for both UV5 (J. Gralla, private communication) and wild-type (J. Majors, private communication) promoters, the fragment of DNA protected from nuclease digestion by RNA polymerase spans the right half of the RNA polymerase site and the operator. The RNA polymerase-protected fragment is about 45 base pairs long, the same size as RNA polymerase binding sites from other promoters (see Pribnow, 1975). The base-pair substitutions of two class II mutations, p^rla (Dickson et al., 1975) and UV5 (J. Gralla, private communication), as well as the homologue of the septanucleotide sequence TATPuATG common to other promoters (Pribnow, 1975), are within the region of the promoter protected by RNA polymerase. Interestingly, this TATGTTG sequence in the wild-type promoter mutates, in the more efficient UV5 promoter, to TATAATG, a precise match of the sequence implicated in formation of tight complexes with RNA polymerase. The UV5 promoter also forms a more stable complex with RNA polymerase *in vitro* than does wild-type promoter (Reznikoff, 1976). The base-pair substitutions of two class II mutations, L241 and L305, are in the left half of the RNA polymerase site, outside the region protected by polymerase (Dickson et al., 1975). These findings distinguish two functional regions of the RNA polymerase site: an entry site and an initiation site. The entry site is about 35 base pairs to the left of the start of *lac* mRNA synthesis; it is not protected from nuclease digestion by RNA polymerase, but does contain promoter mutations, at least of class II. The initiation site covers the site at which transcription starts; it is protected from nuclease digestion by RNA polymerase, and likewise contains promoter mutations, so far of class III. As seems to be the case for other promoters (Schaller, Gray, and Herrmann, 1975; Pribnow, 1975; Walz and Pirrotta, 1975), RNA polymerase shifts along an ~35 base-pair region of DNA from the entry site to the initiation site before it begins transcribing DNA.

The operator site includes the extended operator, the fragment of DNA protected by *lac* repressor protein, and the o^c mutations, all discussed previously. Between the operator site and the first codon of the z gene, there is a space of ten base pairs, which contains part of the sequence encoded in the ribosome binding site on *lac* mRNA. Ribosomes do not protect a unique sequence of *lac* mRNA from digestion by ribonucleases; the size of the protected fragments varies from 29-50 bases long, depending on the enzyme and conditions (Maizels, 1974). In the larger fragments the ribosome binding site includes the right half of the transcribed operator through the first few codons for β-galactosidase.

TRANSCRIPTION OF THE OPERON

Having discussed the individual negative and positive controlling elements, we now consider how they function in concert to regulate expression of the *lac* operon. At present the details of the control mechanism are not fully understood. We will present pertinent results from studies of transcription *in vitro*, and then comment on the more complex situation *in vivo*.

Transcription in vitro

The control of β-galactosidase synthesis by *lac* repressor protein and inducer IPTG, and the stimulatory effect of CAP protein plus cAMP on that synthesis were verified *in vitro* in cell-free systems (Zubay and Chambers, 1971; de Crombrugghe et al., 1971a). However, analysis of the relationship between particular components in the regulation of *lac* mRNA synthesis requires a purified transcription system. De Crombrugghe and coworkers (1971b) established that CAP protein plus cAMP were necessary and sufficient for proper initiation of *lac* mRNA synthesis at the *lac* promoter by RNA polymerase holoenzyme. Consequently, they were able to demonstrate repression of about 80% of *lac* transcription by *lac* repressor protein, the repression being relieved by IPTG and restored by ONPF. Eron and Block (1971) confirmed these findings, and showed that promoter mutations alter the level of *lac* transcription. Depending on conditions, the more efficient p^s and UV5 mutated promoters increase the *lac* mRNA level 3- to 10-fold. *Lac* transcription from the UV5 promoter is substantial in the absence of CAP protein plus cAMP, in agreement with the fact mentioned previously that this mutated promoter has greater affinity for RNA polymerase than wild-type. Further, CAP protein plus cAMP stimulate only slightly *lac* transcription from the L1 promoter, deleted for the CAP site. As stated in the "Introduction," nothing is known about the mechanism of action of CAP protein plus cAMP. One particular theory is that the binding of CAP protein-cAMP complex alters the DNA structure of the adjacent promoter region in such a way to facilitate RNA polymerase binding. Although there is no evidence of CAP protein binding to RNA polymerase, the close proximity of the putative binding site for CAP protein-cAMP complex and entry region for RNA polymerase makes this another tenable hypothesis.

As already predicted from the overlap of the binding sites for RNA polymerase and *lac* repressor protein and from the location of the start of *lac* transcription, the repressor acts by excluding RNA polymerase from its initiation site. The results from *in vitro* transcription experiments in the presence of rifampicin confirm this mechanism. In the cases of the wild-type and UV5 promoters on DNA fragments containing the *lac* promoter-operator region (J. Majors, in preparation cited by Gilbert et al., 1975) and of the p^s promoter on ϕ80d*lac* DNA (Eron and Block, 1971; Chen et al., 1971), repressor binding and formation of RNA polymerase initiation complex are mutually exclusive events. It is not clear why Chen and coworkers (1971) found *lac* repressor and RNA polymerase binding independent in the case of the wild-type promoter on λh80d*lac* DNA.

Although the above-mentioned phenomena are demonstrable in a qualitative fashion, the *in vitro* transcription system does not function efficiently. For example, the ratio of induced to repressed levels is 2- to 4-fold for *lac* mRNA *in vitro* compared to 1,000-fold for β-galactosidase *in vivo*. The quantitation of *in vitro* coupled transcription-translation systems is equally poor. Probing of the more subtle aspects of control of *lac* operon expression requires improved *in vitro* systems.

Expression in vivo

Theoretical analyses of *lac* operon expression *in vivo* so far relate only to the equilibrium aspects of negative control. Two models, a stochastic model and a mass-action model, have been developed that attempt to explain regulation by *lac* repressor protein *in vivo* on the basis of its properties *in vitro*. In both cases the authors assume that the level of β-galactosidase synthesis is a sole function of the fraction of free operator sites. In the stochastic formulation Stuart and Branscomb (1971) consider the effects of the small numbers of repressor molecules (~ 10) and operator sites (~ 1) per cell, and of the variation in the number of repressor molecules between cells, on the average fraction of free operators in the population. Since they treat the case of exponentially growing cells, they make additional assumptions about how repressor is produced during the cell cycle. Although these "small numbers" and "heterogeneity" effects make opposing contributions, they combine to augment the fraction of free operators at low ratios of repressor protein to operator sites in comparison to a conventional mass-action treatment. In this model the basal level can be accounted for either by an affinity of repressor for operator $K_O = 10^{11}$ M^{-1}, a reasonable value for wild-type *lac* repressor at intracellular ionic strengths, or by repressor heterogeneity if one takes larger values for the affinity. In the mass-action formulation von Hippel and coworkers (1974) consider the coupled equilibria of repressor protein, operator sites, and non-operator DNA sites, and the effect of inducer upon these equilibria. They conclude that the nonspecific binding of repressor to DNA plays an essential role in regulation of the operon. In the absence of nonspecific binding, the basal level would be 100-fold lower than the observed level and induction would not occur, assuming an affinity of repressor for operator $K_O = 10^{14}$ M^{-1}.

It is difficult to establish the relative importance of stochastic effects and nonspecific DNA binding on the basis of these two analyses, particularly since the numerical calculations were performed using widely different values of the affinity K_O. In the stochastic model Stuart and Branscomb ignored the weak binding of repressor to non-operator DNA. In the mass-action model the conclusions rest heavily on the assumed affinity $K_O = 10^{14}$ M^{-1}, probably an unrealistic value under physiological conditions. Von Hippel and coworkers show that an affinity $K_O = 10^{11}$ M^{-1} can account for the basal level in the absence of competing non-operator DNA. Lin and Riggs (1975b) make more modest claims regarding nonspecific DNA binding. They point out that 98% of *lac* repressor protein is bound to non-operator DNA, and that inducer merely shifts the repressor from operator to non-operator DNA.

As for comparing induction *in vitro* and *in vivo*, the correlation of the pertinent experimental results, already mentioned in passing, is quite good. In cells growing on glycerol, induction of the *lac* operon by lactose requires the presence of a functional β-galactosidase, which generates the natural inducer by a transgalactosidation reaction (Burstein et al., 1965). The natural inducer of the *lac* operon is allolactose (6-O-β-D-galactopyranosyl-D-glucose), an isomer of lactose, in which the β-1-4 sugar linkage of lactose is changed to a β-1-6 linkage (Jobe and Burgeois, 1972a). The basal level of β-galactosidase serves the purpose of converting lactose into allolactose, a potent inducer with an affinity for *lac* repressor equal to that of IPTG. This shunt guarantees that the cell, when confronted with lactose, will not induce *lac* enzyme synthesis in the absence of a β-galactosidase that can catabolize the sugar. Lactose itself is an anti-inducer (Jobe and Bourgeois, 1973). Although the intracellular concentration of lactose is very high due to the action of the *lac* permease, the affinity of lactose for repressor is so low that it is questionable whether lactose actually represses the operon *in vivo*. As pointed out in a previous section, the *in vivo* induction curve is sigmoidal (see fig. 5*a*), whereas the comparable *in vitro* curve for k_{bapp}, which is proportional to the equilibrium fraction of free operators at constant repressor and ligand concentrations, is hyperbolic (see fig. 6), manifesting no cooperativity. In both curves the half-maximal effect occurs at 2×10^{-4} M IPTG. In a cell-free system the induction curve exhibits some sigmoidicity; however, the half-maximal effect occurs at 5×10^{-5} M IPTG (Zubay and Chambers, 1971). Whether the apparent cooperativity of the *in vivo* response to inducer derives from a subsequent step in transcription or translation is not known.

CONCLUDING REMARKS

The *lac* operon owes its status in molecular biology to its role as a model system for regulation of gene expression. The *lac* repressor, in conjunction with its operator site on DNA and effecting sugars, is the best studied example of negative control. Given the recent advances regarding the CAP protein and the *lac* promoter region, the *lac* system will inevitably provide opportunity for elucidating the general mechanism of positive control by cAMP. Further, the ability to obtain promoter mutations in the RNA polymerase site may facilitate investigation of the multiple steps in initiation of transcription by RNA polymerase. Certainly, the ease of manipulation of the *lac* control system is an important consideration, as is the fortuitous fact that it is probably one of, if not the, most simple regulatory system: there is probably a single binding site for each of the regulatory proteins in the promoter-operator region; the interaction of repressor and operator is highly specific and reversible; and there are a variety of effecting ligands that mediate this interaction. Perhaps most important, there is a wide assortment of mutants already available, or that can be isolated at will, having mutations in the gene for the repressor protein or in the promoter and operator regions.

Beyond the questions central to regulation, the *lac* operon promises a fecund system for studying the physical and chemical bases of protein-nucleic acid interactions, in the interactions of repressor protein with operator and non-operator DNAs. It may also yield insights into conformational transitions, through analysis of the changes in *lac* repressor protein upon binding of effecting ligands, and into protein-protein interactions, by examination of the subunit interactions in the repressor.

Whether any of the particulars of the negative and positive control networks will be relevant to regulatory functions in higher organisms, other than establishing a context for understanding macromolecular recognition processes, remains to be seen. However, the methodology developed to study the *lac* system, such as the membrane filter technique, has already proved useful in biochemical analysis of more complicated systems. Of equal value, perhaps, to investigators in other areas is a feeling for some of the pitfalls that may be encountered, particularly in demonstrating specificity.

ACKNOWLEDGMENTS

We wish to thank the following scientists for making their unpublished results available to us: J. Abelson, P. Bandyopadhyay, W. M. Barnes, C. Brack, A. P. Butler, F. H. C. Crick, R. C. Dickson, J. G. Files, W. Gilbert, J. Gralla, C. Hélène, P. H. von Hippel, J. Hirsh, S. Humphreys, S.-Y. Lin, P. Lu, J. Majors, K. S. Matthews, A. Maxam, J. H. Miller, J. Miwa, B. Müller-Hill, M. Pfahl, A. Revzin, W. S. Reznikoff, T. J. Richmond, A. D. Riggs, J. R. Sadler, R. Schlief, U. Schmeissner, A. Schmitz, T. F. Smith, T. A. Steitz, C.-W. Wu, F. Y.-H. Wu, D. S. Yang. Our work is supported by grants (GM20259, GM20868) and a Career Development Award (to S.B.) from the National Institutes of Health.

REFERENCES

Adam, G., and M. Delbrück. 1968. Reduction of dimensionality in biological diffusion processes. *In* A. Rich and N. Davidson (eds), Structural chemistry and molecular biology. Pp. 198–215. Freeman, San Francisco.

Adler, K., K. Beyreuther, E. Fanning, N. Geisler, B. Gronenborn, A. Klemm, B. Müller-Hill, M. Pfahl, and A. Schmitz. 1972. How *lac* repressor binds to DNA. Nature 237:322–27.

Anderson, W. B., R. L. Perlman, and I. Pastan. 1972. Effect of adenosine 3',5'-monophosphate analogues on the activity of the cyclic adenosine 3',5'-monophosphate receptor in *Escherichia coli*. J. Biol. Chem. 247:2717–22.

Anderson, W. B., A. B. Schneider, M. Emmer, R. L. Perlman, and I. Pastan. 1971. Purification of and properties of the cyclic adenosine 3',5'-monophosphate receptor protein which mediates cyclic adenosine 3',5'-monophosphate-dependent gene transcription in *Escherichia coli*. J. Biol. Chem. 246:5929–37.

Bandyopadhyay, P., and C.-W. Wu. 1975. Structure-function relationship of *lac* repressor from *E. coli*. Biophys. J. 15:302a.

Barkley, M. D., A. D. Riggs, A. Jobe, and S. Bourgeois. 1975. Interaction of effecting ligands with *lac* repressor and repressor-operator complex. Biochemistry 14:1700–1712.

Bauer, W., and J. Vinograd. 1970. Interaction of closed circular DNA with intercalative dyes II. The free energy of superhelix formation in SV40 DNA. J. Mol. Biol. 47:419–35.

Beckwith, J., T. Grodzicker, and R. Arditta. 1972. Evidence for two sites in the *lac* promoter region. J. Mol. Biol. 69:155–60.

Beckwith, J. R., and E. R. Signer. 1966. Transposition of the *lac* region of *Escherichia coli*. J. Mol. Biol. 19:254–65.

Beckwith, J. R., and D. Zipser, eds. 1970. The lactose operon. Cold Spring Harbor Laboratory, Cold Spring Harbor, N.Y.

Beyreuther, K., K. Adler, E. Fanning, C. Murray, A. Klemm, and N. Geisler. 1975. Amino-acid sequence of *lac* repressor from *Escherichia coli*. Eur. J. Biochem. 59:491–509.

Beyreuther, K., K. Adler, N. Geisler, and A. Klemm. 1973. The amino-acid sequence of *lac* repressor. Proc. Nat. Acad. Sci. USA 70:3576–80.

Bourgeois, S. 1966. Sur la nature du répresseur de l'opéron lactose d'*Escherichia coli*. Ph.D. thesis. University of Paris.

Bourgeois, S. 1971a. Methods for studying protein-nucleic acid interaction. *In* B. L. Horecker and E. R. Stadtman (eds.). Current topics in cellular regulation. 4:178–205. Academic Press, New York.

Bourgeois, S. 1971b. Techniques to assay repressors. *In* L. Grossman and K. Moldave (eds.). Methods of enzymology. 21D:491–500. Academic Press, New York.

Bourgeois, S., and A. Jobe. 1970. Superrepressors of the *lac* operon. *In* J. R. Beckwith and D. Zipser (eds.). The lactose operon. Pp. 325–41. Cold Spring Harbor Laboratory, Cold Spring, N.Y.

Bourgeois, S., and M. Pfahl. 1976. Repressors. Adv. Prot. Chem. 30:1–99.

Bourgeois, S., and A. D. Riggs. 1970. The *lac* repressor-operator interaction. IV. Assay and purification of operator DNA. Biochem. Biophys. Res. Commun. 38:348–54.

Bresloff, J. L., and D. M. Crothers. 1975. DNA-ethidium reaction kinetics: Demonstration of direct ligand transfer between DNA binding sites. J. Mol. Biol. 95:103–23.

Brickman, E., L. Soll, and J. Beckwith. 1973. Genetic characterization of mutations which affect catabolite-sensitive operons in *Escherichia coli,* including deletions of the gene for adenyl cyclase. J. Bact. 116:582–87.

Burstein, C., M. Cohn, A. Kepes, and J. Monod. 1965. Rôle du lactose et de ses produits métaboliques dans l'induction de l'opéron lactose chez *Escherichia coli.* Biochim. Biophys. Acta 95:634–39.

Butler, A. P., A. Revzin, and P. H. von Hippel. 1975. Molecular parameters characterizing the interaction of *lac* repressor with inducer and non-operator DNA. J. Mol. Biol.; submitted.

Carter, Jr., C. W., and J. Kraut. 1974. A proposed model for interaction of polypeptides with RNA. Proc. Nat. Acad. Sci. USA 71:283–87.

Caruthers, M. H., D. V. Goeddel, and D. G. Yansura. 1975. Synthesis of lactose operator DNA. Fed. Proc. 34:554.

Chamness, G. C., and C. D. Willson. 1970. An unusual *lac* repressor mutant. J. Mol. Biol. 53:561–65.

Chan, H. W., and R. D. Wells. 1974. Structural uniqueness of lactose operator. Nature 252:205–9.

Chen, B., B. de Crombrugghe, W. B. Anderson, M. E. Gottesman, and I. Pastan. 1971. On the mechanism of action of *lac* repressor. Nature New Biol. 233:67–70.

Chou, P. Y., A. J. Adler, and G. Fasman. 1975. Conformation prediction and circular dichroism studies on the *lac* repressor. J. Mol. Biol. 96:29–45.

Church, G. M., J. L. Sussman, and S. H. Kim. 1975. A detailed model for DNA-protein complexes. Amer. Cryst. Ass. Abstr. 3:17.

Clark, D. J., and A. G. Marr. 1964. Studies on the repression of β-galactosidase in *Escherichia coli.* Biochim. Biophys. Acta 92:85–98.

Crick, F. H. C., and A. Klug. 1975. Kinky helix. Nature 255:530–33.

de Crombrugghe, B., B. Chen, M. Gottesman, I. Pastan, H. E. Varmus, M. Emmer, and R. L. Perlman. 1971a. Regulation of *lac* mRNA synthesis in a soluble cell-free system. Nature New Biol. 230:37–40.

de Crombrugghe, B., B. Chen, W. Anderson, P. Nissley, M. Gottesman, and I. Pastan. 1971b. *Lac* DNA, RNA polymerase and cyclic AMP receptor protein, cyclic AMP, *lac* repressor and inducer are the essential elements for controlled *lac* transcription. Nature New Biol. 231:139–42.

Davidson, N. 1972. Effect of DNA length on the free energy of binding of an unwinding ligand to a supercoiled DNA. J. Mol. Biol. 66:307–9.

Dickson, R. C., J. Abelson, P. Johnson, W. S. Reznikoff, and W. M. Barnes. 1977. Nucleotide sequence changes produced by mutations in the *lac* promoter of *Escherichia coli.* J. Mol. Biol. 110:in press.

Dickson, R. C., J. Abelson, W. M. Barnes, and W. S. Reznikoff. 1975. Genetic regulation: The *lac* control region. Science 187:27–35.

Edelman, P. L., and G. Edlin. 1974. Regulation of the synthesis of the lactose repressor. J. Bact. 120:657–65.

Emmer, M., B. de Crombrugghe, I. Pastan, and R. Perlman. 1970. Cyclic AMP receptor protein of *E. coli:* Its role in the synthesis of inducible enzymes. Proc. Nat. Acad. Sci. USA 66:480–87.

Eron, L., and R. Block. 1971. Mechanism of initiation and repression of *in vitro* transcription of the *lac* operon of *Escherichia coli.* Proc. Nat. Acad. Sci. USA 68:1828–32.

Fanning, T. G. 1975. Iodination of *Escherichia coli lac* repressor. Effect of tyrosine modification on repressor activity. Biochemistry 14:2512–20.

Files, J. G., K. Weber, and J. H. Miller. 1974. Translational reinitiation: reinitiation of *lac* repressor fragments at three internal sites early in the *lac i* gene of *Escherichia coli*. Proc. Nat. Acad. Sci. USA 71:667–70.

Ganem, D., J. H. Miller, J. G. Files, T. Platt, and K. Weber. 1973. Reinitiation of a *lac* repressor fragment at a codon other than AUG. Proc. Nat. Acad. Sci. USA 70:3165–69.

Georgopoulos, C. P., and H. R. Revel. 1971. Studies with glucosyl transferase mutants of the T-even bacteriophages. Virology 44:271–85.

Gierer, A. 1966. Model for DNA and protein interactions and the function of the operator. Nature 212:1480–81.

Gilbert, W. 1972. The *lac* repressor and the *lac* operator. *In* G. E. W. Wolstenholme and M. O'Connor (eds.). Polymerization in biological systems. Pp. 245–59. Associated Scientific Press, Amsterdam, New York.

Gilbert, W., J. Gralla, J. Majors, and A. Maxam. 1975. Lactose operator sequences and the action of *lac* repressor. *In* H. Sund and G. Blauer (eds.). Protein-ligand interactions. Pp. 193–210. Walter de Gruyter, Berlin, New York.

Gilbert, W., and A. Maxam. 1973. The nucleotide sequence of the *lac* operator. Proc. Nat. Acad. Sci. USA 70:3581–84.

Gilbert, W., and B. Müller-Hill. 1966. Isolation of the *lac* repressor. Proc. Nat. Acad. Sci. USA 56:1891–98.

Hamada, F., Y. Ohshima, and T. Horiuchi. 1973. Dissociation of *lac* repressor into subunits. J. Biochem. 73:1299–1302.

von Hippel, P. H., A. Revzin, C. A. Gross, and A. C. Wang. 1974. Non-specific DNA binding of genome regulating proteins as a biological control mechanism: 1. The *lac* operon: equilibrium aspects. Proc. Nat. Acad. Sci. USA 71:4808–12.

von Hippel, P. H., A. Revzin, C. A. Gross, and A. C. Wang. 1975. Interaction of *lac* repressor with non-specific DNA binding sites. *In* H. Sund and G. Blauer (eds.). Protein-ligand interactions. Pp. 270–88. Walter de Gruyter, Berlin, New York.

Hopkins, J. D. 1974. A new class of promoter mutations in the lactose operon of *Escherichia coli*. J. Mol. Biol. 87:715–24.

Horiuchi, T., and A. Novick. 1961. A thermolabile repression system. Cold Spring Harbor Symp. Quant. Biol. 26:247–48.

Humphreys, S. 1975. *Lac* repressor subunit arrangement. J. Mol. Biol.; submitted.

Huston, J. S., W. F. Moo-Penn, K. C. Bechtel, and O. Jardetzky. 1974. Characterization of the *lac* repressor species produced by limited tryptic cleavage. Biochem. Biophys. Res. Commun. 61:441–48.

Ippen, K., J. H. Miller, J. Scaife, and J. Beckwith. 1968. New controlling element in the *lac* operon of *E. coli*. Nature 217:825–27.

Itakura, K., N. Katagiri, and S. A. Narang. 1974. Synthesis of lactose-operator gene fragments by the improved triester method. Can. J. Chem. 52:3689–93.

Jacob, F., and J. Monod. 1961. Genetic regulatory mechanisms in the synthesis of proteins. J. Mol. Biol. 3:318–56.

Jobe, A., and S. Bourgeois. 1972a. *Lac* repressor-operator interaction. VI. The natural inducer of the *lac* operon. J. Mol. Biol. 69:397–408.

Jobe, A., and S. Bourgeois. 1972b. *Lac* repressor-operator interaction. VII. A repressor with unique binding properties: the X86 repressor. J. Mol. Biol. 72:139–52.

Jobe, A., and S. Bourgeois. 1972c. *Lac* repressor-operator interaction. VIII. Lactose is an anti-inducer of the *lac* operon. J. Mol. Biol. 75:303–13.

Jobe, A., A. D. Riggs, and S. Bourgeois. 1972. *Lac* repressor-operator interaction. V. Characterization of super- and pseudo-wild-type repressors. J. Mol. Biol. 64:181–99.

Jobe, A., J. R. Sadler, and S. Bourgeois. 1974. *Lac* repressor-operator interaction. IX. The binding of *lac* repressor to operators containing o^c mutations. J. Mol. Biol. 85:231–48.

Kihara, H. K., and H. Kuno. 1968. Microassay of protein with nitrocellulose membrane filters. Anal. Biochem. 24:96–105.

Krakow, J. S., and I. Pastan. 1973. Cyclic adenosine monophosphate receptor: Loss of cAMP-dependent DNA binding activity after proteolysis in the presence of cyclic adenosine monophosphate. Proc. Nat. Acad. Sci. USA 70:2529–33.

Kuhn, W., and M. Thürkauf. 1961. Biegungsdeformation elastischer Stäbe durch die Wärmebewegung. Z. Elektrochem. 65:307–13.

Laiken, S. L., C. A. Gross, and P. H. von Hippel. 1972. Equilibrium and kinetic aspects of *Escherichia coli lac* repressor-inducer interactions. J. Mol. Biol. 66:143–55.

Lin, S.-Y., and A. D. Riggs. 1972a. *Lac* operator analogues: Bromodeoxyuridine substitution in the *lac* operator affects the rate of dissociation of the *lac* repressor. Proc. Nat. Acad. Sci. USA 69:2574–76.

Lin, S.-Y., and A. D. Riggs. 1972b. *Lac* repressor binding to non-operator DNA: Detailed studies and a comparison of equilibrium and rate competition methods. J. Mol. Biol. 72:671–90.

Lin, S.-Y., and A. D. Riggs. 1974. Photochemical attachment of *lac* repressor to bromodeoxyuridine-substituted *lac* operator by ultraviolet radiation. Proc. Nat. Acad. Sci. USA 71:947–51.

Lin, S.-Y., and A. D. Riggs. 1975a. A comparison of *lac* repressor binding to operator and to non-operator DNA. Biochem. Biophys. Res. Commun. 62:704–10.

Lin, S.-Y., and A. D. Riggs. 1975b. The general affinity of *lac* repressor for *E. coli* DNA: Implications for gene regulation in procaryotes and eucaryotes. Cell 4:107–11.

Lin, S.-Y., and A. D. Riggs. 1976. The binding of *lac* repressor and the catabolite gene activator protein to halogen-substituted analogues of poly[d(A-T)]. Biochim. Biophys. Acta 432:185–91.

Maizels, N. 1973. The nucleotide sequence of the lactose messenger ribonucleic acid transcribed from the UV5 promoter mutant of *Escherichia coli*. Proc. Nat. Acad. Sci. USA 70:3585–89.

Maizels, N. 1974. *E. coli* lactose operon binding site. Nature 249:647–49.

Majors, J. 1975. Specific binding of CAP factor to *lac* promoter DNA. Nature 256:672–74.

Matsuura, M., Y. Ohshima, and T. Horiuchi. 1972. Secondary structure of the *lac* repressor. Biochem. Biophys. Res. Commun. 47:1438–43.

Matthews, K. S. 1974. Ultraviolet difference spectra of the lactose repressor protein. II. Trypsin core protein. Biochim. Biophys. Acta 359:334–40.

Matthews, K. S., H. R. Matthews, H. W. Thielmann, and O. Jardetzky. 1973. Ultraviolet difference spectra of the lactose repressor protein. Biochim. Biophys. Acta 295:159–65.

Maurizot, J.-C., M. Charlier, and C. Hélène. 1974. *Lac* repressor binding to poly [d(A-T)]. Conformational changes. Biochem. Biophys. Res. Commun. 60:951–57.

Myers, G. L., and J. R. Sadler. 1971. Mutational inversion of control of the lactose operon of *Escherichia coli*. J. Mol. Biol. 58:1–28.

Miller, J. H., J. Beckwith, and B. Müller-Hill. 1968. Direction of transcription of a regulatory gene in *E. coli*. Nature 220:1287–90.

Miller, J. H., C. Coulondre, U. Schmeissner, A. Schmitz, and P. Lu. 1975. The use of suppressed nonsense mutations to generate altered *lac* repressor molecules. *In* H. Sund and G. Blauer (eds.). Protein-ligand interactions. Pp. 238–52. Walter de Gruyter, Berlin, New York.

Miwa, J., J. R. Sadler, and T. F. Smith. 1975. A characterization of i^{-d} repressor mutations of the lactose operon. J. Mol. Biol.: submitted.

Müller, W. E. G., Z.-I. Yamazaki, H.-J. Breter, and R. K. Zahn. 1972. Action of bleomycin on DNA and RNA. Eur. J. Biochem. 31:518–25.

Müller-Hill, B. 1971. *Lac* repressor. Angew. Chem. 10:160–72.

Müller-Hill, B. 1975. *Lac* repressor and *lac* operator. Prog. Biophys. Molec. Biol. 30(2/3):227–52.

Müller-Hill, B., L. Crapo, and W. Gilbert. 1968. Mutants that make more *lac* repressor. Proc. Nat. Acad. Sci. USA 59:1259–64.

Müller-Hill, B., T. Fanning, N. Geisler, D. Gho, J. Kania, P. Kathman, H. Meissner, M. Schlotmann, A. Schmitz, I. Triesch, and K. Beyreuther. 1975. The active sites of *lac* repressor. *In* H. Sund and G. Blauer (eds.). Protein-ligand interactions. Pp. 211–27. Walter de Gruyter, Berlin, New York.

Nissley, P., W. B. Anderson, M. Gallo, and I. Pastan. 1972. The binding of cyclic adenosine monophosphate receptor to deoxyribonucleic acid. J. Biol. Chem. 247:4264–69.

Ohshima, Y., T. Horiuchi, M. Yanagida. 1975. Structure of the *lac* repressor studied by negative staining. J. Mol. Biol. 91:515–19.

Ohshima, Y., M. Matsuura, and T. Horiuchi. 1972. Conformational change of the *lac* repressor induced with the inducer. Biochem. Biophys. Res. Commun. 47:1444–50.

Ohshima, Y., T. Mizokoshi, and T. Horiuchi. 1974. Binding of an inducer to the *lac* repressor. J. Mol. Biol. 89:127–36.

Perlman, R. L., and I. Pastan. 1968. Regulation of β-galactosidase synthesis in *Escherichia coli* by cyclic adenosine 3′,5′-monophosphate. J. Biol. Chem. 243:5420–27.

Pfahl, M. 1972. Genetic map of the lactose repressor gene (*i*) of *Escherichia coli*. Genetics 72:393–410.

Pfahl, M. 1976. *Lac* repressor-operator interaction: analysis of the X86 repressor mutant. J. Mol. Biol.; 106:857–69.

Pfahl, M., C. Stockter, and B. Gronenborn. 1974. Genetic analysis of the active sites of *lac* repressor. Genetics 76:669–79.

Platt, T., J. G. Files, and K. Weber. 1973. *Lac* repressor. Specific proteolytic destruction of the NH$_2$-terminal region and loss of the deoxyribonucleic acid-binding activity. J. Biol. Chem. 248:110–21.

Platt, T., K. Weber, D. Ganem, and J. H. Miller. 1972. Translational restarts: AUG reinitiation of a *lac* repressor fragment. Proc. Nat. Acad. Sci. USA 69:897–901.

Pribnow, D. 1975. Nucleotide sequence of an RNA polymerase binding site at an early T7 promoter. Proc. Nat. Acad. Sci. USA 72:784–88.

Reznikoff, W. S. 1976. Formation of the RNA polymerase-*lac* promoter open complex. *In* R.

Losick and M. Chamberlin, eds., RNA polymerase. Pp. 441–54. Cold Spring Harbor Laboratory, Cold Spring Harbor, N.Y.

Reznikoff, W. S., R. B. Winter, and C. K. Hurley. 1974. The location of the repressor binding sites in the *lac* operon. Proc. Nat. Acad. Sci. USA 71:2314–18.

Richmond, T. J., and T. A. Steitz. 1976. Protein-DNA interaction investigated by binding *Escherichia coli lac* repressor protein to poly[d(AU-HgX)]. J. Mol. Biol. 103:25–28.

Richter, P. H., and M. Eigen. 1974. Diffusion controlled reaction rates in spheroidal geometry. Application to repressor-operator association and membrane bound enzymes. Biophys. Chem. 2:255–63.

Riggs, A. D., and S. Bourgeois. 1968. On the assay, isolation, and characterization of the *lac* repressor. J. Mol. Biol. 34:361–64.

Riggs, A. D., S. Bourgeois, and M. Cohn. 1970c. The *lac* repressor-operator interaction. III. Kinetic studies. J. Mol. Biol. 53:401–17.

Riggs, A. D., S. Bourgeois, R. F. Newby, and M. Cohn. 1968. DNA binding of the *lac* repressor. J. Mol. Biol. 34:365–68.

Riggs, A. D., S. Lin, and R. D. Wells. 1972. *Lac* repressor binding to synthetic DNA's of defined nucleotide sequence. Proc. Nat. Acad. Sci. USA 69:761–64.

Riggs, A. D., R. F. Newby, and S. Bourgeois. 1970b. *Lac* repressor-operator interaction. II. Effect of galactosides and other ligands. J. Mol. Biol. 51:303–14.

Riggs, A. D., G. Reiness, and G. Zubay. 1971. Purification and DNA-binding properties of the catabolite gene activator protein. Proc. Nat. Acad. Sci. USA 68:1222–25.

Riggs, A. D., H. Suzuki, and S. Bourgeois. 1970a. *Lac* repressor-operator interaction. I. Equilibrium studies. J. Mol. Biol. 48:67–83.

Sadler, J. R., and A. Novick. 1965. The properties of repressor and the kinetics of its action. J. Mol. Biol. 12:305–27.

Sadler, J. R., and T. F. Smith. 1971. Mapping of the lactose operator. J. Mol. Biol. 62:139–69.

Schaller, H., C. Gray, and K. Herrmann. 1975. Nucleotide sequence of an RNA polymerase binding site from the DNA of bacteriophage fd. Proc. Nat. Acad. Sci. USA 72:737–41.

Schmitz, A., U. Schmeissner, J. H. Miller, and P. Lu. 1976. Mutations affecting the quaternary structure of the *lac* repressor. J. Biol. Chem. 251:3359–66.

Smith, T. F., and J. R. Sadler. 1971. The nature of lactose operator constitutive mutations. J. Mol. Biol. 59:273–305.

Sobell, H. M. 1973. The sterochemistry of actinomycin binding to DNA and its implications in molecular biology. Prog. Nucl. Acid. Res. Mol. Biol. 13:153–90.

Sommer, H., P. Lu, and J. Miller, 1975. Lactose operon repressor interaction with inducer and DNA: Changes in tryptophan fluorescence. Biophys. J. 15:302a.

Sommer, H., P. Lu, and J. H. Miller. 1976. *Lac* repressor: Fluorescence of the two tryptophans. J. Biol. Chem. 251:3774–79.

Steitz, T. A., T. J. Richmond, D. Wise, and D. Engelman. 1974. The *lac* repressor protein: Molecular shape, subunit structure, and proposed model for operator interaction based on structural studies of microcrystals. Proc. Nat. Acad. Sci. USA 71:593–97.

Stuart, R. N., and E. W. Branscomb. 1971. Quantitative theory of *in vivo lac* regulation: significance of repressor packaging. I. Equilibrium considerations. J. Theor. Biol. 31:313–29.

Sung, M. T., and G. H. Dixon. 1970. Modification of histones during spermiogenesis in trout: A molecular mechanism for altering histone binding to DNA. Proc. Nat. Acad. Sci. USA 67:1616–23.

Ullmann, A., and J. Monod. 1968. Cyclic AMP as an antagonist of catabolite repression in *Escherichia coli*. FEBS Letters 2:57–60.

Wallenfels, K., and O. P. Malhotra. 1961. Galactosidases. Adv. Carbohydr. Chem 16:239–98.

Walz, A., and V. Pirrotta. 1975. Sequence of the P_R promoter of phage λ. Nature 254:118–21.

Wang, J. C. 1974. The degree of unwinding of the DNA helix by ethidium. I. Titration of twisted PM2 DNA molecules in alkaline cesium chloride density gradients. J. Mol. Biol. 89:783–801.

Wang, J. C., M. D. Barkley, and S. Bourgeois. 1974. Measurements of unwinding of *lac* operator by repressor. Nature 251:247–49.

Weber, K., T. Platt, D. Ganem, and J. H. Miller. 1972. Altered sequences changing the operator-binding properties of the *lac* repressor: Colinearity of the repressor protein with the *i* gene map. Proc. Nat. Acad. Sci. USA 69:3624–28.

Wu, C.-W., and F. Y.-H. Wu. 1974. Conformational transitions of cyclic adenosine monophosphate receptor protein of *Escherichia coli*. A temperature-jump study. Biochemistry 12:2573–78.

Wu, F. Y.-H., P. Bandyopadhyay, and C.-W. Wu. 1976. Conformational transitions of the *lac* repressor from *Escherichia coli*. J. Mol. Biol. 100:459–72.

Wu, F. Y.-H., K. Nath, and C.-W. Wu. 1974. Conformational transitions of cyclic adenosine monophosphate receptor protein of *Escherichia coli*. A fluorescent probe study. Biochemistry 13:2567–72.

Yang, D. S., and K. S. Matthews. 1975. Modification of the lactose repressor protein with 2-chloromercuri-4-nitrophenol. J. Mol. Biol.; submitted.

Zabin, I., and A. V. Fowler. 1972. The amino acid sequence of β-galactosidase. J. Biol. Chem. 277:5432–35.

Zubay, G., and D. A. Chambers. 1971. Regulating the *lac* operon. *In* D. M. Greenberg (ed.). Metabolic pathways. 5:297–347. Academic Press, New York.

Zubay, G., D. Schwartz, and J. Beckwith. 1970. Mechanism of activation of catabolite-sensitive genes: A positive control system. Proc. Nat. Acad. Sci. USA 66:104–10.

JAMES C. COPELAND

Regulation of Chromosome Replication in Bacteria

4

INTRODUCTION

At the very outset, it can be safely stated that our present knowledge of how chromosome replication is regulated is rudimentary. In fact, a current reviewer of the DNA replication problem (Dressler, 1975) considers understanding of regulation of replication at the level of a mystery. Yet the central role that chromosomes play in cell function forces us to seriously consider this problem. The onset, timing, and control of replication may determine the orderly sequence of events that we know as the cell cycle and may set the process of cell division in motion. Our lack of understanding of this regulation problem is related to our lack of understanding of cell growth and division. For example, we have known since 1858 that cells divide (recognized by Rudolph Virchow), yet our understanding of the cell cycle and the cell division process is to this day in the formative stages. The relationship of chromosome replication and its regulation to the cell cycle and to cell division will be considered (see E. Zeuthen, this volume).

Another factor contributing to our relative lack of insight of this regulation problem is our lack of understanding of how DNA is synthesized. Because the two problems are intimately related, it will be necessary to summarize the current knowledge of DNA replication in this article. The elegant and sophisticated analysis of regulation represented by the Lac operon (Barker and Bourgeois, this volume) and Lambda (Szybalski, this volume) hints at the degree of complexity we might expect to encounter as the solution to this problem of chromosome regulation is reached. As developments with the Lac operon and Lambda have shown, model systems are extremely important to

Department of Microbiology, Ohio State University, Columbus, Ohio 43210.

our understanding of complex biological processes. Bacteria and their phages have proven their value as model systems. So too with regulation of chromosome replication, we can expect that the knowledge gained by studying this problem with bacteria will prove the forerunner for an understanding of the higher forms.

The purpose of this article will be primarily to present an overview of the literature that pertains to regulation of chromosome replication in bacteria and to the particular approaches that have been made to study this problem. Second, it provides an opportunity to present a summary of experiments performed in my laboratory that indicate that regulation of chromosome replication occurs during elongation. Finally, a speculative view of the regulation of chromosome replication will be presented. We will consider the problem in light of the recent developments in regulatory biology and with regard to what is known about the relationships between chromosome replication, the cell cycle, and DNA synthesis.

A number of recent reviews are available that provide an in-depth coverage of topics related to the regulation problem (Gross, 1972; Pato, 1972; Smith, 1973; Matsushita and Kubitschek, 1975; Dressler, 1975; Gefter, 1975).

THE BACTERIAL CHROMOSOME

Chromosomes serve as the central organizers of cell function. Contained within them is all or certainly most of the information that makes an organism what it is. In higher forms the chromosomes are clearly visible with a light microscope during mitosis and meiosis. During other times the chromosomes are not readily observable as distinct structures, and they are found located in the nucleus of the cell. These structures contain DNA and special proteins that are necessary to maintain their structure. By contrast, the bacterial chromosome is much smaller and simpler. In fact, the bacterial cell is often many times smaller than a single chromosome from higher forms. The chromosome contained within the bacterial cell is found highly condensed in a structure called the nuclear body. This nuclear body is equivalent to the nucleus of higher forms, but differs by not being limited by a membrane. This difference is one basis for the distinction made in the terms *prokaryote* and *eukaryote* as applied respectively to bacteria and higher forms.

The Bacterial Nuclear Body

The bacterial nuclear body is a true organelle and can be isolated intact under special conditions that require gentle lysis of cells in high osmotic solutions and sedimentation in sucrose gradients (Stonington and Pettijohn, 1971). In this form the nuclear body is the folded bacterial chromosome. This structure contains, in addition to DNA, both RNA and proteins. The protein is predominantly DNA-dependent RNA polymerase. The RNAs are ribosomal RNA (rRNA) and messenger RNA (mRNA) and possibly a unique RNA responsible for maintenance of this structure. The folded chromosome is stable, and suspensions of nuclear bodies have low viscosity. Upon treatment with RNase or heat, unfolding of the structures results in a dramatic increase in viscosity of the solution. This is not found when the folded chromosomes are treated with DNase. These observations suggest that RNA has a role to play in maintaining the structural integrity of the folded chromosome (Worcel and Burgi, 1972).

The DNA in the folded chromosome is supercoiled (Delius and Worcel, 1974) and may exist as a number of loops (12 to 80) organized about a central RNA core. These folded chromosomes can also be isolated with membrane fragments attached (Pettijohn et al., 1973; Worcel and Burgi, 1974; Ryder and Smith, 1975). This finding agrees with earlier electron microscopic observations that showed the nuclear body and DNA of the chromosome in association with the cell membrane (Ryter and Jacob, 1963). As discussed later, the association of the bacterial chromosome with the cell membrane serves to segregate the chromosome to daughter cells, since bacterial cells lack a mitotic apparatus. Attachment of the chromosome to the membrane also is important in the replication of the chromosome and quite likely in regulation of this replication.

The Bacterial Chromosome as a DNA Molecule

In its unfolded form, the bacterial chromosome is a DNA molecule with its ends covalently bonded together to form a closed circular loop. No proteins or RNA segments are found as integral parts of this structure. The contour length of the DNA molecule ranges from 700 μm to 1300 μm (Cairns, 1963; Bleeken et al., 1966; Wake, 1973), which is over $1,000\times$ greater than the length of the cell that contains it. The volume of the nuclear body is about 10% that of the cell. This fact dramatically illustrates the degree of condensation that occurs to package this DNA molecule into the volume it occupies in the nuclear body within the cell. This condensation is even more impressive when we realize that the nuclear body in a growing cell contains a replicating chromosome and that this chromosome must be utilized to retrieve genetic information to carry out the process of growth.

The molecular weight of the bacterial chromosome is 2.0×10^9 daltons to 2.8×10^9 daltons (Massie and Zimm, 1965, Bak et al., 1970; Klotz and Zimm, 1972; Wake, 1973) in basic agreement with that expected from the length of the DNA molecule. In *Escherichia coli* the amount of DNA in the resting nuclear body corresponds to a single bacterial chromosome (Cooper and Helmstetter, 1968; Kubitschek and Freedman, 1971).

Genetic Maps of the Bacterial Chromosome

Another way to view the bacterial chromosome is by genetically constructing linkage maps of genetic loci (Taylor, 1970; Sanderson, 1974; Young and Wilson, 1975). Genetic maps are circular in arrangement, which agrees with the physical nature of the bacterial chromosome. The very existence of genetic maps suggests that the arrangement of the genetic information in the chromosome must confer selective advantage to the organism. Otherwise, the location of genetic markers would be constantly changing due to translocations and inversions; this would make genetic mapping impossible. It is likely that the arrangement of information in the bacterial chromosome corresponds to its function during the cell cycle, in a way analogous to the organization of genes on the chromosomes of bacteriophage Lambda (Szybalski, 1974) and T4 (Champe, 1974) to their life cycles. Further evidence that the genetic organization of the bacterial chromosome is meaningful is shown by the similarity of genetic maps of different but related organisms such as *E. coli* with *Salmonella typhimurium* (Middleton, 1971) and *B. subtilis* with *B. licheniformis* (Goldberg, Gwinn, and Thorne, 1966).

REPLICATION OF THE BACTERIAL CHROMOSOME

One of the principal acts during cell growth is the duplication of the chromosomes. One complete set is distributed to each daughter cell at cell division, assuring genetic continuity of the progeny cells. In the bacterial cell this segregation process is achieved by attachment of the bacterial chromosome to the cell membrane. Presumably, the duplicated attachment sites grow apart, each pulling with it a copy of the replicated chromosome. Since the bacterial chromosome is a simple structure that in the unfolded form is a DNA molecule, understanding its replication will be greatly enhanced by understanding how DNA is synthesized.

The Process of DNA Replication

DNA synthesis can occur in basically two ways: small fragments of DNA can be synthesized as a part of DNA repair and recombination; or long, extended strands of DNA can be synthesized as a part of the DNA duplication process. DNA duplication can be distinguished from the processes of repair and recombination because the newly made DNA is synthesized semi-conservatively during duplication, and it can be identified under proper conditions in a density gradient. This manner of DNA synthesis is properly called DNA replication.

DNA replication is a complex process. Our appreciation of it has evolved from a simple model of the DNA molecule as a template from which a single enzyme synthesizes an exact copy to an involved model that includes at least four enzymatic functions, a number of proteins, some whose functions are unknown, and a multistepped process. The proper assembly of these components appears to be essential for DNA replication, as illustrated by the requirement for intact, permeabilized cells for *in vitro* DNA replication (Moses and Richardson, 1970). This has led to the idea of an organelle being involved. This organelle is known as a replisome (Bleecken, 1971), and may be intimately associated with the cell membrane.

DNA replication can be subdivided into three distinct processes: initiation, elongation, and termination. Initiation is that part of DNA replication that starts or triggers the beginning of duplication. It is a point of primary control over DNA replication. Once initiated, DNA replication proceeds by synthesizing copies of the parental strands. This is called DNA elongation. It is this process that accounts for the extensive, semi-conservative duplication of the DNA molecule. DNA replication is completed by the termination process, which requires additional protein synthesis in order to replicate the final segment.

The complexity of DNA replication is revealed by a genetic analysis of the process (Gross, 1972; Smith, 1973). In *E. coli* nine distinct genetic loci have been found necessary for DNA replication (Sakai, Hashimoto, and Komano, 1974; Filip et al.; 1974; Beyersman, Messer, and Schlicht, 1974). Also in *B. subtilis* nine genetic loci have been identified (Karamata and Gross, 1970). Four of these genes in *E. coli* are involved with the initiation process (*dna*A, *dna*C (D), *dna*H, and *dna*I; *dna*D has been found to be identical with *dna*C; Wechsler, 1973). Five of these genes are concerned with elongation (*dna*B, *dna*E, *dna*F, *dna*G, and *dna*Z). No distinct mutant has been identified for the termination process; however, it is difficult to distinguish clearly between initiation and termination phenotypes without identifying the chromosomal site involved. Five of the gene products have been purified. Two of these purified products have been identified with known enzymatic functions. Gene *dna*E has been identified with DNA polymerase pol III (Gefter et al., 1971), and gene *dna*F appears to determine a subunit of ribonucleotide reductase (Fuchs et al., 1972), an enzyme that produces substrate deoxyribonucleotides for DNA polymerization. Products for genes *dna*B, *dna*C (D), and *dna*G have been purified, but no enzymatic function has been identified for them as yet. It is likely that other genes essential for DNA replication exist, but mutations for them have not been isolated.

Initiation of DNA Replication

The recognition of a distinct event necessary for beginning DNA replication came from studies that also revealed the regulatory role of this process. These experiments involved starvation of growing cells for required amino acids as a means to study the effect of perturbing protein synthesis on DNA synthesis (Maaløe and Hanawalt, 1961; Lark, Repko, and Hoffman, 1963). They showed that on-going replication continued, but new starts at DNA replication required protein synthesis. This type of experiment also revealed that the site of initiation is unique (Lark et al., 1963). This site represents the origin of replication, and it has been demonstrated by other means as well (Yoshikawa and Sueoka, 1963 a and b). Replication of the bacterial chromosome proceeds sequentially from this origin in a bidirectional manner (Masters and Broda, 1971; Fujisawa and Eisenstark, 1973; Lepesant-Kejzlarova et al., 1975; Harford, 1975). This means that the origin for replication and the terminus are not structurally associated. The origin and terminus are both membrane-bound (Sueoka and Quinn, 1968; Yahara, 1972). The exact role that membrane attachment plays in initiation is not known, but it could serve a regulatory function.

The events that lead to initiation are separable in time during the cell cycle (Lark and Renger, 1969). One event that is sensitive to low concentrations of choloramphenicol occurs about 5 to 10 minutes after restart of growth following amino acid starvation. This event is probably the synthesis of a protein on ribosomes. Another amino acid-requiring but chloramphenicol-resistant event, which is essential for initiation, occurs about 15 minutes after restart of growth. This event may respresent the non-ribosomal addition of amino acids to membrane, which could be involved in attachment of DNA to the membrane. A third event is indicated since initiation does not occur until 15 minutes after completion of the second step. It has been pointed out recently that ordering of events during the initiation process according to their chloramphenicol sensitivity may be misleading (Cooper and Wensthoff, 1971; Cooper, 1974), so this sequence of events remains to be firmly established.

The initiation process requires transcription (Lark, 1972a). Initiation will not occur if transcription is blocked by rifampicin or streptolidigin, drugs that specifically affect DNA-dependent RNA polymerase. This step in initiation is specific for transcription and does not require subsequent protein synthesis, since removal of the block to RNA polymerase while simultaneously blocking protein synthesis by chloramphenicol addition allows initiation to occur. A likely role for this RNA transcript in initiation is to serve as a primer from which DNA pol III can begin to synthesize DNA. A model accounting for a required RNA transcript to initiate DNA replication of the Lambda chromosome has been proposed (see Szybalski, this volume). However, before we can safely extrapolate a mechanism for initiation from one system to another, we must recognize that different modes of DNA replication exist (theta, Cairns, 1963; sigma or rolling circle, Gilbert and Dressler, 1968; D-loop in mitochondria, Kasamatsu, Robberson, and Vinograd, 1971; replication of a linear DNA molecule for T7, Dressler, Wolfson, and Magazin, 1972; and single-strand to replicative form in ØX174, Sinsheimer, 1968). A distinct mechanism for initiation of DNA replication could exist for each of these replication modes making extrapolation of a mechanism from one to another unwarranted. It seems likely that the mechanisms for initiation of DNA replication within a given mode will be the same. Where studied in sufficient detail, it has been found that replication of bacterial chromosomes is by the theta mode.

Initiation of chromosome replication may take place even through DNA replication is blocked (Sueoka et al., 1973). This was shown by starving thymine requiring *B. subtilis* cells and then using them as toluenized cells for the *in vitro* synthesis of DNA. Thymine starvation is known to prematurely induce initiation of chromosome replication (Pritchard and Lark, 1964). However, it is also known that toluenized cells are incapable of initiating chromosome replication (Burger, 1971; Matsushita, White, and Sueoka, 1971). Yet the cells starved for thymine showed multiple rounds of replication for a marker located near the origin when used in the *in vitro* assay for DNA synthesis. This could only come about if initiation of replication could occur in the cells while DNA replication was blocked by thymine starvation. These initiated origins could then serve as sites for continued DNA replication in the toluenized-cells.

Elongation of DNA During Replication

Once initiated, chromosome replication proceeds by a process not fully understood today. During the past few years, sufficient detail about elongation has been obtained to show that it is complex and multistepped. The key observations have been the finding that DNA replication is discontinuous (Sakabe and Okasaki, 1966); the finding of the mutant *pol*A deficient in DNA pol I, (DeLucia and Cairns, 1969), which made possible the isolation of pol II and pol III (Kornberg and Gefter, 1971); the isolation and characterization of the *dna* mutants (Kohiyama et al., 1963); and finally, the recognition of the need for structural integrity of the replication system (Schekman, Weiner, and Kornberg, 1974), or replisome, which led to the development of the *in vitro* DNA replication system as represented by toluene treated cells (Moses and

Richardson, 1970). As with DNA segregation and initiation, the cell membrane plays a role in DNA elongation, for nascent DNA is found associated with the membrane. The cell membrane, in particular the mesosome, may be the site of replisome assembly and function (Ryter and Jacob, 1963).

Discontinuous DNA elongation. Nascent DNA is synthesized in short pieces about 1,000 nucleotides long that are then joined to form long, extended segments (Okazaki et al., 1968). Discovery of this manner of synthesizing DNA resolved one of the paradoxes for DNA synthesis, namely, how to synthesize DNA in the 3' to 5' direction when all of the known polymerases synthesize 5' to 3'. Resolution of one paradox by discontinuous DNA synthesis created another. Since DNA polymerases are incapable of starting synthesis *de novo* and require a primer, a need was created to explain how each fragment of DNA began. This problem appears to be solved by the discovery of a short RNA strand covalently bonded to the nascent DNA fragments (Sugino, Hirose, and Okazaki, 1972). DNA-dependent RNA polymerase is capable of starting synthesis *de novo,* and DNA polymerases can add onto the 3' end of RNA strands. The RNA primer is subsequently cleaved from the nascent DNA fragment, and the resulting gap is filled in, probably by pol I. Adjacent 5' and 3' ends of these extended fragments are covalently joined by DNA ligase. The need for RNA primers to continue DNA elongation may provide a control point for regulating DNA replication (Lark, 1972b). It should be noted that the RNA transcript for initiation is distinct from the RNA primers needed to continue DNA elongation. The initiation transcript is sensitive to rifampicin (Lark, 1972a), whereas the RNA primers are not (Sugino et al., 1972).

The existence of these RNA primers for synthesis of nascent DNA fragments is not without question (Nath and Hurwitz, 1974). Their detection is subject to artifact and they have not always been unambiguously found. However, recent work directed to these criticisms continues to support the existence of elongation RNA primers and further solidifies this model (Okazaki et al., 1975; Kurosawa et al., 1975).

It has not been resolved whether one or both strands of nascent DNA are synthesized discontinuously in *E. coli* (Okazaki et al., 1968; Herrman, Huf, and Bonhoeffer, 1972), but for *B. subtilis* the results show that only one strand is synthesized discontinuously (Kainuma and Okazaki, 1970; Ganesan et al., 1976). Possibly, discontinuous synthesis can occur on both strands if progress of the DNA polymerase in the 5' to 3' direction is retarded (Olivera and Bonhoeffer, 1972). Then transcription events ahead of the polymerase could serve as primers for further DNA synthesis. On the other hand, if DNA polymerase movement is unaffected, then progress in the 5' to 3' direction of synthesis might be fast enough to preclude the need for RNA primers. Under all circumstances DNA synthesized in the 3' to 5' direction would always require RNA primers.

DNA polymerases. For our purposes a brief description of the DNA polymerases will be sufficient. The reader is referred to reviews that provide an in-depth coverage of these enzymes (Kornberg, 1974; Gefter, 1975). It is important to recognize that these polymerases are similar in their enzymatic properties and that some of them also possess other enzymatic functions, such as exonuclease activity, in addition to their polymerase function.

The first discovered DNA polymerase, pol I, is primarily involved in the repair and recombination processes (DeLucia and Cairns, 1969). Its role in DNA replication cannot be ruled out, because available *pol* A mutants have residual pol I activity that may be sufficient to satisfy an essential role (Lehman and Chien, 1973). In support of pol I being involved with DNA replication is the finding that *pol* A *rec* A double mutants are inviable (Gross, 1972). Also, a conditional *pol* A mutant that lost the 5' to 3' exonuclease activity but retained polymerase activity at the non-permissive temperature was found to be lethal (Konrad and Lehman, 1974). The pol I enzyme is admirably suited for the gap-filling process described for discontinuous DNA synthesis. These observations bring into focus the interrelationships between DNA replication, repair, and recombination.

Pol II is a distinct DNA polymerase that probably is involved in repair or recombination processes too (Moses and Richardson, 1970). No essential role for this enzyme has been found. Conceivably, it could function as a back-up system for pol I.

The pol III polymerase is distinct from the other DNA polymerases and has been demonstrated to be essential for DNA replication. The *dna*E locus has been shown to determine the pol III polymerase (Kornberg and Gefter, 1971). Recent developments that are important to our consideration of regulation involve studies with the purified polymerase *in vitro*. A purified preparation of this enzyme was found to be inactive for the *in vitro* synthesis of bacteriophage M13 and ØX174DNA. This led to the discovery of a protein factor that associates with the pol III enzyme to make an active complex called pol III*. In addition a second protein factor called copolymerase, copol III*, has been found (Wickner and Kornberg, 1974; Hurwitz and Wickner, 1974). This factor is required together with RNA primer, ATP and Mg+ at the first stage of elongation. The second stage of the elongation process is independent of copol III* and ATP. These findings establish the role for ATP in DNA elongation. ATP is required to synthesize the RNA primer, and it is necessary for the function of the pol III* complex. It is important to note that non-enzymatic protein factors like these described for the pol III* complex often play a role in regulation.

Nucleases, ligase, and other protein factors. Nuclease activity associated with the polymerases appears to be essential for DNA replication. A recently isolated conditional mutant in *E. coli, polAexl,* has normal pol I polymerizing activity but is deficient in 5′ to 3′ exonuclease activity at the non-permissive temperature. Unlike other *pol* A mutants, the *polAexl* mutation is lethal at the nonpermissive temperature (Konrad and Lehman, 1974).

The *rec*BC enzyme (exonuclease V) is an ATP-dependent exonuclease involved in recombination and repair. Recently it has been found to possess an unwinding activity also requiring ATP (Linnard MacKay, 1974). Possibly this enzyme is also involved in DNA replication.

Polynucleotide ligase closes nicks in DNA strands by forming bonds between 3′-OH and 5′-PO$_4$ groups on adjacent nucleotides (Lehman, 1974). The role of this enzyme in discontinuous DNA synthesis is quite apparent.

DNA-binding proteins that promote DNA strand separation are essential for phage T4 replication and recombination. Such binding proteins have been found in uninfected *E. coli* and in mammalian cells (Alberts, 1968). The DNA-denaturing activity of these proteins could be essential for DNA replication in bacteria, although this function has not been proved yet.

Finally, another protein factor that could also be involved in DNA replication is the omega protein (Wang, 1971). This protein has been shown to unwind supercoiled DNA, and could serve as a swivel protein during DNA replication.

Termination of DNA Replication

Since replication of the bacterial chromosome is bidirectional, the site where replication ends is far removed from the site where it began. This terminus is specifically associated with the cell membrane. Completion of chromosome replication appears to be a distinct and separate process from initiation of chromosome replication and chromosome elongation. This was demonstrated in a study of DNA synthesis in a temperature-sensitive *dna*A initiation mutant in *E. coli* (Marunochi and Messer, 1973). These cells were starved for required amino acids. DNA synthesis occurred during starvation and then stopped, as is characteristic for a block at the initiation step. Next, the cells were shifted to non-permissive temperature, to prevent any initiation of DNA replication, and amino acids were added back. A short burst of DNA synthesis ensued, which indicated that chromosome replication was not completed for all cells during the amino acid starvation. Further study indicated that a terminal segment, about 0.5 percent of the entire chromosome was not replicated in the absence of protein synthesis. Apparently, replication of this terminal segment and protein synthesis late in the cell cycle are required to start the cell division process in *E. coli*. The requirement for protein synthesis to terminate chromosome replication, suggests that this process is regulated (Winston and Matsushita, 1976).

The Replication Fork

What have been described in the previous sections as separate events in reality all occur together in the replication forks that are characteristic for the replicating bacterial chromosome. Autoradiographic experiments show these replication forks to move away from a common origin at apparently equal rates (Wake, 1973). It is at the replication fork that nascent DNA is synthesized and that the unreplicated portion of the chromosome is separated from the replicated part. The replication fork represents the accumulation of events that lead to initiation, elongation, and eventually termination of chromosome replication. These processes occur in association with the cell membrane (Ganesan and Lederberg, 1965; Smith and Hanawalt, 1967) and require an assemblage of enzymes and protein factors that is now recognized as the replisome.

BACTERIAL CHROMOSOME REPLICATION AND THE CELL CYCLE

The period of time between cell divisions, or the cell cycle, can be made to vary in bacteria as a function of nutrient energy source. In nutritionally rich medium, where amino acids, vitamins, nucleobases, and glucose are supplied, bacterial cells may have a generation time as short as 20 minutes. When grown in nutritionally defined medium, such as mineral salts, required growth factors, and glucose, bacterial cells will grow with generation times in the range of 40 to 70 minutes. If the energy source is other than glucose, the generation time in this defined medium can be very long and, depending on the energy source, may be 200 minutes or even longer.

Bacteria grown in the rich, complex medium are much larger than bacteria grown in defined media, 1.3 μm^3 compared to 0.3 μm^3. The larger cells contain many ribosomes that enable them to synthesize proteins rapidly enough to keep pace with the fast growth rate. The large bacterial cell also contains more nuclear bodies than the small cell. Fast-growing cells with a 20-minute generation time will contain as many as four nuclear bodies. Those growing at intermediate rates, such as a 60-minute generation time, will have two nuclear bodies. Bacteria growing at very slow generation times may have only one nuclear body (Maaløe and Kjeldgaard, 1966).

The DNA Cycle

The rate of chromosome elongation is the sum of the rates of travel at each replication fork. The rate of replication appears to be the same for each fork.

This conclusion is made from the observation that the terminus of replication is equidistant from the origin (Masters and Broda, 1971; Lepesant-Kejzlarova et al., 1975; Harford, 1975). Direct measurements of the distance that replication forks travel, taken from autoradiographs, are consistent with this view (Wake, 1973). At 37C in *E. coli* the length of time to complete replication of the chromosome is about 40 minutes (Cooper and Helmsteffer, 1968). Measurement of the distance that replication forks travel early and late during the DNA cycle show them to be different (Wake, 1974). The rate of chromosome elongation appears to slow down toward the latter part of the DNA cycle. The average rate of synthesis at each replication fork approaches 1,000 nucleotide-pairs polymerized per second.

Coordination of the DNA and Cell Cycles

Since the bacterial cell cycle can be made to vary over a wide range of generation times, an obvious problem is to understand how the DNA cycle is coordinated with the cell cycle. General agreement exists for bacterial cells growing at moderate to fast generation times, but conflicting observations have been made for cells growing at slow generation times.

At moderate generation times, where the cell cycle is as long or longer in duration than the DNA cycle, a single set of replication forks traverse the bacterial chromosome in time to complete replication before division occurs. A particular relationship of the DNA cycle to the cell cycle has been found (Cooper and Helmstetter, 1968). At moderate and fast generation times, the period of the DNA cycle is constant. This has been defined as the C period. Furthermore, another constant relationship was observed between the ending of the DNA cycle and cell division. This period lasts 20 minutes and is identified as the D period. In *E. coli* a number of observations indicate that the timing of cell division is dependent upon the termination of chromosome replication. Treatments that block DNA replication before termination also block cell division (Pierucci and Helmstter, 1969). Apparently a tight connection between the cycles is not always essential, because in *B. subtilis* it is possible to block DNA replication without stopping subsequent cell division (Donachie, Martin, and Begg, 1971). This results in anucleate cells being produced. We know that the DNA cycle can be dissociated from the cell cycle by mutation in both *E. coli* and *B. subtilis* (Hirota et al., 1968; Mendelson, 1972).

When bacterial cells are grown in nutritionally rich medium, the cell cycle becomes shorter than the DNA cycle (Helmstetter and Cooper, 1968). This creates the obvious problem of there being too little time to complete the DNA cycle. Since the DNA cycle is constant at moderate and fast generation times, it appears that DNA synthesis is proceeding at its maximal rate and cannot be further increased. One manner by which more DNA can be synthesized in the same period of time is by introducing additional replication forks on the chromosome before the first set has reached the terminus. This was found and is called dichotomous replication (Oishi, Yoshikawa, and Sueoka, 1964; O'Sullivan and Sueoka, 1967). In this situation the bacterial chromosome begins to replicate a second time before it has completed replicating the first time. During this second DNA cycle, replication proceeds from both origins of the already replicating chromosome. For dichotomous replication the DNA cycle started in one cell cycle is not completed until the next cell cycle. It was found that the D period, the time between the end of the DNA cycle and the end of the next cell cycle, or cell division, was always the same. Clearly, the coordination of the DNA cycle with the cell cycle is regulated.

Under conditions where the DNA cycle is blocked, subsequent cell division may be blocked, but cell growth may continue. When the block to the DNA cycle is released, multiple initiations of chromosome replication ensue (Pritchard and Lark, 1964; Lark and Bird, 1965; Worcel, 1970). Generally, only one arm of the replicating chromosome is used to initiate additional replication forks. This indicates that a functional difference exists between origins of a replicating chromosome. Stable replication, not requiring chromosome initiation, is also possible following a block to the DNA cycle (Kogoma and Lark, 1970; Lark, 1972). During this block of DNA synthesis, protein synthesis must be allowed to occur. Then release of the DNA cycle, but now with protein synthesis being inhibited, results in stable DNA synthesis. Study of this stable replication, which is continuous in the absence of protein synthesis, indicates that only one arm of the replicating chromosome is being repeatedly used. Again, this is evidence that a functional difference exists between origins of a replicating chromosome. To account for dichotomous replication, the origin on both arms of the replicated chromosome must become functional at some time during the DNA cycle. It has been suggested that only one of the two newly made origins is attached to the cell membrane (Marvin, 1968), but later during the DNA cycle the other origin also becomes attached. This event could have regulatory significance during the normal cell cycle.

At growth rates greater than 90 minutes, the coordination of the DNA cycle with the cell cycle is not so well understood. Contributing to this problem is the difficulty of maintaining slowly growing cells in balanced growth, an essential requirement for studies of the bacterial cell cycle. The observations fall into two categories. The first show that the DNA cycle, or the C period, is constant and that the relationship between the DNA cycle and the cell cycle, or the D period, remains the same at all growth rates (Kubitschek and

Freeman, 1971; Chandler, Bird, and Caro, 1975). This means that as the cell cycle becomes longer the DNA cycle occupies less of it and occurs during the latter part of the cell cycle. In contrast to this model, the second category of observations indicate that the DNA cycle is not constant for slowly growing cells, but that the DNA cycle becomes increasingly extended as the cell cycle is lengthened (Eberle and Lark, 1967; Cooper and Helmstetter, 1968; Bird and Lark, 1970; Gudas and Pardee, 1974). Furthermore, the relationship of the DNA cycle to the cell cycle may change, since the DNA cycle is found to start during the first half of the cell cycle for these slowly growing cells. The source of these disagreements for slowly growing cells may involve lack of balanced growth for the cultures used or perturbation of the relationship between the cell and DNA cycles by manipulations used to obtain synchronized cells. A resolution of these differences is important to a complete understanding of the coordination of the DNA cycle with the cell cycle.

APPROACHES TO THE STUDY OF REGULATION
OF BACTERIAL CHROMOSOME REPLICATION

Several distinct approaches have been made to elucidate the control of chromosome replication. Some are integrative in design, that is, the experiments measure a systematic adjustment of many cell components to a new physiological situation. The shift of growing cells from one growth condition to another falls into this category. Another approach is to simply measure the relationship of the DNA cycle to the cell cycle for cells grown under different conditions. This generally requires the use of cell populations synchronized for cell growth and cell division, although use of randomly growing populations for cell cycle studies can be employed under certain conditions to be explained later. An attempt to specifically identify the regulatory relationship between protein synthesis and DNA replication was made in amino acid starvation experiments or through the use of protein synthesis inhibitory agents. The most specific approach to determine the role of a particular gene in the regulation of chromosome replication is by the use of conditional DNA mutants. Each of these methods has contributed to our understanding of regulation of chromosome replication in some unique way. As already pointed out, these approaches often involve the study of DNA replication and/or the cell cycle as the primary attribute being observed. But regulatory characteristics of chromosome replication can be identified in these studies. Some of this information has been discussed in previous sections. What follows will be a brief discussion of the particular strengths and limitations of these approaches to a resolution of the regulatory problem and a recognition of the contribution each approach has made.

Nutritional Shift Experiments

Cells grown in a particular medium will display traits characteristic of that medium such as rate of growth, cell size, and rate of macromolecular synthesis. From a nutritionally complex medium to a minimal medium, these traits may differ by four fold or more. The intent of nutritional shift experiments was to study the transition period when cells grown in one medium were shifted to another. During this time after the shift, cells have to readjust to the new growth conditions. The order and rates of change of macromolecular synthesis during this transition revealed some fundamental aspects of macromolecular regulation (Schaechter, 1961; Maaløe and Kjeldgaard, 1966).

Nutritional shifts may be made either from a defined, minimal medium to a medium nutritionally richer in composition, a shift-up, or in the opposite direction, a shift-down. In the shift-up type of experiment, it was found that the rate of DNA and protein synthesis remained constant while the rate of RNA synthesis showed an immediate and dramatic increase. Later during the transition, the rate of protein synthesis increased followed by an increased rate of DNA synthesis. At this time the rates of macromolecular synthesis were adjusted to the new rate of growth for that medium. A nutritional shift-down produced the opposite effect. RNA and protein synthesis slowed down immediately, whereas DNA synthesis continued at a slowly decreasing rate. By the end of the transition period, RNA and protein synthesis had resumed at reduced rates and the rate of DNA synthesis had adjusted to that characteristic for cells in this minimal medium.

These nutritional shift experiments showed that changes in patterns and rates of macromolecular synthesis were specific for each type of macromolecule. This showed that distinct controls existed for DNA synthesis when compared with RNA and protein synthesis. Furthermore, the shift-up experiments indicated that the primary regulation over macromolecular synthesis existed at the start or initiation of synthesis. In particular, the rates of transcription and translation for individual macromolecules appear to be the same for slowly growing cells compared with fast growing cells. The patterns and shifts in rates of macromolecular synthesis in going from one nutritional condition to another were consistent with either stopping any new initiations of macromolecular synthesis or in stimulating additional initiations (Maaløe and Kjeldgaard, 1966). This principle of macromolecular regulation remains valid and has greatly influenced much of the thinking in regulatory biology today.

Cell Cycle Experiments

The relationship of the DNA cycle to the cell cycle has already been described (Helmstetter and Cooper, 1968; Cooper and Helmstetter, 1968). In this type of experiment, usually some means is employed to synchronize cell growth and division. This may be done by collecting bacterial cells on a nitrocellulose filter, inverting the filter, and eluting newly divided cells from the filter. The age of the cells collected in this fashion is directly related to their age in the cell cycle when the cells were randomly mixed in culture. For example, progeny of cells that were late in the cell cycle just before filtering will be among the earliest eluted off the filter; whereas those earlier in the cell cycle will be eluted off the filter at later times. This method of obtaining cells according to their position in the cell cycle is useful, since cells growing randomly can be radioisotopically labeled and then later separated to determine the ability to incorporate that labeled compound as a function of cell age in the cell cycle. The method is not without its problems and may give a distorted cell cycle due to delayed elution of newly divided cells (Matsushita and Kubitschek, 1975).

Velocity sedimentation of randomly grown cells in a sucrose gradient has been used to selectively obtain small cells, which are the newly divided cells (Kubitschek and Freedman, 1971). The resulting population of small cells grows and divides synchronously for two or three cell cycles. Another method that has been used successfully to obtain synchronized bacterial populations involves diluting cells into fresh growth medium as they approach stationary phase (Cutler and Evans, 1966). Repeated cycling of cells in this way leads to a population that is synchronized for subsequent growth and division.

Relationships between the DNA cycle and the cell cycle have also been studied with randomly growing cells. Cells in balanced growth can be pulse labeled with ^{3}H-thymine, and the number of cells actively synthesizing DNA at that time can be determined by autoradiographic means (Eberle and Lark, 1967). The proportion of the cell cycle occupied by the DNA cycle is directly proportional to the fraction of total cells labeled with ^{3}H-thymine, provided the cell cycle is not shorter than the DNA cycle.

The results obtained from these studies have explicitly shown that chromosome replication is regulated during the cell cycle. Clearly, the initation event is controlled and appears to be the major means of regulating chromosome replication in rapidly growing cells, a conclusion also supported by results obtained by nutritional shift experiments. The role of dichotomous replication in maintaining the proper relationship of chromosome replication to cell division in these rapidly growing cells was made clear from such studies. The relationship between termination of chromosome replication and subsequent cell division was also determined from these experiments. Finally, conflicting results were obtained for slowly growing cells, and it remains uncertain whether the rate of chromosome elongation in these cells is slower than in faster growing cells. Also, the exact relationship of the DNA cycle to the cell cycle in slowly growing cells remains to be determined. The primary limitation of the study of cell cycles, as well as the nutritional shift experiment, is the lack of specificity they have for identifying the mechanisms that underlie macromolecular control.

Amino Acid Starvation and
Inhibitory Agents for Protein Synthesis

Chemical inhibitors and amino acid starvation have been used to determine the specific effect that perturbation of protein synthesis has on DNA replication (Pardee and Prestidge, 1956; Maaløe and Hanawalt, 1961; Lark, Repko, and Hoffman, 1963). For amino acid starvation, mutants requiring particular amino acids are shifted from a defined medium containing these amino acids to one lacking them. Generally, starvation has been carried out for a number of amino acids simultaneously. When this is done, DNA replication slows gradually and finally stops. Further analysis indicates that the chromosome population replicates to the terminus region and becomes aligned. A similar result is obtained when a specific protein inhibitor, such as chloramphenicol, is used to treat growing cells.

The use of amino acid starvation or chloramphenicol addition (Lark and Lark, 1964) coupled with means for measuring DNA synthesis or replication has provided data for a number of important concepts concerning DNA replication and its regulation. It has been demonstrated that the origin of chromosome replication is unique (Lark, Repko, and Hoffman, 1963). Alignment of chromosome replication by amino acid starvation also provided data to show that replication was sequential (Lark, Repko, and Hoffman, 1963). The response of DNA replication to amino acid starvation shows that protein synthesis is not necessary for on-going DNA synthesis, but that a protein is required to initiate a subsequent round of chromosome replication (Maaløe, 1961). Since amino acids are not direct precursors of nucleobases, the postulated role of a protein in starts at chromosome replication was that of a regulatory, protein initiator.

Amino acid starvation has proved very useful for studying chromosome replication and its regulation. However, some simplifying assumptions used to interpret these experiments are now known to be in error, and the effects that amino acid starvation has on DNA replication must be reconsidered. For example, many early amino acid starvation experiments did not differentiate among the amino acids used. Most experiments employed multiple amino acid starvation. This use implies that each amino acid is alike in the effect it will have on DNA replication when a mutant requiring that amino acid is starved for it. Subsequent work has shown that starvation for different amino acids can produce different effects on DNA replication. Furthermore, early amino acid starvation experiments were interpreted solely in terms of the effect on DNA replication brought about by blocking protein synthesis through amino acid starvation. We now know that amino acid starvation has multitudinous effects on the cell (Copeland, Phillips, and Mao, 1977), not all of which are mediated by blocking protein synthesis. All of these effects should be considered when accounting for amino acid starvation-induced changes in DNA replication. Finally, chromosome termination as a distinct process of chromosome replication is operationally indistinguishable from initiation blocks when DNA synthesis or measurement of chromosome alignment are used as the only criteria, as they often are. Possibly some effects of amino acid starvation that are attributed to affecting initiation may in fact be affecting chromosome termination.

Mutants Affecting DNA Replication

Mutations that specifically block DNA replication offer the best chance for determining the mechanisms for regulation of the process (Gross, 1972). This approach is being widely exploited at this time. Conditional DNA mutants fall into two major groups. One group includes those that stop DNA replication immediately when shifted to non-permissive conditions. Mutations that block synthesis of precursors of DNA affect elongation factors or enzymes, or affect regulation during elongation would be included in this group. The other major group of conditional DNA mutants are those that stop DNA synthesis some time after being shifted to the non-permissive condition. This group would include mutants that have altered initiation factors and/or are affected in some aspect of regulation of the initiation process. Since termination of chromosome replication appears to be a distinct process, this group of late shut-off mutants would also include those affected in the termination process. As already described, four genes, *dna*A, *dna*C (D), *dna*H, and *dna*I, are known to be involved in the initiation process.

Measurement of Chromosome Replication

The earliest experiment measuring chromosome replication in bacteria involved labeling with heavy isotopes (Messelson and Stahl, 1958). This design was further refined in the double-labeling experiment in which a radioactive isotope and a density isotope were used to identify portions of the bacterial chromosomes that replicate at different times (Lark, Repko, and Hoffman, 1963). The latter approach provided sufficient resolution of the replication process to identify the uniqueness of the origin of replication. The double-label experiment was modified to take advantage of genetic transformation and to use genetic markers as a substitute for the radioisotopic marker (Yoshikawa and Sueoka, 1963b). The principle advantage of this genetic adaptation is a very high degree of resolution, which is limited only by the number of genetic markers available and the ability to discriminate among them by mapping techniques. Another genetic technique that provides a measure of chromosome configuration is the marker frequency experiment (Yoshikawa and Sueoka, 1963a). This experiment also uses genetic transformation and reflects the frequency of markers, usually near the origin, relative to a common reference marker near the terminus. Chromosome populations that have completed replication to the terminal marker can be distinguished from those that have not. The use of genetic markers to study chromosome replication and configuration provides a degree of specificity not available by other approaches. This is an important consideration if one wants to determine whether the initiation or termination process has blocked further chromosome replication. It should be remembered that a synchronous wave of initiation following a given treatment does not prove that all chromosomes had terminated because of that treatment.

PROPOSED MODELS FOR REGULATION OF
BACTERIAL CHROMOSOME REPLICATION

Attempts to explain regulation have focused on the initiation process. Possibly this is because most of the work on replication and regulation of the bacterial chromosome has been done with cells growing at moderate to fast growth rates. Under these conditions the rate of replication is maximal and constant, and, therefore, consideration of other regulatory mechanisms has seemed unnecessary. Regulation of the initiation event could account for the results of shift-up experiments, the relationship of the DNA cycle to the cell cycle for moderate- and fast-growing cells, dichotomous replication, and the response of auxotrophic mutants to amino acid starvation. The timing of the initiation event would set in motion the replication process, which would run its course until the bacterial chromosome was duplicated. This constituted a round of replication. Another cycle would begin only when the initiation process was started again (Maaløe, 1961). Thus control over the initiation event constituted control over chromosome replication. The most far-reaching model to explain how this control functioned to regulate the self-replicating bacterial chromosome, as well as other self-duplicating DNA entities, was the replicon model (Jacob and Brenner, 1963). As more has become known about DNA replication and its relationship to the cell cycle, other mechanisms have been proposed to explain control of the initiation process and the relationship of the DNA cycle to the cell cycle. The principle features of these proposals make up the material in this section.

The Replicon Model

This model went beyond explaining just control over the initiation of replication (Jacob and Brenner, 1963). It described the essential features of self-duplicating entities or replicons. To possess this property of self-duplication, a replicon must contain all of the information that directs its duplication and regulates the process. It was proposed that replicons are closed, circular DNA molecules. Since the time of this proposal nearly all prokaryote replicons studied have been found to be circular DNA molecules during their replication. The exceptions are RNA genomes of certain bacteriophages (Hindley, 1973) and the DNA genome of bacteriophage T7, which replicates in a linear form (Dressler, Wolfson, and Magazin, 1972). The bacterial chromosome behaves as a single replicon.

According to this model, the signal to start the replication of a replicon is a protein molecule coded by a gene resident in the replicon. This protein molecule, or initiator, interacts with a specific recognition site in the replicon called the replicator. It is this interaction that triggers the replication process. Once started, replication continues until the whole structure is duplicated. Another round of replication requires another specific initiation signal to set the replication process in motion again.

The interaction of the initiator with its replicator would be highly specific, such that an initiator would recognize only one kind of replicator. Also, the regulation proposed was the positive type, which was thought to fit best with evidence for a diffusible initiator that was obtained with a temperature sensitive F-factor unable to replicate at the non-permissive temperature (Jacob, Brenner, and Cuzin, 1963).

Another important feature of this model was the attachment of the replicon to the cell membrane. This attachment served to explain the regular segregation of the duplicated replicons to daughter cells.

The replicon model is as useful today as it was when first proposed. Modification to bring it in line with new facts does not significantly change the model's essential features. For example, we now know that the initiation process is more complex than just the interaction of the initiator with its replicator. Yet this proposed interaction still could explain the regulation of the initiation process. We also know that the replicator of the replicon is equivalent to the origin of replication of the bacterial chromosome. And we now know that the bacterial chromosome replicates bidirectionally from this origin.

As further verification of the replicon model, it has been found that the insertion of one replicon into another, such as the F-factor into the bacterial chromosome, can serve to suppress temperature sensitive mutations that affect initiation at the non-permissive temperature (Nishimura et al., 1971).

Under this non-permissive condition, the initiation process of the bacterial replicon is inoperative. Yet, the integrated F-replicon is functional and can serve to initiate its replication and go on to replicate the bacterial chromosome attached to it. This is called integrative suppression. Normally, the integrated F-replicon appears to be recessive to the bacterial replicon during cellular growth, and it remains inactive and is passively replicated as a part of the bacterial replicon. The F-replicon becomes activated during the bacterial mating process. Integrative suppression can also occur with the bacteriophage P1 in *E. coli* (Lindahl, Hirota, and Jacob, 1971).

Negative Control of the Initiation Process

Another possible form of regulation of the initiation process could be negative control (Pritchard, Barth, and Collins, 1969; Rosenberg, Cavalieri, and Ungers, 1969). That is, the initiation process could be normally repressed during the cell cycle. This could be accomplished by the classical scheme for repression whereby a protein repressor molecule interacts with the replicator and blocks any transcription from that site. A transcription event is known to be required for the initiation process. Interaction with a small-molecule inducer could inactivate the repressor and allow transcription of the region to occur. Once the RNA primer molecule is formed, the subsequent events required to complete the initiation process could take place.

In some proposals the amount of repressor in the cell is thought to vary during the cell cycle (Pritchard et al., 1969). According to this account, repressor is made soon after initiation of chromosome replication in an amount sufficient to inactivate further initiations. No further repressor is synthesized during the cell cycle. As the cell grows, the repressor concentration decreases to a critical level that is no longer sufficient to block the initiation process; then initiation ensues.

The exact type of regulation over the initiation process remains to be determined. Experience from studies of other regulatory systems would suggest caution in arriving at a conclusion ahead of definitive results. For example, a regulatory series like that observed in fungi (Marzluf, this volume) might serve to control the initiation process. In that case a negative controller of initiation might itself be negatively controlled, the net result giving the appearance of positive regulation. Other networks could be imagined to produce the appearance of over-all negative regulation.

Regulation of the Initiator

Recently it was recognized that if a positive initiator was involved with controlling the initiation process, then some manner of control of the initiator itself was needed (Sompayrac and Maaløe, 1973). Control of the initiator could be achieved if it were a part of an operon, the only other gene being an autorepressor (see Goldberger and Deely, this volume). As cell volume increases from growth, then the concentration of the autorepressor is lowered, which derepresses the operon. Under this derepressed condition, both initiator and autorepressor are produced. The increased concentrations of initiator leads to initiation of chromosome replication, thereby consuming initiator molecules. The increased concentration of the autorepressor acts to repress the operon, thus shutting off further synthesis of both the autorepressor and the initiator. Cell division and further growth reduces the concentration of the autorepressor, which in turn derepresses the operon to start the whole cycle again. Computer modeling of this system indicated that only 250 molecules of the autorepressor would be necessary to obtain a stable system if regulation of initiation is the positive type. But as many as 1,500 molecules of the autorepressor would be needed to achieve the same stability and precision if regulation of initiation was negative, according to the inhibitor dilution model (Pritchard, Barth, and Collins, 1969).

Initiation Control as a Function of Cell Mass or Size

By studying the relationship of initiation to the cell cycle, it was realized that the frequency of initiation correlated well with cell mass or size (Donachie and Begg, 1970). This gave rise to the concept of a critical cell mass or size, the unit cell, which somehow determined the timing and frequency of initiation. Lately, this idea has been further refined to explain the relationship of the cell cycle and DNA cycle (Donachie, 1974). The principle feature of this model is that unit cell doubling sets into motion two independent cycles, the cell cycle and the DNA cycle. The exact mechanism that triggers the onset of these cycles is unspecified. Perhaps the most unique aspect of this model is that the cell cycle is a period of 60 minutes independent of the growth rate. Each time a doubling of the unit cell occurs, the DNA and cell cycles begin, and 60 minutes later cell division takes place. This cell cycle can be further subdivided into two functional periods. The first period lasts 40 minutes, and during this time protein synthesis must occur. The requirement for protein synthesis is independent of the rate of protein synthesis. The second period occupies the remaining 20 minutes, and during this time there appears to be no requirement for DNA, RNA, or net protein synthesis. However, there is a need for a protein whose synthesis is dependent upon the replication of a terminal segment of the chromosome. Presumably, this 20-minute period of the cell cycle is required to assemble previously synthesized components required for the cross-septum and for cell division. The duration of the DNA cycle is about 40 minutes as determined previously.

The best way to appreciate the significance of the requirement for an invariant 60-minute cell cycle is to first consider a unit cell growing in a medium where the growth rate is equal to or greater than 60 minutes. For the time being, we will exclude very slowly growing cells from consideration. This unit cell starts the cell cycle and DNA cycle simultaneously. At 40 minutes the DNA cycle is completed and concomitantly the first period of the cell cycle. Replication of the chromosome terminus triggers the synthesis of a specific protein required to complete the cell division process. During the remaining 20 minute period, the unit cell doubles and cell division soon follows. At the doubling of the unit cell, new cell and DNA cycles are initiated. This process would repeat itself again and again, as long as the cells remained in this medium. However, if this unit cell is transferred to a medium where growth rate is considerably shorter than 60 minutes, say 30 minutes, then the following events will occur according to this model. First we start with the unit cell that has begun both the cell and the DNA cycles. The cell is growing at a rate that will double the unit cell in 30 minutes. At that time of doubling, a second set of cell and DNA cycles are put into motion. Because the first DNA cycle is not completed by 30 minutes, the chromosome will contain two sets of replication forks and be replicating dichotomously. At 40 minutes the first DNA cycle and the first period of that cell cycle will be completed. At 60 minutes the unit cell will have doubled again. This sets in motion still another round of cell and DNA cycles. Also at this time the first cell cycle period is complete, and cell division occurs. What we now have are two cells each twice the original unit cell size and each involved in two sets of cell and DNA cycles. Note that each subsequent cell division will occur at 30-minute intervals, exactly equal to the rate of growth. But the time between the onset and the completion of each cell cycle is a constant 60-minute period. This same relationship between the rate of cell growth and the cell cycle would hold true for other growth rates as well. Note that the faster-growing cell will be larger at the time of cell division than the slower-growing cell. This size difference will be proportional to the difference in growth rates, in agreement with observations made on cell size and mass at different growth rates (Donachie, 1968). This model nicely accounts for many of the known attributes of the DNA and cell cycles for moderate- to fast-growing cells. An independent analysis of DNA and cell cycle data supports the notion that these are intrinsically independent cycles and that the cell cycle is not timed by the DNA cycle (A. Koch, this volume). The two cycles are normally coupled, at least in *E. coli,* by the requirement for the termination protein for cell division. This termination protein is in turn dependent on the replication of a terminal chromosome segment. However, the inherent timing of the cell cycle does not depend on the DNA cycle but on some property of, or correlated to, the unit cell.

As discussed in the section on the cell cycle, observations on slowly growing cells are not in agreement. The validity of extending the unit cell model to explain the relationship between DNA and cell cycles for slowly growing bacteria is presently uncertain.

Membrane Attachment as a Mechanism to Regulate Chromosome Replication

As already mentioned, the bacterial chromosome is known to be intimately associated with the cell membrane in a number of ways. The origin and terminus of the chromosome appear to be permanently attached to the membrane (Sueoka and Quinn, 1968; Yamaguchi and Yoshikawa, 1973; Sueoka and Hammers, 1974). The replication fork also is found associated with cell membrane. Other more transient associations of the bacterial chromosome with the cell membrane are known to exist (Ivarie and Pene, 1973). DNA attachment to the cell membrane, and in particular to the mesosome, has been observed with the electron microscope (Ryter and Jacob, 1963; Van Iterson et al., 1975). Of particular importance to our consideration of regulation, has been the finding that normally both origins on the arms of a duplicated chromosome serve as starting sites for additional replication when the chromosome is being duplicated dichotomously (Quinn and Sueoka, 1970). However, when chromosome replication is prematurely induced by thymine starvation, then only one of the two origins serve as a site for the additional replication (Pritchard and Lark, 1964). This finding suggests that soon after formation the two origins are functionally different. This difference may involve the attachment of the origin to the cell membrane. The original origin would be attached in order to serve as the site for initiation of replication, but the newly made origin may not attach until later in the cell cycle. Premature initiation would then occur from the origin site attached to the cell membrane, whereas dichotomous initiation would occur later in the cell cycle when both origins are membrane-attached (Quinn and Sueoka, 1970).

In support of this concept of membrane involvement is the finding that a chloramphenicol-resistant and amino acid-requiring event is necessary for initiation, and that this event takes place late in the sequence leading to initiation (Lark and Renger, 1969).

The model has been proposed which suggests that the attachment of DNA to the membrane serves as a mechanism to regulate the initiation of chromosome replication (Marvin, 1968). According to this model the number of attachment sites for the bacterial chromosome are limited. Only when the chromosome is attached can it be replicated. The formation of a site on the membrane is itself determined by the rate of growth of the cell, thereby tying the two processes of cell growth and chromosome initiation together. Recent studies of the cell cycle and DNA cycle and their perturbation by treatments or agents specific for protein synthesis, DNA synthesis, or membrane, support the idea of membrane attachment of the chromosome as being a regulatory event during initiation (Helmstetter, 1974).

The Replisome Model

We know that DNA replication is a complex process requiring a number of proteins and at least one transcriptional event. Also we know that membrane attachment of the bacterial chromosome is probably very important. A wholistic model to explain regulation of chromosome replication has taken into account these facts. This model proposes that an organelle, or replisome, is necessary for chromosome replication (Bleecken, 1971). Until this organelle is completely assembled, replication cannot begin. Maturation of the replisome, a protein-RNA complex, takes place on a particular site of the bacterial chromosome, called the replisome region, presumably the origin. Since this is a unique site, only one replisome can be assembled for each unreplicated chromosome. Complete assembly of the replisome leads to initiation of chromosome replication. The replisome serves as the growing point for DNA elongation. According to this model the origins would be available for replisome maturation immediately after being duplicated. The rate of replisome maturation is proportional to the rate of protein synthesis, which would directly relate the timing of maturation and initiation to cell growth for cells in balanced growth. Finally, the replisome is attached to the cell membrane. This model could be made compatible with either a positive or negative type of control over initiation of chromosome replication.

The array of proposals to account for regulation of chromosome replication all deal with initiation events. They include both positive and negative types of regulation, control of initiation determined by cell size or mass, and the role of membrane attachment to control of replication. Finally, the complexity of the replication process is recognized in the replisome model, which requires the complex apparatus to be completely assembled before replication can ensue. This assembly of the complex serves to regulate the replication process. We will reconsider the problem of regulation of chromosome replication in its entirety in a later section. At that time we can attempt to organize and bring some understanding to this multitude of proposed models as they relate to the process of control of chromosome replication in bacteria.

AMINO ACID STARVATION AND ITS EFFECT ON CELLS

Amino acid starvation experiments were the first type to provide specific information about regulation of chromosome replication. From these studies it was concluded that protein synthesis was necessary for renewed DNA replication. DNA synthesis in progress was apparently unaffected by amino acid starvation. Other important properties of the bacterial chromosome, its regulation during the cell cycle and its replication, were studied either directly or indirectly through the use of amino acid starvation or its counterpart, specific inhibition of protein synthesis by drugs such as chloramphenicol.

Throughout the early experiments two basic assumptions about the effect of amino acid starvation of the bacterial cell were made or implied, as revealed by the conclusions drawn from those experiments. First, it was thought that the principle effect of amino acid starvation is to block protein synthesis, since amino acids are the direct precursors of the proteins. As we shall see, this is true, but the intricate involvement of protein synthesis with the whole economy of the cell makes that simple statement inaccurate. The other underlying assumption often made from these amino acid starvation experiments was that all amino acids were equivalent in their effect on regulation of chromosome replication. Simultaneous starvations for several amino acids were performed. This was done to obtain a more complete block over subsequent DNA replication. But we now know that amino acids differ greatly in their roles in proteins and in regulatory processes. Our purpose in this section will be to briefly examine the effect of amino acid starvation on bacterial cells, so that we can better evaluate the impact of starvation on regulation of chromosome replication.

Effect of Amino Acid Starvation on Protein Synthesis

Starvation of an amino acid auxotroph for a required amino acid soon stops net protein synthesis. However, we now know that protein synthesis continues in starved cells due to protein turnover (Mandelstam, 1957; Borek, Pontecorvo, and Rittenberg, 1958; Brumschede and Bremer, 1971; Rafeli-Eshkol, Epstein, and Hershko, 1974). In the absence of growth it occurs at rates of up to 8 percent of the protein per hour. When bacterial cells are starved for nitrogen or carbon sources, as much as 40 percent of the total protein may be degraded (Nath and Koch, 1971). This extensive protein turnover itself requires protein synthesis. These studies showed that protein turnover is a routine process of cell behavior and may be greatly increased in times of stress. This latter observation signifies that turnover of proteins is regulated. Also, we should be aware that turnover of particular proteins may differ in rates and control.

In amino acid-starved stringent cells (RelA[+]) inducible or repressible proteins can be made. For example, ornithine transcarbamylase is made at derepressed rates in amino acid starved *E. coli* (Gallant et al., 1970). Functional proteins are not synthesized in amino acid starved relaxed cells (RelA⁻) presumably because of faulty protein synthesis associated with this phenotype (Brumschede and Bremer, 1971). Amino acid starvation also affects particular proteins differently. For example, the level of ribosomal proteins is lower in amino acid starved, relaxed cells than in stringent cells (Goodman, Manor, and Rombants, 1969). Also the specific amino acid synthetase for the amino acid being starved is rapidly inactivated and its synthesis derepressed during starvation (Williams and Neidhardt, 1969).

We can see that amino acid starvation does block over-all net protein synthesis, but any prediction we make about a particular protein could be in error. Amino acid starvation can affect the turnover and the synthesis of individual proteins differently. Turnover of proteins is stimulated by stress, and the amino acids supplied by this process are sufficient to allow for inducible or derepressible enzyme synthesis at elevated rates. The low level of protein synthesis during amino acid starvation might be sufficient to supply the low numbers of a regulatory protein to maintain control in a starved cell.

Effect of Amino Acid Starvation on RNA Synthesis

The fact that amino acid starvation affects RNA synthesis at all is evidence for a regulatory relationship, since the majority of amino acids are not direct or immediate precursors for nucleic acid synthesis (Gallant and Cashel, 1967). One of the important facts of this regulatory situation is that RNA control is non-coordinate (Edlin et al. 1968); Nierlich, 1968; Winslow and Lazzarini, 1969). The synthesis of stable RNAs, ribosomal and transfer RNAs, is immediately affected by amino acid starvation, but messenger RNA synthesis is not. A genetic locus was found to affect RNA control during amino acid starvation, the *rel*A gene (Stent and Brenner, 1961). Wild-type cells (RelA⁺) are stringent in response to amino acid starvation, which means that stable RNA synthesis is reduced during starvation. Mutant cells (RelA⁻) are relaxed during starvation and allow stable RNA synthesis to continue. By study of this mutant, the putative role of guanosine tetraphosphate (ppGpp) as an effector molecule was discovered (see M. Cashel, this volume). The importance of the effects on RNA control to our discussion is that they illustrate the specificity of amino acid starvation on the regulation process. Also, RNA control, as affected by amino acid starvation, does not appear to require a protein regulator molecule whose synthesis is blocked by the starvation.

Effect of Amino Acid Starvation on Other Cellular Processes

Numerous roles for amino acids can now be catalogued. Among them is the unique role of methionine, as formyl methionine, for initiating polypeptide synthesis in bacteria (Clark and Marcker, 1965; 1966). Methionine also serves as a methyl donor (Gold, Hurwitz, and Anders, 1963) and methylation of nucleic acids is thought to have a regulatory role (Craddock, 1970; Adams, 1973; Degen and Morris, 1973). Methionine was found to be required for normal maturation of ribosomal RNA in *Saccharomyces cerevisiaie* (Wejksnora and Haber, 1974). A unique role for methionine starvation as it affects DNA replication has been demonstrated (Billen and Hewitt, 1966; Billen, 1968; Lark, 1968). Methionine starved *E. coli* did not immediately replicate DNA made during methionine starvation when auxotrophs were released from starvation. The DNA made during methionine starvation was methyl-deficient and was first methylated before it could be used as a template for further DNA synthesis.

Amino acid starvation effects can be mediated through their respective tRNAs, as illustrated by the RNA control studies. It is known that tRNAs have many regulatory roles in addition to their function during the translation process (Littaner and Inouye, 1973). Only a few will be mentioned here. The pleiotrophy of *his*T mutants in regulating the histidine, leucine, isoleucine, and valine pathways is due to a loss of pseudouridine adjacent to the anticodon in the corresponding tRNAs (Cortese et al., 1974). In another case the major host leucine tRNA is cleaved by a phage T4 nuclease, and a phage coded leucine tRNA appears during infection of *E. coli* (Kano-Sueoka and Sueoka, 1966; Scherberg and Weiss, 1970; Yudelevich, 1971). It also is interesting to note that tRNAs are involved in non-ribosomal amino acid additions to peptides found in the cell membrane and wall (Soffer, Horinishi, and Leibowitz, 1969).

The major involvement of tRNAs in regulatory function greatly enhances the regulatory possibilities for amino acid starvation. The existence of multiple tRNA species for one amino acid suggests a regulatory role for those additional tRNAs (Blank and Soll, 1971). With this in mind, a consideration of the number of codon assignments for amino acids reveals some interesting relationships. The amino acids methionine and tryptophan each have only one codon assignment; the amino acids leucine, serine, and arginine each have six codon assignments; all other amino acids have codon assignments intermediate to these extremes. If multiple codon assignments increase the possibilities for regulatory roles, then the amino acids leucine, arginine, and serine are particularly well suited for a regulatory role.

The uniqueness of amino acids in their regulatory involvement is obvious from this discussion. It follows that each amino acid should be considered individually for its possible role in affecting the regulation of chromosome replication during amino starvation. It cannot be assumed that each amino acid will behave like every other amino acid.

EFFECT OF AMINO ACID STARVATION ON
CHROMOSOME REPLICATION IN *BACILLUS SUBTILIS*

I chose leucine for my first study of amino acid starvation effects on chromosome replication because leucine auxotrophs in my *B. subtilis* stock culture collection gave the most immediate shut-off of DNA synthesis (Copeland, 1969). The starved cells retained their viability and resumed growth without delay when leucine was added back. Leucine-starved cells did not complete chromosome replication to the terminus, as was expected if replication was controlled solely at the initiation event. It was later found that the leucine effect could be demonstrated in both of the commonly used strains of *B. subtilis* (Copeland, 1971a; 1971b). A detailed marker frequency analysis confirmed that chromosome replication was not completed to the terminus in leucine-starved cells. The following is a brief summary of the current status of leucine starvation effects on chromosome replication in *B. subtilis*.

Amino Acid Survey

A number of *B. subtilis* amino acid auxotrophs were starved individually for a particular amino acid. Each auxotroph used was judged from plate tests not to be leaky for its mutational block. The period of starvation was long enough to ensure that each mutant completed all the DNA replication of which it was capable. A number of paramaters were measured such as increase in optical density, viable cell number, amount of DNA, and chromosome configuration. This latter measurement was made by marker frequency analysis. If chromosomes have completed replication to the terminus, then the ratio of a genetic marker near the origin to one located near the terminus would be 1.0. If all chromosomes had started replication but none had completed it, then the ratio would become 2.0. Intermediate ratios would indicate a mixed population of completed and incompleted chromosomes. Remember, according to the initiation control model, if chromosome replication is regulated only at the initiation event and amino acid starvation only blocks the synthesis of a protein initiator, then DNA replication will complete to the terminus when allowed to run its course during any amino acid starvation. The results shown in table 1 give the amount of DNA synthesized during starvation for the amino acid indicated and the resulting marker frequency ratio. These results have been arranged into two groups according to the outcome of the marker frequency test. For those amino acids in the top group, starved *B. subtilis* replicated nearly all of their chromosomes to the terminus. In no case did the marker frequency ratio indicate totally complete alignment, although some values were not significantly different from a value of 1.0. The probable reason for this lack of complete alignment is the extent of protein turnover that occurs during starvation. For those amino acids comprising the second group, leucine and methionine, starved *B. subtilis* did not complete replication to the terminus for a significantly greater number of chromosomes. The three determinations for leucine were for different cell lines or strains and will be described in greater detail later.

When the amino acids were grouped according to the degree of chromosome alignment resulting from starvation, the degree of alignment did not correlate with the amount of DNA made, amino acid biosynthetic families, amino acid chemical types, or the number of codon assignments for the amino acids. Thus there are two groups that can be discerned: those amino acids that allow chromosome replication to be completed, in agreement with the initiation control model; and those that lead to a significantly greater number of partially replicated chromosomes.

Kinetics of DNA Synthesis in Leucine-Starved B. subtilis

Three *B. subtilis* leucine auxotrophs had been found to synthesize different amounts of DNA, yet they all had a significantly large number of incomplete chromosomes. The kinetics for total DNA synthesis in these auxotrophs are shown in figure 1. Kinetics of total DNA synthesis are difficult to determine, because chemical DNA determinations are subject to losses and considerable variation. However, chemical determinations are not subject to other interpretation, as are determinations based only on radioisotopically labeled precursor incorporation. BC29, a 168 strain, synthesized the least amount of DNA. The kinetics are probably best expressed by a curve with a single plateau. The second auxotroph, BCW503, a W23 strain, synthesized 30 to 35% additional DNA during leucine starvation. This was done with a decreasing rate, and DNA synthesis stopped with a single plateau. The third auxotroph, BC200, a 168 strain, made the most DNA during leucine starvation. It synthesized as much as 60 to 70% additional DNA and did it in two stages. The first plateau was reached after 30 to 35% increase in DNA was realized. Then DNA synthesis started again and doubled in amount to the 60–70% range. For all three cell-lines growth and net protein synthesis stopped very soon upon starvation for leucine. All cell lines retained viability throughout starvation.

For cells in balanced growth, the amount of DNA needed to complete the randomly replicating chromosomes is a function of the growth rate. If all chromosomes are replicating with a single set of replication forks, then the amount of the expected increase is nearly 40% (Maaløe and Hanawalt, 1961). Since *B. subtilis* grown in defined glucose-salts medium has a growth rate of 70 to 80 minutes, it is unlikely that all chromosomes are replicating, so the expected amount of DNA needed to complete replication to the terminus will

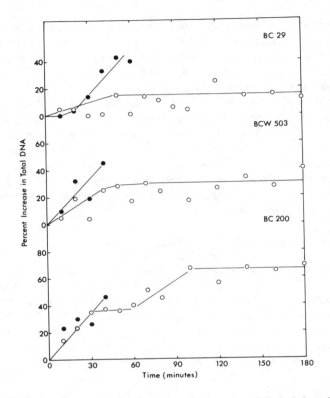

Fig. 1. Kinetics of total DNA change during leucine starvation. Cells in balanced growth in glucose, mineral-salts medium plus required growth factors. Leucine removed by filtering and washing cells. Total DNA determined by diphenylamine reaction. Results are the average of four or more experiments. Solid cricles = filtered cells to which leucine was added back; open circles = leucine-starved cells.

be less than 40%. The 30–35% additional DNA synthesized by BCW503 would seem to be close to the amount needed for completion under these circumstances. In any event, BC29 synthesized less than the amount needed to complete chromosome replication, and BC200 synthesized more than enough DNA. To account for the second plateau in DNA synthesized by BC200 according to the initiation control model, it would be necessary to restrict reinitiation to a limited number of chromosomes and to accomplish this in the absence of net protein synthesis. Clearly, the kinetics of DNA synthesis in these three cell-lines of *B. subtilis* when starved for leucine are not fully consistent with predictions made from the initiation control model.

Chromosome Configuration in Amino Acid-Starved B. subtilis

A detailed marker frequency analysis was done on DNA isolated from BCW503 cells that had been starved for leucine (Copeland, 1971a). The results are presented in figure 2. It was found that those markers closest to the origin had the largest marker frequency ratio, and as the map position of the test marker approached the terminus, the marker frequency ratio declined. These results clearly show that the chromosomes in BCW503 starved for leucine have not replicated to the terminus. About 60% of the chromosome population is incomplete in this experiment. Furthermore, the gradual decrease in marker frequency ratio for markers approaching the terminus indicates that replication forks have stopped in a random way between origin and terminus. This detailed analysis eliminates the interpretation that only the terminus segment was unreplicated, a posssibility if only origin and terminus markers are compared.

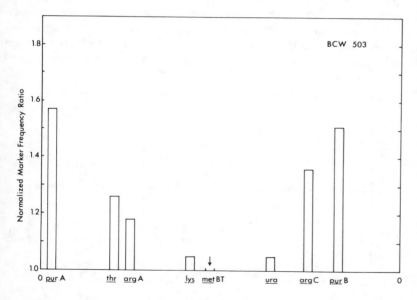

Fig. 2. Marker frequency analysis of leucine-starved BCW503. Cells were grown and starved as indicated in the legend to figure 1. DNA sample for analysis taken after 150 minutes of starvation. All marker frequency ratios relative to the late replicating *met*B marker. Ratios normalized to ratios for same marker pair using spore DNA. Results are the average of four or more determinations. Markers are arranged according to their position on the bidirectionally replicating map for *B. subtilis*. "O" designates the origin of replication, and would be joined on a circular map. "T" designates the terminus where replication stops:

Another interesting and important observation is derived from the work with BCW503. This cell-line gave the amount and kinetics of DNA synthesis consistent with those expected for completion of chromosome replication to the terminus. Oftentimes the amount of DNA synthesized and the kinetics of synthesis in response to amino acid starvation have been used as indicators that DNA replication has gone to completion at the terminus. The marker frequency analysis of BCW503 shows that amount and kinetics of DNA synthesis are inaccurate indicators for chromosome configuration. This conclusion was supported recently by independent means (Evans and Eberle, 1975).

Another way in which chromosome configuration can be determined is by the density transfer experiment. The outcome of such an experiment is shown in figure 3. BC200 cells grown in a defined, H_2O medium were starved for leucine until DNA synthesis stopped. They were then transferred to complex, D_2O medium where growth and DNA synthesis were restarted. A DNA sample was taken after a 17% increase in total DNA. The sample was fractionated on a cesium chloride gradient and the fractions assayed genetically for transforming activity. If all chromosomes had completed replication to the terminus during leucine starvation, then subsequent replication in such an early sample would have been highly synchronized for the markers located

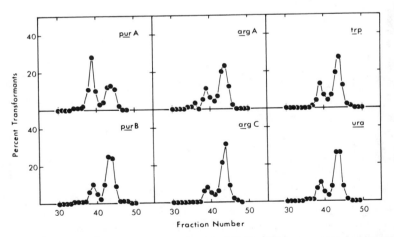

Fig. 3. Density-transfer analysis of leucine-starved BC200. Cells were grown and starved as indicated in the legend to figure 1. After 180 minutes of starvation, cells were transferred to a complex D_2O medium. DNA was isolated from a sample taken after a 17 percent increase. DNA was fractionated on a CsCl gradient and the fractions assayed for marker transformation activity. Markers are arranged as to their direction of replication; counterclockwise-top panels, clockwise-bottom three panels, and their order of replication; early-leftmost panels, intermediate-middle panels, late-rightmost panels on the *B. subtilis* genetic map.

TABLE 1

EFFECTS OF INDIVIDUAL AMINO ACID STARVATIONS
ON CHROMOSOME REPLICATION

Cell-Line[a]	Amino Acid	Percentage of DNA Increase[b]	Marker Frequency Ratio[c]
BC29	Tryptophan	73 (6)[d]	1.19 (.02)
BC67	Histidine	54 (1)	1.08 (.02)
BC67	Cysteine	34 (6)	1.27 (.06)
BC88	Arginine	39 (4)	1.17 (.07)
BC94	Isoleucine	102 (1)	1.07 (.05)
Average for group			1.16 (.06)
BC29	Leucine	17 (2)	1.32 (.01)
BC200-C	Leucine	45 (2)	1.38 (.06)
BCW503	Leucine	29 (3)	1.45 (.07)
BC88	Methionine	106 (10)	1.48 (.02)
Average for group			1.41 (.03)

[a]BC designations are for 168 strains; BCW designates a W23 strain.

[b]Total DNA measured by diphenylamine reaction. Cells grown in glucose–mineral salts medium plus required growth factors. Samples taken after 2 generation-time equivalents of starvation compared to samples taken at start of starvation.

[c]Marker frequency ratio compares an early replicating marker, $purA16$, to a late replication marker, $metB5$. Samples taken after 2 generation-time equivalents of starvation. Transformations carried out with DNA at 2 μg/ml. All ratios normalized to ratios determined with spore DNA.

[d]Values in parentheses are standard errors of the mean. Each determination made three or more times.

TABLE 2

DENSITY TRANSFER ANALYSIS OF LEUCINE- OR
TRYPTOPHAN-STARVED BC29[a]

Genetic Markers[c]	Percentage Replicated One or More Times[b]	
	Leucine-Starved[d]	Tryptophan-Starved[e]
Counterclockwise		
$PurA$	27	37
$argA$	13	2
ile	16	3
Clockwise		
$purB$	11	4
$argC$	11	3
ura	25	7

[a]Cells in balanced growth in glucose-mineral salts medium filtered and washed of either tryptophan or leucine. After 120 minutes of starvation, the cells were transferred by filtration to a complex D_2O medium. Samples were taken and analyzed as indicated in the legend to figure 3.

[b]Determined from the distribution of transforming activity for a given marker in the fractions according to:

$$[(LH-HH) /2 + HH/2] \div [LL + (LH - HH)/2 + HH/2] \times 100$$

where LL is equivalent to the transforming activity in the light fraction, LH with that in the hybrid fraction, and HH with that in the heavy fraction.

[c]Counterclockwise and clockwise refer to the direction of replication and the order of markers according to their relative position on the genetic map for B. subtilis.

[d]Sampled after a 15 percent increase in total DNA.

[e]Sampled after a 17 percent increase in total DNA.

near the origin and markers further away would not have replicated at all. In contrast, it was found that all of the markers assayed had replicated to about the same extent except for the marker closest to the origin. The greater amount of replication about this origin site indicates that the population of chromosomes is mixed, containing some completed and others incompleted, which agrees with the marker frequency result for this strain (see table 1).

The results of a density transfer experiment for BC29 starved for either leucine or tryptophan are shown in table 2. Recall that tryptophan is one of the amino acids of the group that allow completion of replication during starvation. The results from the leucine-starved cells are again consistent with a large number of chromosomes being incomplete following starvation. In contrast, the tryptophan-starved cells show a pattern of replication that indicates that the great majority of those chromosomes had completed replication during starvation. Only the marker closest to the origin was replicated to a significant degree in this early sample from tryptophan-starved cells.

The conclusions drawn from these experiments on chromosome configuration following amino acid starvation are that significantly greater numbers of chromosomes have not completed replication to the terminus when cells are starved for leucine, in contrast to the result for tryptophan-starved cells. It appears that about half of the chromosomes are incomplete after leucine starvation. The replication forks have stopped in a random order between the origin and the terminus on these incompleted chromosomes. These stopped forks appear to continue replication when growth is restarted following leucine starvation.

Is the Leucine Starvation Effect on DNA Replication Regulated?

There can be a number of ways in which amino acid starvation could interfere with chromosome replication other than by a regulatory circuit. A number of experiments have been done to test for that possibility. It has been found that leucine-starved cells are quite normal in all chraacteristics measured. They retain viability during starvation and resume growth almost immediately upon restoration of leucine. The cells appear normal, as viewed with a phase contrast microscope, during and following leucine starvation. There are no indications of abnormal growth or abnormal cell divisions. Protein turnover in the three cell-lines studied is about the same and does not exceed 10% in 90 minutes of leucine starvation. These strains continue to respire during leucine starvation. RNA control in each of these cell-lines during leucine starvation is stringent (Thomas and Copeland, 1973). This would eliminate from consideration faulty protein synthesis during starvation, since faulty protein synthesis occurs only in relaxed cells and not in stringent cells. The amount of ppGpp accumulation in each of these cell lines is the same during leucine starvation (Thomas and Copeland, 1973). Each of these observations eliminates a possible indirect cause for prematurely blocking chromosome replication before it could reach the terminus (Copeland, Phillips, and Mao, 1977).

Other observations of a more positive nature also support the hypothesis that leucine starvation affects regulation of chromosome replication. First, the change in DNA/mass ratios during and following leucine starvation are regular and consistent with a regulated response. The DNA/mass ratio increases during starvation proportionately with the amount of DNA synthesized. The final ratios reached are multiples of the lowest one for these three cell-lines studied. Upon restart of growth the DNA/mass ratios decrease toward values for cells in blanced growth. DNA synthesis begins again only after a reduction in the DNA/mass ratio (Copeland, Phillips, and Mao, 1977).

The leucine starvation effect is itself genetically determined. This is shown by the characteristic response that each of the three cell-lines exhibits to leucine starvation. But other genetic loci have been identified that modify the leucine starvation effect by changing the amount of DNA that is synthesized. Only when a methionine mutation is combined with those leading to thymine requirement will *B. subtilis* starved for leucine make the highest amount of DNA, ie., 60 to 70%. One possible connection between these mutant loci involves methylation, since methionine serves as a methyl donor and thymine-requiring mutants are blocked in their ability to methylate deoxyuridine to make thymidine. Whether this modifying influence of the *met* and *thy* loci on the leucine starvation effect is a part of a general mechanism that affects DNA replication during leucine starvation or a separate one remains to be determined (Copeland, Phillips, and Mao, 1977).

The studies of individual amino acid starvation in *B. subtilis* have shown that amino acids can differ in their effect on chromosome replication. The largest group of the amino acids tested belongs to a class in which starvation leads to the great majority of chromosomes being completed. This response is entirely consistent with the initiation control model. Starvation for leucine and methionine produce a significant increase in numbers of incompleted chromosomes. A close examination of the leucine starvation effect shows that about half of the chromosomes are incomplete and that the replication forks have stopped in a random order between origin and terminus on the chromosome. Replication can continue from these forks when the missing amino acid leucine is restored. These observations and kinetics of DNA synthesis all are incompatible with the initiation control model. Examination of other ways that might account for premature termination of chromosome replication have shown that the leucine starvation effect is specific, under genetic control, and appears to be regulated. Further experiments need to be done to test beyond doubt the regulated aspect of this leucine starvation effect, but the present evidence is substantial enough to warrant a working model that leucine starvation is affecting regulation of chromosome replication. The stage of DNA replication most likely to be affected by leucine starvation is DNA elongation.

REGULATION OF CHROMOSOME REPLICATION IN BACTERIA

The purposes of regulation are manifold, but at least two main reasons for regulation can be identified. One is to maintain a steady state in cells. This is particularly important in prokaryotes, which are sometimes subject to sudden and drastic changes in environment. Multicellular eukaryotes tend to maintain a constant environment about their cell and organ systems that subjects their cells to generally less drastic or sudden changes. The second reason for regulation is to provide a switching device to stop and start processes. These switching events serve to maintain order rather than steady states, although some regulatory systems could do both. The switch control may act only once during a cell cycle, or only in response to certain situations. In developmental systems some switch controls may act only once during the lifetime of an organism. Regulation makes it possible for an organism to maximize its existence. It provides the most economical way for life.

Regulation can be carried out at two levels. The genetic level of regulation serves to control the activity of the chromosome. Generally this is done by a specific molecule recognizing a particular site on the chromosome. Binding of that molecule to that site can either stimulate or prevent further interaction by other molecules at that or at other nearby sites on the chromosome. In this way the retrieval of information from the chromosome is controlled. The other level of regulation is at the functional level whereby the activity of a molecule is controlled by interaction with other specific molecules. Generally, the functional molecules in the cell are the protein enzymes. Those that serve in a regulatory capacity are allosteric and have a site for enzymatic function and one for a regulatory function. In the case of autogenous regulation (see Goldberger and Deely, this volume), the functional molecule or enzyme also serves as the regulatory effector molecule that acts at the genetic level to control its own synthesis. The regulation of chromosome replication is a special case of autogenous regulation where the functional molecule, the DNA chromosome, serves to regulate itself. Our consideration of the regulation of chromosome replication will be simplified if we discuss each stage of DNA replication in turn.

Regulation of Chromosome Initiation

At this time initiation control is the only well-documented form of control over the replication process. In slowly growing cells regulation of the initiation process can serve as a switch control to set the process of chromosome duplication in motion during the cell cycle. In this form it serves to keep the proper order of chromosome replication within the cell cycle. Initiation control would only operate once per cell cycle, and then it would have no further regulatory role for the remainder of the DNA cycle or cell cycle. However, in rapidly growing cells initiation control serves to maintain steady state conditions. When bacterial cells grow rapidly, the rate of chromosome replication is at a maximum, and an increase rate of DNA synthesis cannot be obtained by increasing the rate of DNA elongation at the forks. Yet, the rapid rate of cell growth demands a rate of DNA synthesis beyond that possible at a set of replication forks. Without a means to increase DNA synthesis, balanced growth would not be possible at rapid growth rates, and cell growth would outpace chromosome duplication. This balanced growth is accomplished by introducing additional sets of replication forks into an already replicating chromosome, a process of dichotomous chromosome replication.

Regulation of the initiation event is certainly at the genetic level, since a specific site on the chromosome, the origin, is involved. But control of the initiation event may be at the functional level too. For example, consider the replisome model where the regulation of the initiation event is determined by the completion of the replisome.

Numerous models to account for regulation of initiation have been proposed. Some involve a protein, the initiator, which is responsible for regulating the initiation process. Certainly, at least one ribosomally synthesized protein is required for the initiation process, and it could be the initiator described in these models. The action of the initiator has been described as being positive or negative. Not enough is known about initiation to make a choice between these two variations of the model. It would be wise to consider even the possibility of a series of regulators to control initiation (see Marzluf, this volume). Under some conditions initiation control may appear negative, but the combination of two negative regulators acting in series could give the appearance of a positive type of control. The advantage of this kind of regulation complex may be to make the initiation event responsive to a number of different cellular processes.

Another model of initiation control proposes that the attachment of the origin to the membrane serves to regulate the process (Marvin, 1968). The evidence for a chloramphenicol-resistant, amino acid-requiring event in the initiation process supports the idea of membrane involvement (Lark and Renger, 1969), since it is known that amino acids are added to membrane sites without the use of ribosomes (Soffer et al., 1969). Also, the finding that prematurely induced initiation occurs only on one of the two origins of a newly replicated chromosome (Pritchard and Lark, 1964), whereas dichotomous replication proceeds from both origins (Sueoka and Quinn, 1970) suggest that one of the newly made origins is functionally different from the other. Presumably this difference could involve membrane attachment.

Finally, the third type of initiation control model proposes that some structural element such as the replication complex or replisome needs to be assembled before replication can proceed (Bleecken, 1971), and that it is the completion of this replisome that serves to regulate the initiation event. Although this model may account for some aspects of the initiation process, it cannot account for the successive rounds of premature initiations without some difficulty.

An RNA transcription event is required for the initiation process (Lark, 1972a). It may be this event that is regulated (Lark, 1972b), if the RNA transcript serves as the primer for DNA synthesis. However, an RNA core has been proposed as a structural element that maintains the integrity of the folded chromosome (Worcel and Burgi, 1972). If the folded chromosome configuration is necessary for replication, then control of this RNA element may regulate the initiation event. This latter type of model would then be grouped together with the replisome model.

It may be more than fortuitous that a model describing initiation control exists for each of the steps in the process leading to initiation. Evidence in support of each model may reflect the point of view of the experiment relative to the initiation process. It seems likely that an event as important as initiation of chromosome replication, would be controlled in more than one way. Multiple control over initiation would serve to tie chromosome replication to the events of the cell cycle, both in terms of timing and steady state, and to the process of chromosome segregation. Possibly a single mechanism of control would not suffice for all of these functions.

Regulation of Chromosome Elongation

There is little evidence to conclusively demonstrate regulation of the elongation process of chromosome replication. The role of regulation at this stage of chromosome duplication would be to maintain steady state conditions. As pointed out in the previous section, control of initiation serves to maintain steady-state conditions for rapidly growing cells. When cells grow slowly, regulation of initiation serves as a switch control. It is under these conditions of slow growth that an elongation control mechanism, separate from that of initiation control, might be expected to operate and to be most easily demonstrated. The results obtained for slowly growing cells are not in agreement on this point. If the period of the DNA cycle, the C period, is progressively longer for slowly growing cells, then this would be evidence for elongation control. Because it is difficult to maintain slowly growing cells in balanced growth when working with batch cultures, experiments of this type are difficult to perform. This may account for the lack of agreement on the timing of the DNA cycle for slowly growing cells.

Elongation control would operate at the functional level. There is a large number of possible steps during chromosome elongation where control could be maintained. The finding of two protein factors associated with the active form of DNA polymerase pol III is the strongest indication for regulation of elongation (Wickner and Kornberg, 1973; Wickner et al., 1973). Protein cofactors of this type are often involved in regulatory functions. Recently it was found that the V_{max} of cytoplasmic DNA polymerase from bone marrow cells could be affected by ATP (Byrnes, Downey, and So, 1974). If prokaryote DNA polymerase, pol III, were similarly affected, then one mechanism for DNA elongation control would be established. This could account in part for the role of ATP in DNA replication. This control of elongation could be effected through the formation of the putative RNA primers necessary for Okazaki fragment synthesis or by the need for ATP and copol III* to activate polymerization by pol III*.

There are several other ways that the elongation process could be controlled. For example, it is known that the DNA unwinding protein is essential to DNA replication of the bacteriophage T4 (Alberts, 1968). Furthermore, the extent of DNA replication is proportional to the number of DNA unwinding proteins present. There are nucleases, ligase, and possibly a swivel protein and other unknown factors that are involved with DNA elongation, anyone of which could serve as a point for regulation of the elongation process.

Our results with the leucine starvation effect on chromosome replication in *B. subtilis* are compatible with a regulatory role during the elongation process. Only further work will test the validity of this assumption and determine the mechanism by which this putative control operates.

Regulation of elongation of chromosome replication seems mandatory. The chromosome is very large DNA molecule in bacteria, being about 2×10^9 daltons in molecular weight and about 3×10^6 base pairs in length. Control only at the initiation event would commit a cell to synthesizing all of this DNA in the advent of a sudden, drastic perturbation in environment. This would seem unlikely. Also, elongation control could serve as the fine-tuning mechanism needed to keep chromosome replication in line with other events during the cell cycle. As with our consideration of initiation control, it seems likely to me that more than one mechanism of elongation control would ensure a close coupling of the replication process with the numerous and diverse events that occur during cell growth.

Regulation of Chromosome Termination

Some of the considerations made for regulation of the initiation event are equally applicable when discussing regulation of the termination process. In fact, without specifically associating the regulated event with the site of the chromosome, it would not be possible to differentiate between regulation of initiation from regulation of termination. Some of the putative temperature-sensitive initiation mutants instead could be termination mutants (Schubach, Whitmer, and Davern, 1973).

Regulation of chromosome termination could serve as a switch control or as a steady-state control of chromosome replication exactly as proposed for initiation control. Control of chromosome termination is at the genetic level, since a particular site on the chromosome is involved. At this time a protein seems to be necessary in order to replicate this terminal site (Marunochi and Messer, 1973). It is not known whether this control acts in a positive or negative way. Regulation of chromosome termination may serve the sole purpose of tying chromosome replication to cell division, but the absence of such a tight couple in *B. subtilis* makes this idea less attractive (Donachie and Begg, 1970). An understanding of the termination event in chromosome replication and its regulation will have to await further work. Future studies will have to carefully differentiate between events at the initiation step and the termination step of chromosome replication so as to avoid considerable confusion in the literature.

Regulation of Chromosome Replication in Retrospect

I believe that through this discourse I have proved my opening statement that our understanding of chromosome replication in bacteria is truly rudimentary, but I hope that it is now less of a mystery. To bring our understanding of the regulation of chromosome replication process to the elegant and sophisticated level achieved with the *Lac* operon and with bacteriophage Lambda is clearly for the future, but it is a future with promise of many exciting and rewarding discoveries for those who care to take this path.

ACKNOWLEDGMENT

James C. Copeland is the recipient of a Public Health Service Career Development Award (1-K4-GM-70300).

REFERENCES

Adams, R. L. P. 1973. Delayed methylation of DNA in developing sea urchin embryos. Nature New Biol. 244:27–29.

Alberts, B. M., F. J. Amodio, M. Jenkins, E. D. Butman, and F. L. Ferris. 1968. Studies with DNA-cellulose chromatography. I. DNA-binding proteins from *Escherichia coli*. Cold Spring Harbor Symp. Quant. Biol. 33:289–305.

Bak, A. L., C. Christiansen, and A. Stenderup. 1970. Bacterial genome sizes determined by DNA renaturation studies. J. Gen. Microbiol. 64:377–80.

Beyersmann, D., W. Messer, and M. Schlicht. 1974. Mutants of *Escherichia coli* B/r defective in deoxyribonculeic acid initiation: *dna*I, a new gene for replication. J. Bacteriol. 118:783–89.

Billen, D., and R. Hewitt. 1966. Influence of starvation for methionine and other amino acids on subsequent bacterial deoxyribonucleic acid replication. J. Bacteriol. 92:609–17.

Billen, D. 1968. Methylation of the bacterial chromosome: An event at the "replication point." J. Mol. Biol. 31:477–86.

Bird, R. E., and K. G. Lark. 1970. Chromosome replication in *Escherichia coli* 15T at different growth rates: Rate of replication of the chromosome and the rate of formation of small pieces. J. Mol. Biol. 49:343–66.

Blank, H. U., and D. Soll. 1971. Purification of five leucine transfer ribonucleic acid species from *Escherichia coli* and their acylation by heterologous leucyl-transfer ribonucleic acid synthetase. J. Biol. Chem. 246:4947–50.

Bleecken, S., G. Strohbach, and E. Sarfert. 1966. Autoradiography of bacterial chromosomes. Zeitschrift Allg. Microbiol. 6:121–23.

Bleecken, S. 1971. "Replisome" controlled initiation of DNA replication. J. Theor. Biol. 32:81–92.

Borek, E., L. Pontecorvo, and D. Rittenberg. 1958. Protein turnover in microorganisms. Proc. Nat. Acad. Sci. USA 44:369–74.

Brumschede, H. and H. Bremer. 1971. Synthesis and breakdown of proteins in *Escherichia coli* during amino acid starvation. J. Mol. Biol. 57:35–57.

Burger, R. M. 1971. Toluene-treated *Escherichia coli* replicate only that DNA which was about to be replicated *in vivo*. Proc. Nat. Acad. Sci. USA 68:2124–26.

Byrnes, J. J., K. Downey, and A. G. So. 1974. Metabolic regulation of cytoplasmic DNA sythesis. Proc. Nat. Acad. Sci. USA 71:205–8.

Cairns, J. 1963. The bacterial chromosome and its manner of replication as seen by autoradiography. J. Mol. Biol. 6:208–13.

Cairns, J. 1963. The chromosome of *Escherichia coli*. Cold Spring Harbor Symp. Quant. Biol. 28:43–46.

Champe, S. P. 1974. Linkage map of bacteriophage T4. *In* A. I. Laskin and H. A. Lechevalier (eds.). Handbook of microbiology. Pp. 644–47. CRC Press.

Chandler, M., R. E. Bird, and L. Caro. 1975. The replication time of *Escherichia coli* chromosome as a function of cell doubling time. J. Mol. Biol. 94:127–32.

Clark, B. F. C., and K. A. Marcker. 1965. Coding response of N-formyl-methionyl-sRNA to UUG. Nature 207:1038–39.

Clark, B. F. C., and K. A. Marcker. 1966. The role of N-formylmethionyl-sRNA in protein biosynthesis. J. Mol. Biol. 17:394–406.

Cooper, S., and C. E. Helmstetter. 1968. Chromosome replication and the division cycle of *Escherichia coli* B/r. J. Mol. Biol. 31:519–40.

Cooper, S., and G. Wensthoff. 1971. Comment on the use of chloramphenicol to study the initiation of deoxyribonucleic acid synthesis. J. Bacteriol. 106:709–11.

Cooper, S. 1974. A criterion for using chloramphenicol to define different processes in the initiation of DNA synthesis in bacteria. J. Theor. Biol. 46:117–27.

Copeland, J. C. 1969. Regulation of chromosome replication in *Bacillus subtilis*. Effects of amino acid starvation in strain 168. J. Bacteriol. 99:730–36.

Copeland, J. C. 1971a. Regulation of chromosome replication in *Bacillus subtilis*. Marker frequency analysis after amino acid starvation. Science 172:159–61.

Copeland, J. C. 1971b. Regulation of chromosome replication in *Bacillus subtilis*. Effects of amino acid starvation in strain W23 J. Bacteriol. 104:595–603.

Copeland, J. C., S. J. Phillips, and M. W. H. Mao. 1977. Effects of amino acid starvation on chromosome replication in *Bacillus subtilis*. *In* D. Schlessinger (ed.). Microbiology 77. Amer. Soc. Microbiol., in press.

Cortese, R., R. Landsberg, R. A. Vonder Haar, H. E. Umbarger, and B. N. Ames. 1974. Pleiotrophy of *his*T mutants blocked in pseudo-uridine synthesis in tRNA: Leucine and isoleucine-valine operons. Proc. Nat. Acad. Sci. USA 71:1857–61.

Craddock, V. M. 1970. Transfer RNA methylases and cancer. Nature 228:1264–68.

Cutler, R. G. and J. E. Evans. 1966. Synchronization of bacteria by a stationary-phase method. J. Bacteriol. 91:469–76.

Degnen, S. T., and R. Morris. 1973. Deoxyribonucleic acid methylation and development in *Caulobacter* bacterioides. J. Bacteriol. 116:48–53.

Delius, H., and A. Worcel. 1974. Electron microscopic visualization of the folded chromosome of *Escherichia coli*. J. Mol. Biol. 83:107–9.

DeLucia, P., and J. Cairns. 1969. Isolation of an *Escherichia coli* strain with a mutation affecting DNA polymerase. Nature 224:1164–66.

Donachie, W. D. 1968. Relationship between cell size and time of initiation of DNA replication. Nature 219:1077–78.

Donachie, W. D., and K. J. Begg. 1970. Growth of the bacterial cell. Nature 227:1220–24.

Donachie, W. D., D. T. M. Martin, and K. J. Begg. 1971. Independence of cell division and DNA replication in *Bacillus subtilis*. Nature New Biol. 231:274–76.

Donachie, W. D. 1974. Cell division in bacterial. *In* A. R. Kolber and M. Koniyama (eds.). Mechanism and regulation of DNA replication. Pp. 431–45. Plenum Publishing, New York.

Dressler, D., J. Wolfson, and M. Magazin. 1972. Initiation and reinitiation of DNA synthesis during replication of bacteriophage T7 Proc. Nat. Acad. Sci. USA 69:998–1002.

Dressler, D. 1975. The recent excitement in the DNA growing point problem. Ann Rev. Microbiol. 29:525–59.

Eberle, H. and K. G. Lark. 1967. Chromosome replication in *Bacillus subtilis* cultures growing at different rates. Proc. Nat. Acad. Sci. USA 57:95–101.

Edlin, G., G. S. Stent, R. F. Baker, and C. Yanofsky. 1968. Synthesis of a specific messenger RNA during amino acid starvation of *Escherichia coli*. J. Mol. Biol. 37:257–68.

Evans, I. M., and H. Eberle. 1975. Accumulation of the capacity for initiation of deoxyribonucleic acid replication in *Escherichia coli*. J. Bacteriol. 121:883–91.

Filip, C. C., J. S. Allen, R. A. Gustafson, R. G. Allen and J. R. Walker. 1974. Bacterial cell division regulation: Characterization of the *dna*H locus of *Escherichia coli*. J. Bacteriol. 119:443–49.

Fuchs, J. A., H. O. Karlstrom, H. R. Warner, and P. Reichard. 1972. DNA synthesis-detective gene product in *dna*F mutant of *Escherichia coli*. Nature New Biol. 238:69–71.

Fujisawa, T. and A. Eisenstark, 1973. Bidirectional chromosomal replication in *Salmonella typhimurium*. J. Bacteriol. 115:168–76.

Gallant, F., and M. Cashel. 1967. On the mechanism of amino acid control of ribonucleic acid biosynthesis. J. Mol. Biol. 25:545–53.

Gallant, J., H. Erlich, B. Hall, and T. Laffler. 1970. Analysis of the RC function. Cold Spring Harbor Symp. Quant. Biol. 35:397–405.

Ganesan, A. T., and J. Lederberg. 1965. A cell membrane bound fraction of bacterial DNA. Biochem. Biophys. Res. Com. 18:824–35.

Ganesan, A. T., J. J. Anderson, J. Luh, and M. Effron. 1976. DNA metabolism in *Bacillus subtilis* and its phage SPPI. *In* D. Schlesinger (ed.). Microbiology 76. Pp. 319–25. Amer. Soc. Microbiol.

Gefter, M. L., Y. Hirota, T. Kornberg, J. A. Wechsler, and C. Barnoux. 1971. Analysis of DNA polymerases II and III in mutants of *Escherichia coli* thermosensitive for DNA synthesis. Proc. Nat. Acad. Sci. USA 68:3150–53.

Gefter, J. L. 1975. DNA replication. Ann. Rev. Biochem. 44:45–78.

Gilbert, W., and D. Dressler. 1968. DNA replication: the rolling circle model. Cold Spring Harbor Symp. Quant. Biol. 33:473–84.

Gold, M., J. Hurwitz, and M. Anders. 1963. The enzymatic methylation of RNA and DNA. II. On the species specificity of the methylating enzymes. Proc. Nat. Acad. Sci. USA 50:164–69.

Goldberg, I., D. D. Gwinn, and C. B. Thorne. 1966. Interspecies transformation between *Bacillus subtilis* and *Bacillus licheniformis* Biochem. Biophys. Res. Comm. 23:543–48.

Goodman, D., H. Manor, and W. Rombants. 1969. Ribosomal protein synthesis during and after amino acid starvation in relaxed and stringent bacteria. J. Mol. Biol. 40:247–60.

Gross, J. D. 1972. DNA replication in bacteria. Curr. Top. Microbiol. and Immunol. 57:39–74.

Gudas, L. J., and A. B. Pardee, 1974. Deoxyribonucleic acid synthesis during the division cycle of *Escherichia coli:* a comparison of strains B/r, K-12, 15, and 15T$^-$ under conditions of slow growth. J. Bacteriol. 117:1216–23.

Harford, N. 1975. Bidirectional chromosome replication in *Bacillus subtilis* 168. J. Bacteriol. 121:835–47.

Helmstetter, C. E., and S. Cooper, 1968. DNA synthesis during the division cycle of rapidly growing *Escherichia coli* B/r. J. Mol. Biol. 31:507–18.

Helmstetter, C. E. 1974. Initiation of chromosome replication in *Escherichia coli* II. Analysis of the control mechanism. J. Mol. Biol. 84:21–36.

Herrmann, R., J. Huf, and F. Bonhoeffer. 1972. Cross hybridization and rate of chain elongation of the two classes of DNA intermediates. Nature. New Biol. 240:235–37.

Hindley, J. 1973. Molecular structure and function in RNA phages. Brit. Med. Bull. 29:236–40.

Hirota, Y., F. Jacob, A. Ryter, G. Buttin, and T. Nakai. 1968. On the process of cellular division in *Escherichia coli*. I. Asymmetric cell division and production of deoxyribonucleic acid-less bacteria. J. Mol. Biol. 35:175–92.

Hurwitz, J., and S. Wickner. 1974. Involvement of two protein factors and ATP in *in vitro* DNA synthesis catalyzed by DNA polymerase III of *Escherichia coli*. Proc. Nat. Acad. Sci. USA 71:6–10.

Ivarie, R. D., and J. J. Pene. 1973. Association of many regions of the *Bacillus subtilis* chromosome with the cell membrane. J. Bacteriol. 114:571–76.

Jacob, F., and S. Brenner. 1963. On the regulation of DNA synthesis in bacteria: The replicon hypothesis. Compt. Rend. Acad. Sci. 256:298–300.

Jacob, F., S. Brenner, and F. Cuzin. 1963. On the regulation of DNA replication in bacteria. Cold Spring Harbor Symp. Quant. Biol. 28:329–48.

Kano-Sueoka, T., and N. Sueoka. 1966. Modification of leucyl-sRNA after bacteriophage infection. J. Mol. Biol. 20:183–209.

Kasamatsu, H., D. L. Robberson, and J. Vinograd. 1971. A novel closed circular mitochondrial DNA with properties of a replicating intermediate. Proc. Nat. Acad. Sci. USA 68:2252–57.

Klotz, L. C., and B. H. Zimm. 1972. Size of DNA determined by visco-elastic measurements: Results on bacteriophages, *Bacillus subtilis*, and *Escherichia coli*. J. Mol. Biol. 72:779–800.

Kogoma, T., and K. G. Lark. 1970. DNA replication in *Escherichia coli:* Replication in absence of protein synthesis after replication inhibition. J. Mol. Biol. 52:143–64.

Kohiyama, M., H. Lanfrom, S. Brenner, and F. Jacob. 1963. Modifications de fonctions indispensables chez des mutants thermosensibles d'*Escherichia coli*. Sur une mutant empêchant la replication du chromosome bacterien. Compt. Rend. Acad. Sci. 257:1979–81.

Konrad, E. B., and I. R. Lehman. 1974. A conditional lethal mutant of *Escherichia coli* K-12 defective in the 5′ to 3′ exonuclease associated with DNA polymerase I. Proc. Nat. Acad. Sci. USA 71:2048–51.

Kornberg, A. 1974. *DNA Synthesis*, p. 399. San Francisco, W. H. Freeman.

Kornberg, T. and M. L. Gefter. 1971. DNA synthesis in cell free extracts: purification and properties of DNA polymerase II. Proc. Nat. Acad. Sci. USA 68:761–64.

Kubitschek, H. E., and M. L. Freedman. 1971. Chromosome replication and the division cycle of *Escherichia coli* B/r. J. Bacteriol. 107:95–99.

Kurosawa, Y., T. Ogawa, S. Hirose, T. Okazaki, and R. Okazaki. 1975. Mechanism of DNA chain growth. X V. RNA-linked nascent DNA pieces in *Escherichia coli* strains assayed with spleen exonuclease. J. Mol. Biol. 96:653–64.

Lark, C., and K. G. Lark. 1964. Evidence for two distinct aspects of the mechanism regulating chromosome replication in *Escherichia coli*. J. Mol. Biol. 10:120–36.

Lark, C. 1968. Studies on the in vivo methylation of DNA in *Escherichia coli* 15 T. J. Mol. Biol. 31:389–99.

Lark, K. G., T. Repko, and E. J. Hoffman. 1963. The effect of amino acid deprivation on subsequent deoxyribonucleic acid replication. Biochim. Biophys. Acta 76:9–24.

Lark, K. G., and R. Bird. 1965. Premature chromosome replication induced by thymine starvation: Restriction of replication to one of the two partially completed replicas. J. Mol. Biol. 13:607–10.

Lark, K. G., and H. Renger. 1969. Initiation of DNA replication in *Escherichia coli* 15T. Chronological dissection of three physiological processes required for initiation. J. Mol. Biol. 42:221–36.

Lark, K. G. 1972a. Evidence for the direct involvement of RNA in the initiation of DNA replication in *Escherichia coli*. J. Mol. Biol. 64:47–60.

Lark, K. G. 1972b. Genetic control over the initiation of the synthesis of the short deoxynucleotide chains in *Escherichia coli*. Nature New Biol. 240:237–40.

Lehman, I. R., and J. R. Chien. 1973. Persistence of deoxyribonucleic acid polymerase I and its 5′ to 3′ exonuclease activity in Pol A mutants of *Escherichia coli* K12. J. Biol. Chem. 248:7717–23.

Lehman, I. R. 1974. DNA ligase: Structure, mechanism, and function. Science 186:790–97.

Lepesant-Kejzlarova, J., J.-A. Lepesant, J. Walle, A. Billualt, and R. Dedonder. 1975. Revision of the linkage map of *Bacillus subtilis* 168. Indications for circularity of the chromosome. J. Bacteriol. 121:823–34.

Lindahl, G., Y. Hirota, and F. Jacob. 1971. On the process of cellular division in *Escherichia coli:* Replication of the bacterial chromosome under control of prophage P2. Proc. Nat. Acad. Sci. USA 68:2407–11.

Littaner, U. Z., and H. Inouye. 1973. Regulation of tRNA. Ann. Rev. Biochem. 42:439–70.

Maaløe, O. 1961. The control of normal DNA replication in bacteria. Cold Spring Harbor Symp. Quant. Biol. 26:45–52.

Maaløe, O., and P. C. Hanawalt. 1961. Thymine deficiency and the normal DNA replication cycle I. J. Mol. Biol. 3:144–55.

Maaløe, O., and N. O. Kjeldgaard. 1966. Control of macromolecular synthesis. W. A. Benjamin, Menlo Park, Calif. 284 pp.

MacKay, V., and S. Linn. 1974. The mechanism of degradation of duplex deoxyribonucleic acid by the recBC enzyme of *Escherichia coli* K12. J. Biol. Chem. 249:4286–94.

Mandelstam, J. 1957. Turnover of protein in starved bacteria and its relationship to the induced synthesis of enzyme. Nature 179:1179–81.

Marunouchi, T., and W. Messer. 1973. Replication of a specific terminal chromosome segment in *Escherichia coli* which is required for cell division. J. Mol. Biol. 78:211–28.

Marvin, D. A. 1968. Control of DNA replication by membranes. Nature 219:485–86.

Massie, H. R. and B. H. Zimm. 1965. Molecular weight of the DNA in the chromosome of *Escherichia coli* and *Bacillus subtilis*. Proc. Nat. Acad. Sci. USA 54:1636–41.

Masters, M., and P. Broda. 1971. Evidence for the bidirectional replication of the *Escherichia coli* chromosome. Nature New Biol. 232:137–40.

Matsushita, T., K. P. White, and N. Sueoka. 1971. Chromosome replication in toluenized *Bacillus subtilis* cells. Nature New Biol. 232:111–14.

Matsushita, T. and H. E. Kubitschek, 1975. DNA Replication in bacteria. Adv. Microbiol. Physiol. 12:247–327.

Mendelson, N. H. 1972. Deoxyribonucleic acid distribution in *Bacillus subtilis* independent of cell elongation. J. Bacteriol. 111:156–62.

Middleton, R. B. 1971. The genetic homology of *Salmonella typhimurium* and *Escherichia coli*. Genetics 69:303–15.

Moses, R. E., and C. C. Richardson. 1970. Replication and repair of DNA in cells of *Escherichia coli* treated with toluene. Proc. Nat. Acad. Sci. USA 67:674–81.

Nath, K. and A. L. Koch. 1971. Protein degradation in *Escherichia coli*. II. Strain differences in the degradation of protein and nucleic acid resulting from starvation. J. Biol. Chem. 246:6956–67.

Nath, K. and J. Hurwitz. 1974. Covalent attachment of ribonucleotides at 3′-hydroxyl ends of deoxyribonucleic acid catalyzed by deoxyribonucleic acid-dependent ribonucleic acid polymerase of *Escherichia coli*. J. Biol. Chem. 249:2605–15.

Nierlich, D. P. 1968. Amino acid control over RNA synthesis: A re-evaluation. Proc. Nat. Acad. Sci. USA 60:1345–52.

Nishimura, Y., L. Caro, C. M. Berg, and Y. Hirota. 1971. Chromosome replication in *Escherichia coli*. IV. Control of chromosome replication and cell division by an integrated episome. J. Mol. Biol. 55:441–56.

Oishi, M., H. Yoshikawa, and N. Sueoka. 1964. Synchronous and dichotomous replication of the *Bacillus subtilis* chromosome during spore germination. Nature 204:1069–73.

Okazaki, R., T. Okazaki, K. Sakabe, K. Sugimoto, R. Kainuma, A. Sugino, and N. Iwatsuki. 1968. *In vivo* mechanism of DNA chain growth. Cold Spring Harbor Symp. Quant. Biol. 33:129–43.

Okazaki, R., S. Hirose, T. Okazaki, T. Ogawa, and Y. Kurosawa. 1975. Assay of RNA-linked nascent DNA pieces with polynucleotide kinase. Biochem. Biophys. Res. Comm. 62:1018–24.

Olivera, B. M., and F. Bonhoeffer. 1972. DNA replication—Two size classes of intermediates from discontinuous replication. Nature New Biol. 240:233–35.

O'Sullivan, A., and N. Sueoka. 1967. Sequential replication of the *Bacillus subtilis* chromosome. J. Mol. Biol. 27:349–68.

Pardee, A., and L. Prestidge. 1956. The dependence of nucleic acid synthesis on the presence of amino acids in *Escherichia coli*. J. Bacteriol. 71:677–83.

Pato, M. L. 1972. Regulation of chromosome replication and the bacterial cell cycle. Ann. Rev. Microbiol. 26:347–68.

Pettijohn, D. E., R. M. Hecht, O. G. Stonington, and T. D. Stamato. 1973. Factors stabilizing DNA folding in bacterial chromosomes. *In* R. D. Wells and R. B. Inman (eds.). DNA synthesis *in vitro*. Pp. 145–62. Baltimore, University Park Press.

Pierucci, O. and C. E. Helmstetter. 1969. Chromosome replication, protein synthesis, and cell division in *Escherichia coli*. Fed. Proc. 28:1755–60.

Pritchard, R. H., and K. G. Lark, 1964. Induction of replication by thymine starvation at the chromosome origin in *Escherichia coli*. J. Mol. Biol. 9:288–307.

Pritchard, R. H., P. T. Barth, and J. Collins. 1969. Control of DNA synthesis in bacteria. Symp. Soc. Gen. Microbiol. 19:263–97.

Quinn, W. G. and N. Sueoka. 1970. Symmetric replication of the *Bacillus subtilis* chromosome. Proc. Nat. Acad. Sci. USA 67:717–23.

Rafaeli-Eshkol, D., D. Epstein, and A. Hershko. 1974. Roles of protein synthesis and tRNA aminoacylation in the regulation of intracellular protein breakdown in *E. coli* Biochem. Biophys. Res. Comm. 61:899–905.

Rosenberg, B. H., L. G. Cavalieri, and G. 'Ungers. 1969. The negative control mechanism for *Escherichia coli* DNA replication. Proc. Nat. Acad. Sci. USA 63:1410–17.

Ryder, O. A. and D. W. Smith. 1975. Properties of membrane-associated folded chromosomes of *E. coli* related to initiation and termination of DNA replication. Cell 4:337–45.

Ryter, A., and F. Jacob. 1963. Etude au microscope electronique des relations entre mesosomes et noyaux chez *Bacillus subtilis*. Comp. Rend. Acad. Sci. 257:3060–63.

Sakai, H., S. Hashimoto, and T. Komano. 1974. Replication of deoxyribonucleic acid in *Es-*

cherichia coli C mutants temperature sensitive in the initiation of chromosome replication. J. Bacteriol. 119:811–20.

Sakabe, K., and R. Okazaki. 1966. A unique property of the replicating region of chromosomal DNA. Biochim. Biophys. Acta. 129:651–54.

Sanderson, K. E. 1974. The current linkage map of Salmonella typhimurium. In A. I. Laskin and H. A. Lechevalier (eds.). Handbook in microbiology. Condensed ed., Pp. 295–307. CRC Press.

Schaechter, M. 1961. Patterns of cellular control during unbalanced growth. Cold Spring Harbor Symp. Quant. Biol. 26:53–62.

Schekman, R., A. Weiner, A. Kornberg. 1974. Multienzyme systems of DNA replication: Proteins required for chromosome replication are resolved with the aid of a simple viral DNA template. Science 186: 987–93.

Scherberg, N. H., and S. B. Weiss. 1970. Detection of bacteriophage T4 and T5 coded transfer RNAs. Proc. Nat. Acad. Sci. USA 67:1164–71.

Schubach, W. H., J. D. Whitmer, and C. I. Davern. 1973. Genetic control of DNA initiation in *Escherichia coli*. J. Mol. Biol. 74:205–21.

Sinsheimer, R. 1968. Bacteriophage φχ174 and related viruses. Prog. Nucl. Acid Res. Mol. Biol. 8:115–69.

Smith, D. W. and P. C. Hanawalt. 1967. Properties of the growing point region in the bacterial chromosome. Biochim. Biophys. Acta 149:519–31.

Smith, D. W. 1973. DNA synthesis in prokaryotes: replication. Prog. Biophys. Molec. Biol. 26:321–408.

Soffer, R. L., H. Horinishi, and M. I. Leibowitz. 1969. The aminoacyl tRNA transferases. Cold Spring Harbor Symp. Quant. Biol. 34:529–33.

Sompayrac, L. and D. Maaløe. 1973. DNA replication-autorepressor model. Nature New Biol. 241:133–35.

Stent, G. S. and S. Brenner. 1961. A genetic locus for the regulation of ribonucleic acid synthesis. Proc. Nat. Acad. Sci. USA 47:2005–15.

Stonington, O. G., D. E. Pettijohn. 1971. The folded genome of *Escherichia coli* isolated in a protein-DNA-RNA complex. Proc. Nat. Acad. Sci. USA 68:6–9.

Sueoka, N., and W. G. Quinn. 1968. Membrane attachment of the chromosome replication origin in *Bacillus subtilis*. Cold Spring Harbor Symp. Quant. Biol. 33:695–705.

Sueoka, N., T. Matsushita, S. Ohi, A. O'Sullivan, and K. White. 1973. *In vivo* and *in vitro* chromosome replication in *Bacillus subtilis*. *In* R. D. Wells and R. B. Inman (eds.). DNA synthesis *in vitro*. Pp. 385–404. Baltimore, University Park Press.

Sueoka, N., and J. M. Hammers. 1974. Isolation of DNA-membrane complex in *Bacillus subtilis*. Proc. Nat. Acad. Sci. USA. 71:4787–91.

Sugino, A., S. Hirose, and R. Okazaki. 1972. RNA linked nascent DNA fragments in *Escherichia coli*. Proc. Nat. Acad. Sci. USA 69:1863–67.

Szybalski, W. 1974. Genetic and molecular map of *Escherichia coli* bacteriophage Lambda (λ). *In* A. I. Laskin and H. A. Lechevalier (eds.). Handbook of microbiology. Condensed ed., Pp. 650–57. CRC Press.

Taylor, A. L. 1970. Current linkage map of *Escherichia coli*. Bacteriol. Rev. 34:155–75.

Thomas, J., and J. C. Copeland. 1973. Effects of leucine starvation on control of ribonucleic acid synthesis in strains of *Bacillus subtilis* differing in deoxyribonucleic acid regulation. J. Bacteriol. 116:938–43.

Van Iterson, W., P. A. M. Michels, F. Vyth-Dreese, and J. A. Aten. 1975. Nuclear and cell division in *Bacillus subtilis:* Dormant nucleoids in stationary-phase cells and their activation. J. Bacteriol. 121:1189–99.

Wake, R. G. 1972. Visualization of reinitiated chromosome in *Bacillus subtilis*. J. Mol. Biol. 68:501–9.

Wake, R. G. 1973. Circularity of the *Bacillus subtilis* chromosome and further studies on its bidirectional replication. J. Mol. Biol. 86:223–31.

Wake, R. G. 1974. Termination of *Bacillus subtilis* chromosome replication as visualized by autoradiography. J. Mol. Biol. 86:223–31.

Wang, J. C. 1971. Interaction between DNA and an *Escherichia coli* protein W. J. Mol. Biol. 55:523–33.

Wechsler, J. A. 1973. Complementation analysis of mutations of the *dna*B, *dna*C, and *dna*D loci. *In* R. D. Wells and R. B. Inman (eds.). DNA synthesis *in vitro*. Pp. 375–83. University Park Press, Baltimore.

Wejksnora, P. J., and J. E. Haber. 1974. Methionine dependent synthesis of ribosomal ribonucleic acid during sporulation and vegetative growth of *Saccharomyces cerevisiae*. J. Bacteriol. 120:1344–55.

Wickner. W., and A. Kornberg. 1974. A holoenzyme form of deoxyribonucleic acid polymerase III. Isolation and properties. J. Biol. Chem. 249:6244–49.

Williams, L. S., and F. C. Neidhardt. 1969. Synthesis and inactivation of aminoacyl-transfer RNA synthetases during growth of *Escherichia coli*. J. Mol. Biol. 43:529–50.

Winslow, R. M., and R. A. Lazzarini. 1969. Amino acid regulation of the rates of synthesis and chain elongation of ribonucleic acid in *Escherichia coli*. J. Biol. Chem. 244:3387–3414.

Winston, S., and T. Matsushita. 1977. Protein synthesis and the release of the replication terminus from the cell membrane in *Bacillus subtilis*. *In* D. Schlessinger (ed.). Microbiology 77. Amer. Soc. Microbiol., in press.

Worcel, A. 1970. Induction of chromosome re-initiation in a thermo-sensitive DNA mutant of *Escherichia coli*. J. Mol. Biol. 52:371–86.

Worcel, A., and E. Burgi. 1972. On the structure of the folded chromosome of *Escherichia coli*. J. Mol. Biol. 71:127–47.

Worcel, A., and E. Burgi. 1974. Properties of a membrane attached form of the folded chromosome of *Escherichia coli*. J. Mol. Biol. 83:91–105.

Yahava, I. 1972. On the attachment of the replication origin to membrane in *Escherichia coli*. Jap. J. Genet. 47:45–51.

Yamaguchi, K., and H. Yoshikawa. 1973. Bacterial chromosome replication-topology of chromosome membrane junction in *Bacillus subtilis*. Nature New Biol. 244:204–6.

Yoshikawa, H. and N. Sueoka. 1963a. Sequential replication of *Bacillus subtilis* chromosome. I. Comparison of marker frequencies in exponential and stationary growth phases. Proc. Nat. Acad. Sci. USA 49:559–66.

Yoshikawa, H. and N. Sueoka. 1963b. Sequential replication of the *Bacillus subtilis* chromosome. II. Isotopic transfer experiments. Proc. Nat. Acad. Sci. USA 49:806–13.

Young, F. E., and G. A. Wilson. 1975. Chromosomal map of *Bacillus subtilis*. *In* P. Gerhardt, R. N. Costilow, and H. L. Sadoff (eds.). Spores VI. P. 596–614. Amer. Soc. Microbiol.

Yudelevich, A. 1971. Specific cleavage of an *Escherichia coli* leucine transfer RNA following bacteriophage T4 infection. J. Mol. Biol. 60:21–29.

ROBERT F. GOLDBERGER AND ROGER G. DEELEY

Autogenous Regulation of Gene Expression

5

INTRODUCTION

The essence of autogenous regulation is that a protein encoded in a given structural gene has not only a primary function, such as that of an enzyme or structural protein, but also a regulatory function, controlling expression of its own gene. By this mechanism a protein regulates the rate of synthesis of additional copies of that same protein as well as the rate of synthesis of any other protein encoded in the same operon. We will not be concerned here with the questions of whether the autogenous regulatory protein is a repressor or an activator, whether it is the product of an inducible gene or of a repressible gene, whether its gene is responsive to catabolite repression, or even whether it exerts control at the level of transcription or translation. We will discuss regulation within the framework of the idea, presented by Jacob and Monod (1961), that a regulatory macromolecule controls expression of all genetically regulated systems, keeping in mind that if a system is to be controlled autogenously, then the regulatory macromolecule must be specified by one of the structural genes of the operon that it regulates.

Perhaps the first clear proposal for autogenous regulation as a theoretical concept was that of Maas and McFall (1964). They suggested that the first and allosteric enzyme of a metabolic pathway may play a role in regulating expression of the operon in which its structural gene resides. However, such a mechanism had been hinted at previously (Vogel, 1957), and was developed subsequently by Gruber and Campagne (1965), Englander and Page (1965), Cline and Bock (1966), Koshland and Kirtley (1966), Mehta (1973), and others. All of these suggestions had a similar idea in mind: they envisaged some form of control, often at the level of translation, that was exerted by a

Laboratory of Biochemistry, National Cancer Institute, National Institutes of Health, Bethesda, Maryland 20014.

protein, often a nascent polypeptide chain, that regulated the synthesis of additional copies of that very protein.

In the past five years evidence for an autogenous regulatory mechanism has been obtained in a large number of systems in a wide variety of organisms (Goldberger, 1974). In this review we will make no attempt to catalogue the large number of autogenously regulated systems or even to discuss selected examples in any depth. Rather, we will discuss the criteria required for identifying an autogenously regulated system, the differences in the structures of autogenously and classically regulated systems, the evolution of regulatory mechanisms, the differences in the functional behavior of autogenously and classically regulated systems, and the possible role of autogenous regulation in constitutive gene expression.

CRITERIA FOR IDENTIFYING AUTOGENOUS REGULATION

It is often difficult to determine whether a regulatory mechanism is indeed autogenous. One of the problems is that it is not sufficient to know that there is a close linkage between a regulatory gene and the operon controlled by the product of that gene. One must show that the regulatory gene in question is actually part of the operon that its product controls. For example, the gene that specifies the repressor of the lactose operon of *Escherichia coli* is in juxtaposition to the *lac* operon, but is not under control of the same promoter and operator genes. Thus the *lac* operon of *E. coli* is not autogenously regulated, even though the regulatory gene lies adjacent to the operon. Another problem in determining whether a system is autogenously regulated is that a protein specified by one of the structural genes of an operon may affect expression of that operon only indirectly. For example, any mutation in the gene for an enzyme of a metabolic pathway that limits the activity of the enzyme may alter expression of the operon by altering the intracellular concentration of a coeffector for the operon, such as the substrate, an intermediate, or the end product of the metabolic pathway. Such a mutation may even cause an alteration in expression of the operon simply by changing the growth rate of the organism. In the case of microorganisms it is often possible to determine whether a protein exerts a direct effect on expression of an operon or an indirect, metabolic, effect. The most rigorous proof rests with the demonstration that a purified preparation of the protein encoded in one of the structural genes of an operon directly regulates transcription or translation of that operon *in vitro*. In the case of higher organisms we must be less demanding for the time being. But at the very least one would have to show that a mutation in a given structural gene leads to an altered differential rate of synthesis of that protein. Furthermore, if the protein is an enzyme, it would be helpful if one could show that the mutant enzyme has the same V_{max} and the same K_m as does the wild-type enzyme. Otherwise, one could not rule out the possibility that the altered enzyme affects expression of its structural gene only through some indirect, metabolic mechanism. However, even with higher organisms, it may sometimes be possible to obtain evidence from *in vitro* experiments. For example, Stevens and Williamson (1973) have shown that immunoglobulin specifically inhibits translation of the messenger-RNA that specifies the heavy chain of this protein.

STRUCTURAL DIFFERENCES BETWEEN AUTOGENOUSLY REGULATED
SYSTEMS AND CLASSICALLY REGULATED SYSTEMS

The differences between autogenous regulation and classical regulation are more easily understood when one examines schematic models for these two mechanisms in their various modes. For example, figure 1 depicts the modern form in which the 1961 model of Jacob and Monod is understood, greatly

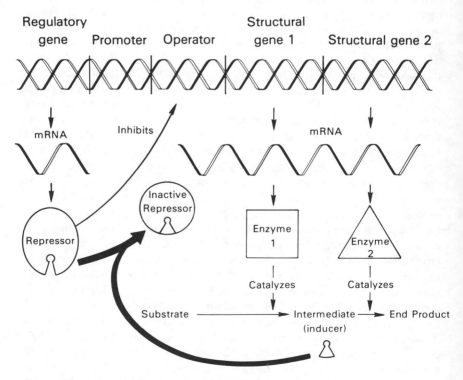

Fig. 1. Schematic model for a classically inducible system.

simplified in the convention adopted for this scheme. It shows a regulatory gene next to an operon that consists of a promoter, an operator, and structural genes. In this classically regulated, inducible system the operon specifies the enzymes of a catabolic pathway. Next to the operon, but not part of it, lies the structural gene for the repressor. This protein, which is synthesized constitutively, interacts with the operator gene with a high degree of specificity and a high affinity and this interaction results in a diminished frequency of transcription of the operon. The inducer in the example shown in figure 1 is the first intermediate of the catabolic pathway. When this small molecule interacts with the repressor, it renders the repressor inactive, allowing an increased rate of transcription of the operon.

In general, an inducible mechanism involving a repressor, such as that shown schematically in figure 1, is utilized to regulate catabolic systems, and functions in an adaptive capacity. Such systems allow the organism to utilize energy-rich substrates not usually present in the environment, while sparing the organism the waste of manufacturing the enzymes necessary to metabolize rare substrates when a more common one is available. The lactose operon may serve as an example. When glucose is available in the medium, the organism utilizes this sugar, and the enzymes for uptake and catabolism of lactose are repressed. When glucose is depleted from the medium, however, and lactose is present, then lactose enters the cell, is converted in one step to allolactose, and this compound acts as inducer of the lactose operon (Jobe and Bourgeois, 1972). Allolactose binds to the *lac* repressor, removing it from the operator gene, thereby causing a greatly increased frequency of transcription of the operon. The intracellular levels of the proteins involved in lactose utilization rise dramatically, and the organism thrives in its new environment, utilizing lactose as its source of energy.

Now if we draw the same scheme for an autogenously regulated system, we see (figure 2) that there is no longer a separate regulatory gene. Instead, there is a closed regulatory loop, in which the repressor *is* the enzyme catalyzing one of the steps of the catabolic pathway—in this case, the first enzyme. In all other respects, the two systems (figures 1 and 2) are the same. The autogenous system, in contrast to the classical one shown in figure 1, requires that the protein specified by one of the genes of the operon have a dual function. One feature of such a system is immediately obvious: the system is buffered against great overswings in gene expression as the organism reacts to new environmental conditions. The reason for this is that any perturbation of the system that tends to cause increased expression of the operon will also cause an increase in the intracellular concentration of the repressor that tends to oppose the response. Thus the reaction of the cell to the original signal for increased expression will be damped out by the response to that signal. The

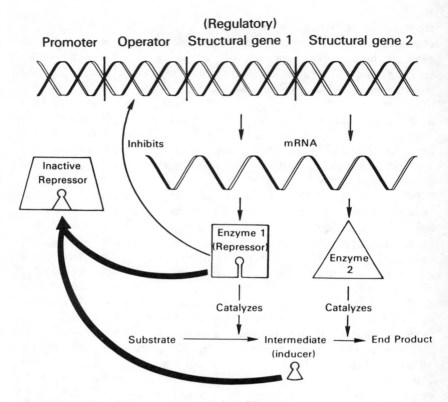

Fig. 2. Schematic model for an autogenously inducible system.

result must be a compromise, which can be computed on the basis of the strengths of interaction of the various macromolecules involved.

Figure 3 uses the same convention to illustrate a classically repressible system. The classical regulatory gene is again located outside the operon. It specifies a protein that is not active by itself. It is called an *aporepressor*. It takes on the ability to act as a repressor only when it interacts with the end product of the biosynthetic pathway catalyzed by the enzymes specified by the structural genes of the operon. The end product is referred to as the *corepressor*. Such systems have an economic function. They spare the organism from overproducing the end products of biosynthetic pathways, because when a sufficient amount of end product has been accumulated, the aporepressor is converted to active repressor, which, in turn, results in a decrease in the production of more end product.

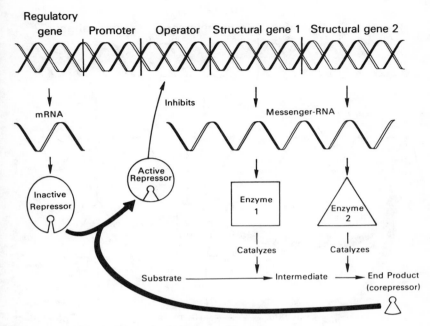

Fig. 3. Schematic model for a classically repressible system.

The same convention has been used to present the equivalent, but autogenously controlled, system in figure 4. Once again, the system forms a closed regulatory loop, with the regulatory gene now one of the structural genes contained within the operon. The protein specified by this gene is the first enzyme of the biosynthetic pathway. It interacts with the end product (corepressor) to form active repressor, and thereby takes on the ability to inhibit further transcription of the operon.

Similar schemes can be drawn for systems controlled by positive regulators (or activators). Figure 5 shows such a system. It is modeled on the regulatory mechanism proposed by Englesberg for the arabinose operon (Englesberg, Squires, and Meronk, 1969). In this scheme there is an additional genetic element, the initiator gene, the site at which the positive activator binds to facilitate transcription of the operon. In the classical system shown in figure 5 the product of the regulatory gene is, by itself, a repressor. However, upon binding the substrate or an intermediate of the catabolic pathway, the inducer, it can no longer function as a repressor. Instead, it takes on a new activity— that of an activator required for transcription of the operon.

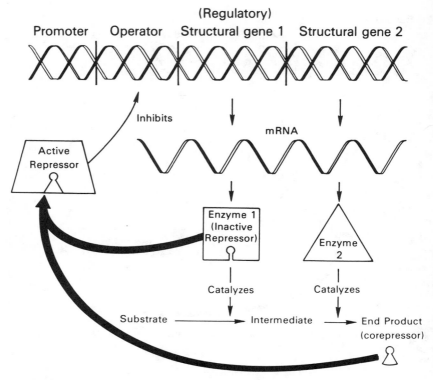

Fig. 4. Schematic model for an autogenously repressible system.

The analogous autogenous system is shown in figure 6. Once again, there is essentially the same arrangement of the parts of the regulatory system, except that the now familiar closed regulatory loop is formed.

Considering the schemes presented in figures 1–6, it is clear that an important difference between classical and autogenous regulation is the mode of synthesis of the regulatory macromolecule. In autogenously regulated systems synthesis of this macromolecule is itself regulated, whereas in classically regulated systems it is not. Even if one postulates a second macromolecule to regulate the synthesis of the classical regulatory protein, the system remains an open regulatory circuit. In contrast, in autogenously regulated systems the regulatory macromolecule regulates the rate of its own synthesis and thus forms a closed regulatory loop. It is this closed regulatory loop that endows autogenously regulated systems with properties that are quantitatively and in

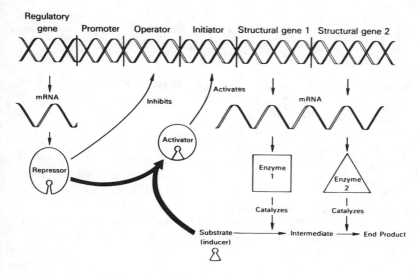

Fig. 5. Schematic model for a classically activated system.

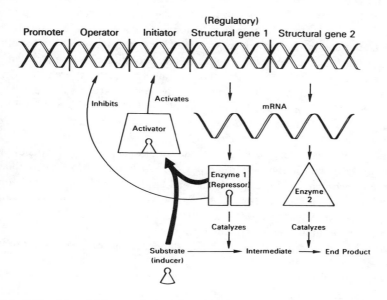

Fig. 6. Schematic model for an autogenously activated system.

some cases qualitatively different from those of comparable classically regulated systems. These differences are discussed more fully in a later section.

EVOLUTION OF REGULATORY SYSTEMS

About three years ago, D. J. Cove (1974) called attention to the evolutionary significance of the bifunctionality of certain proteins and to the fact that autogenous regulatory proteins are a specialized case of such bifunctional proteins. For example, Cove cited studies that suggested that in *Saccharomyces cerevisiae* one iso-cytochrome *c* regulates the rate of synthesis of another iso-cytochrome *c* (Sels et al., 1965; Clavilier, Péré, and Slonimski, 1969). Indeed, Cove himself had presented evidence that in *Aspergillus nidulans*, nitrate reductase acts not only as an autogenous regulator but also regulates the rate of synthesis of several catabolic enzymes not encoded in the same operon (Cove, 1972). The existence of such bifunctional proteins may provide some insight into the ancient history of biological regulation.

It is widely accepted that early in the evolutionary process the synthesis of enzymes was not regulated. Cove (1974) has pointed out that regulated synthesis of an enzyme may involve the evolution of a protein with two different activities: (1) the ability to recognize those environmental conditions under which the enzyme would be required; and (2) the ability to influence expression of the gene in which the enzyme was encoded. Therefore, this protein would have to be able not only to recognize changes in the level of the substrate or end product of the enzyme but also to regulate the rate of synthesis of the enzyme. Cove (1974) suggested that evolution of a single protein in a manner that would simultaneously generate two such different activities would be highly improbable. However, the probability would be greatly increased if the protein already had one of the two activities and could be modified through the evolutionary process to acquire the second activity as well. In the case of an inducible system, this primeval protein could have been any one that would recognize the substrate (or closely related compound) of a catabolic pathway. In the case of a repressible system this protein could have been any one that would recognize the end product (or closely related compound) of a biosynthetic pathway. According to this idea, regulatory systems began to evolve by starting with a protein that already was capable of interacting with some molecule in a pathway catalyzed by the enzymes to be regulated. What better candidate could one imagine than one of the enzymes of the metabolic pathway itself?

Cove (1974) has also pointed out that in some cases in which the evolutionary process selected for a modified catalytic protein with a regulatory function, the result may have been a defective protein either for catalysis or for regulation or for both. If that were the case, a different evolutionary pathway would be preferable: duplication of the gene that specified the enzyme. This would provide the starting point from which each gene could be modified so that one characteristic of the protein could be selected independent of the other. Such an evolutionary pathway would end with regulatory proteins that appear to have no relationship to the enzymes of the metabolic pathways they regulate. It is possible, however, that amino acid analyses might show some evidence of the ancient identity of the regulatory protein and one of the enzymes of the metabolic pathway.

Thus autogenous regulation may have been the first form of regulation to evolve. Later, through gene duplication and translocation, regulatory genes may have become separated from the operons that their products controlled. But even in the case of classical regulation, such as that exemplified by the *lac* operon of *E. coli,* we may find close linkage between a regulatory gene and the operon its product regulates. Therefore, there must be some advantage for the organism to maintain all the elements required for expression of a given operon, and for its regulation, in one relatively compact region of the chromosome. Still later in evolution, and perhaps under other selective pressures, regulatory genes may have become more widely separated from the operon whose expression they controlled, resulting in those classically regulated systems, such as the galactose operon of *E. coli,* in which the regulatory gene or genes are not contiguous with the regulated operon.

One of the questions to be answered if one accepts the idea that autogenous regulation was the first form of regulation to evolve is, Why was it preserved in certain cases and not preserved in others. As mentioned above, one possible reason for evolving an autogenous system into a classically regulated system is that the original bifunctional protein may not have been sufficiently potent in either one or both of its two functions. Another possibility is that some specific attributes of autogenous regulation are suited for certain cellular functions better than is classical regulation, whereas classical regulation may be suited better for other cellular functions. The following section is devoted to a detailed consideration of the latter possibility.

FUNCTIONAL DIFFERENCES BETWEEN AUTOGENOUSLY REGULATED SYSTEMS AND CLASSICALLY REGULATED SYSTEMS

In this section we consider two principal questions: (1) does autogenous regulation offer selective advantages over an otherwise identical system regulated by a constitutively synthesized regulator, and (2) does autogenous regulation offer possible modes of control that cannot be accomplished with systems involving constitutively synthesized regulators? These questions are difficult to answer on the basis of physiological evidence alone since one would have to compare regulatory systems that are identical in all respects except their mode of regulation. Michael Savageau (1974, 1975), however, has derived mathematical expressions describing both autogenously regulated systems and otherwise identical systems controlled by constitutively synthesized regulatory molecules. These mathematical models have allowed him to compare, on the basis of several functional criteria, the behavior of inducible and repressible systems that differ solely in their mode of regulation.

Repressible systems have been compared on the basis of their ability to: (1) maintain a constant level of end product while demand for that end product varies; (2) reduce enzyme synthesis when the end product is supplied exogenously; (3) respond to changes in the availability of substrate; (4) reestablish a new steady state when the system is perturbed; (5) respond rapidly to changes in the availability of substrate or the demand for end product; and (6) continue to function despite internal perturbations, such as might occur when the activity of an enzyme changes as a result of mutation. Inducible systems have been compared on the basis of the same criteria, except the first and second ones have been replaced by: (1) a sharp threshold in the concentration of the substrate of a metabolic pathway required for induction; and (2) the ability to make the most metabolic end product available to the organism for a given change in substrate concentration.

The results that Savageau (1974, 1975) obtained by comparing both constitutively regulated and autogenously regulated systems on the basis of several of these functional criteria have been summarized in figure 7. This figure is divided into quadrants. The area above the horizontal axis describes inducible systems, and the farther up from the horizontal axis, the greater is the strength of induction by substrate (or by an intermediate of a pathway). The area below the horizontal axis describes the repressible systems, and the lower down from the horizontal axis, the greater is the strength of repression by end product. The area to the left of the vertical axis describes systems involving an autogenously regulated repressor, and the farther to the left from the vertical axis, the greater is the strength of repression by this autogenous regulator. The area to the right of the vertical axis describes systems involving an autogenously regulated activator, and the farther to the right from the vertical axis, the greater is the strength of activation by this autogenous regulator. It is clear that any point on this whole plot represents a system with certain characteristics. For example, any system represented by a point that lies *on* the vertical axis will not be autogenously regulated at all; it will be classically regulated, since the autogenous contribution to its regulation is zero.

An absolute requirement of all regulated systems is that they be stable. In other words, they must be able to reestablish a steady state after they have

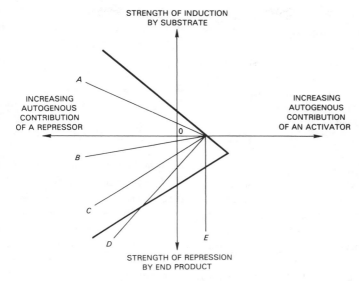

Fig. 7. Two-dimensional plot, redrawn from Savageau (1974, 1975) with permission of the author.

been perturbed. Systems with such stability are represented by the points that lie within the pie-shaped area bordered by the heavy lines in figure 7. Savageau (1974, 1975) refers to these lines as the "boundary of instability." Systems represented by points outside this boundary are unstable and therefore are not considered further. For those systems that lie within the pie-shaped area of stability, the most stable systems will be those that are defined by points farthest away from the boundary of instability.

Systems defined by the points along any particular line, such as A, B, C, D, or E, are systems with behavior that is identical with respect to several criteria. Two criteria that Savageau (1974) has selected as primary in their importance for inducible systems are a sharp threshold in the concentration of substrate required for induction and an ability to make the most product available from a given change in substrate concentration (in other words, the degree to which genetic expression is altered). The inducible systems defined by the points along line A behave identically in terms of these two criteria. It is important to note that lines such as line A diverge toward the left from the boundary of instability. The first conclusion that can be drawn is that for systems such as those along line A, as the autogenous contribution of the repressor increases, the system becomes more stable. Thus systems like these, involving autogenously regulated repressors, are inevitably more stable than systems that utilize a constitutively synthesized regulatory molecule. However, inspection of line A to the right of the vertical axis reveals that systems involving autogenously regulated activators become less stable as the autogenous contribution of the activator increases. Similar reasoning (by considering line D, for example) leads to the conclusion that repressible systems, such as those for amino acid biosynthesis, are more stable if they are controlled by an autogenous activator than if they are controlled by a classical regulatory molecule.

Savageau (1974, 1975) has also examined another set of parameters of regulated systems. He studied the speed with which systems respond to changes in the concentration of substrate or end product and the time taken to establish a new steady state after such a perturbation. From his calculations Savageau concludes that an autogenous repressor provides inducible systems with greater temporal responsiveness than does a classical repressor and that an autogenous activator provides repressible systems with greater temporal responsiveness than does a classical activator. Thus autogenous regulation of inducible systems controlled by repressors provides greater stability and a faster response to changes in substrate concentration than does classical regulation, whereas autogenous regulation of repressible systems controlled by activators provides greater stability and a faster response to changes in end product concentration than does classical regulation.

Up to this point we have considered autogenously regulated systems for which it is possible to describe comparable systems involving constitutively synthesized regulatory molecules. Autogenous regulation can, however, provide a system with properties for which there are no counterparts in a classically regulated system. For example, line E of figure 7 does not cross the ordinate; therefore, systems defined by the points along this line cannot be controlled by classical regulators. They are ideally buffered. That is to say, when the demand for end product changes, the system will provide end product or utilize substrate at a new rate but will reestablish a steady state level of end product identical to the level that existed prior to the perturbation. Such ideal buffering cannot be obtained when the regulatory molecule is synthesized constitutively. In classically regulated systems, for example, when there is an increased demand for end product, increased gene expression can be maintained only by maintaining a decreased concentration of end product.

Savageau (1974, 1975) has pointed out that although his theoretical treatment is straightforward and leads to some interesting conclusions, the validity of those conclusions depends partly upon the relative weight assigned to each of the criteria used in assessing the performance of a particular system. Such assignments will inevitably improve as more and more regulatory systems are understood at the molecular level. It should also be pointed out that we have been considering regulated systems in isolation from one another. Actually, in order to understand cellular metabolism it may be necessary to deal with the question of how regulation of one system is integrated with that of other regulated systems that impinge upon it. Moreover, it now appears that in some systems the same regulatory protein may function as both a repressor *and* an activator, depending upon the binding of specific ligands. An example of such a case is the *araC* protein of the arabinose operon (Englesberg et al., 1969). Other cases of such dual control are beginning to come to light.

OTHER ROLES FOR AUTOGENOUS REGULATION

Recently, Kourilsky and Gros (1974) have discussed various combinations of simple regulatory mechanisms, some of which result in closed regulatory loops. Autogenous regulation, in which a protein directly regulates the rate of its own synthesis, is the simplest form of the closed regulatory loop. The general form of the closed regulatory loop involves two regulatory proteins, each of which controls the rate of synthesis of the other. Kourilsky and Gros (1974) have discussed closed regulatory loops in terms of the various possible combinations of regulatory proteins—repressors and activators without the participation of any inducer or corepressor. They suggest that a combination of two activators results in mutual amplification of expression of the two genes; a combination of two repressors may result in a switch mechanism, by which expression of a gene (or a group of genes) may be inhibited very severely and for a prolonged period of time. Actually, Eisen et al. (1970) have used an example of such a mechanism in the bacteriophage lambda as a model for differentiation in its simplest form. A simple example is shown schematically in figure 8. In this autogenously activated system initial activation leads to amplification of operon expression, providing that the rate of expression of the operon is sufficient to produce an increasing concentration of activator despite the dilution that results from cell growth. Such a mechanism would be suitable only for a system in which an irreversible commitment to a maximal rate of gene expression is desirable. Figure 9 shows a model for an autogenously repressed system that is not influenced by any co-effector. In this case the degree to which the operon will be expressed will depend upon the affinity of this repressor for its operator. If the affinity, for example, is very high, only a few molecules of repressor per cell will suffice to keep the operon repressed, and consequently a steady state will be reached in which the intracellular concentration of repressor will be very low. If the affinity of the repressor for its operator is several orders of magnitude lower, however, the steady state that will be reached will be one in which the intracellular concen-

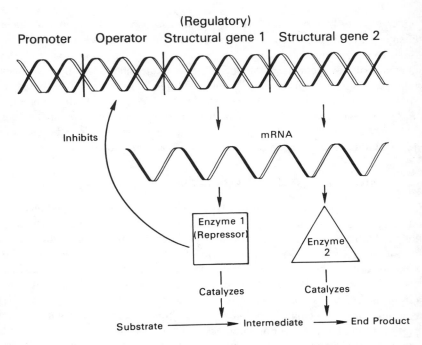

Fig. 8. Schematic model for an autogenously activated system not influenced by any inducer or corepressor.

tration of the repressor is much higher. Whatever the affinity may be, an interesting feature of this mechanism is that it will maintain the regulatory protein at a relatively constant concentration, regardless of growth rate and regardless of cell size.

Although the renaissance in molecular biology in the past twenty years is closely identified with the development of our understanding of regulation of gene expression in bacteria, much thought has also gone into the mechanism of constitutive gene expression in prokaryotes. It has not been difficult to eliminate certain possibilities for explaining constitutive gene expression. For example, it cannot result from a single transcription occurring with each chromosomal replication; if that were the case, then differences among the numbers of molecules of the various proteins in the cell would have to be explained solely by differences in the rates of degradation of the proteins or of their corresponding messenger-RNA molecules. While some variation in stability has been found, the magnitude of this variation is not sufficient to explain the very widely differing intracellular concentrations of the various

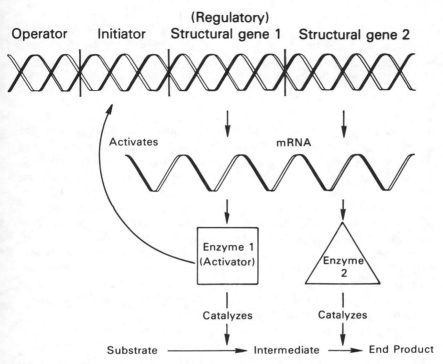

Fig. 9. Schematic model for an autogenously repressible system not influenced by any inducer or corepressor.

cellular proteins. A more popular concept has been the idea that the rate of transcription of a constitutively expressed gene is dependent only upon the affinity of the promoter of that gene for the RNA polymerase. However, this mechanism does not provide a means for keeping the concentration of a protein constant under all conditions; when the chromosome is being replicated and the number of genes for a particular protein doubles, the rate of synthesis of that protein would double. On the other hand, there are conditions under which autogenous regulation can result in a nearly constant intracellular concentration of a protein, regardless of the rate at which the chromosome is being replicated. These conditions are those in which the autogenous regulatory protein is a repressor of its own structural gene and does not interact with any co-effector (see figure 9). A wide variety of structural genes could be regulated in this fashion; the intracellular concentrations of the gene products would remain constant throughout the life of the cell, and would be set at a level determined by the affinity of each protein for its operator. At the present time there is no evidence to indicate how widespread this mechanism may be. We want to point out, however, that this is a viable theoretical possibility, and to suggest that it is likely to be found both in prokaryotes and in higher organisms.

SUMMARY

In this theoretical discussion we have presented models that describe the characteristics of autogenous regulation in its various modes and that contrast these characteristics with those of comparable classically regulated systems. We have discussed studies in which such a contrast has brought into clear relief the quantitative, and in some cases qualitative, differences between autogenous and classical regulation. In certain cases autogenous regulation provides greater stability and temporal responsiveness than does classical regulation. Unlike classical regulation, autogenous regulation can also provide a mechanism for buffering the response of the regulated system to a change in the environment, and for maintaining a constant intracellular concentration of a protein regardless of growth rate. In addition, autogenous regulation may be utilized for amplication of gene expression and for severe and prolonged inhibition of gene expression.

The characteristics of autogenous regulation described above may suffice to explain why it has persisted through the evolutionary process. The question of how regulation of gene expression evolved in the first place is a much more difficult one to answer. However, as we have argued, the question is greatly simplified if one assumes that autogenous regulation preceded classical regulation. Thus we suggest that autogenous regulation may have been the first mechanism for regulating gene expression, and that the special characteristics of autogenous regulation are responsible for the persistence of this mechanism in certain systems.

REFERENCES

Clavilier, L., G. Péré, and P. P. Slonimski. 1969. Mise en évidence de plusieurs loci indépendants impliqués dans la synthèse de l'iso-2-cytochrome *c* chez la levure. Mol. Gen. Genet. 104:195–218.

Cline, A. L., and R. M. Bock. 1966. Translational control of gene expression. Cold Spring Harbor Symp. Quant. Biol. 31:321–33.

Cove, D. J. 1972. The control of nitrogen metabolism in *Aspergillus nidulans*. Heredity 29:119.

Cove, D. J. 1974. Evolutionary significance of autogenous regulation. Nature 251:256.

Eisen, H., P. Brachet, L. Pereira da Silva, and F. Jacob. 1970. Regulation of repressor expression in λ. Proc. Nat. Acad. Sci. USA 66:855-62.

Englander, S. W. and L. A. Page. 1965. Interpretation of data on sequential labeling of growing polypeptides. Biochem. Biophys. Res. Commun. 19:565–70.

Englesberg, E., C. Squires and F. Meronk, Jr. 1969. The L-arabinose operon in Escherichia coli B/r: A genetic demonstration of two functional states of the product of a regulator gene. Proc. Nat. Acad. Sci. USA 62:1100–1107.

Goldberger, R. F. 1974. Autogenous regulation of gene expression. Science 183:810–16.

Gruber, M., and R. N. Campagne. 1965. Regulation of protein synthesis: An alternative to the repressor-operator hypothesis. Koninkl. Ned. Acad. Wetenschap. Proc. Ser. C 68:270–76.

Jacob, F., and J. Monod. 1961. Genetic regulatory mechanisms in the synthesis of proteins. J. Mol. Biol. 3:318–56.

Jobe, A., and S. Bourgeois. 1972. *Lac* repressor-operator interaction. VI. The natural inducer of the *lac* operon. J. Mol. Biol. 69:397–408.

Koshland, D. E., Jr., and M. E. Kirtley. 1966. Protein structure in relation to cell dynamics and differentiation. *In* M. Locke (ed.). Major problems in developmental biology. Pp. 217–49. Academic Press, New York.

Kourilsky, P., and F. Gros. 1974. Prokaryote models for regulation of gene expression: Genetic control of transcription. *In* M. Harris and B. Thompson (eds.). Regulation of gene expression in eukaryotic cells. Pp.17-41. Fogarty International Center Proceedings no. 25. DHEW Pub. No. (NIH) 74–648.

Maas, W., and E. McFall. 1964. Genetic aspects of metabolic control. Ann. Rev. Microbiol. 18:95–110.

Mehta, N. G. 1973. A model for the regulation of repressor synthesis. J. Sci. and Indus. Res. 32:1–7.

Savageau, M. A. 1974. Comparison of classical and autogenous systems of regulation in inducible operons. Nature 252:546–49.

Savageau, M. A. 1975. Significance of autogenously regulated and constitutive synthesis of regulatory proteins in repressible biosynthetic systems. Nature 258:208–14.

Sels, A. A., H. Fukuhara, G. Péré, and P. P. Slonimski. 1965. Cinétique de la biosynthèse induite de l'iso-1-cytochrome *c* et de l'iso-2-cytochrome *c* au cours de l'adaptation à l'oxygène. Biochim. Biophys. Acta 95:486–502.

Stevens, R. H., and A. R. Williamson. 1973. Isolation of messenger RNA coding for mouse heavy-chain immunoglobulin. Proc. Nat. Acad. Sci. USA 70:1127–31.

Vogel, H. J. 1957. Repression and induction as control mechanisms in enzyme biogenesis: The "adaptive" formation of acetylornithinase. *In* W. D. McElroy and B. Glass (eds.), The chemical basis of heredity. Pp. 276–89. Johns Hopkins University Press, Baltimore.

GEORGE A. MARZLUF

Regulation of Gene Expression in Fungi

6

"One side will make you grow taller, and the other side will make you grow shorter." "One side of what? The other side of what?" thought Alice to herself. "Of the mushroom," said the Caterpillar, just as if she had asked it aloud. Alice remained looking thoughtfully at the mushroom for a minute, trying to make out which were the two sides of it; and, as it was perfectly round, she found this a very difficult question.[1]

A complete understanding of the regulation of gene expression may reveal why a mushroom is indeed perfectly round. Certainly one of the primary long-term objectives of inquiry concerning gene expression is an explanation of the processes of differentiation and morphogenesis. Regulation of gene expression in fungi, most frequently studied with *Neurospora, Aspergillus,* and yeast, is often viewed as a model for understanding control in eukaryotic organisms. Hopefully, many of the principles of regulation gleaned from such studies with fungi can be extrapolated in varying degrees to higher organisms. The fungi are truly higher organisms (eukaryotes) in terms of their cellular structure and genetic organization. They possess a larger and more structured cell than prokaryotes and also contain mitochondria, ribosomes, and plasma membranes characteristic of higher forms. Most important, the fungi possess authentic chromosomes and nuclei and undergo the familiar processes of mitosis and meiosis. In short, their genetic organization appears to be identical to, or to closely resemble, that of higher eukaryotes. *Neurospora* and yeast have about ten-times as much DNA as does *Escherichia coli* and about

Department of Biochemistry, Ohio State University, Columbus, Ohio 43210.

20% of the amount of DNA found in the haploid genome of *Drosophila*. However, since these fungi contain only approximately 1% of the DNA found in mouse or man, caution must accompany and temper any conceptual jumps from fungi to man. Nevertheless, many attributes of the fungi do suggest that they may be valuable models for the study of eukaryotic regulation.

Neurospora contains histones (Hsiang and Cole, 1973), repetitive DNA sequences (Brooks and Huang, 1972: Dutta, 1974), and both *Neurospora* and yeast have been shown to possess multiple RNA polymerase species (Timberlake and Turian, 1974; Adman, Schultz, and Hall, 1972). Furthermore, Poly-A sequences have been found in messenger RNA of yeast (Reed and Wintersberger, 1973) and *Neurospora* (Russell, unpublished data). Adenylate cyclase (Flawia and Torres, 1972), cyclic-AMP, and c-AMP phosphodiesterase (Scott and Solomon, 1973) have been found in *Neurospora* and implicated in morphogenesis (Scott, Mishra, and Tatum, 1973). Finally, these fungi undergo a limited but significant amount of cell differentiation and development, accompanied by differential and phase-specific gene activity (Matsuyama, Nelson, and Siegel, 1974).

Because of their simple growth requirements, the fungi are easily manipulated. The availability of relatively sophisticated genetic systems permits a parallel biochemical and genetic dissection of fungal regulatory systems, much as has been used with prokaryotes, but which is unavailable for any other higher organisms with the possible exception of *Drosophila*. This review will not even attempt to cover all the interesting studies of gene regulation in fungi, but instead will focus attention on particular aspects of regulation that have been clarified by studies with fungi and in some cases have been carefully examined only in fungi.

COMPARTMENTATION AS A REGULATORY DEVICE

The large size and highly organized structure of the eukaryotic cell has consequences for regulatory systems. Metabolic reserves are also commonly found in eukaryotic cells, thus providing for greater metabolic stability than found in prokaryotes. However, pools of stored compounds must somehow be confined so as not to interfere with the familiar patterns of feedback inhibition and repression exerted by the smaller, genuine catabolic or biosynthetic pools of such metabolites.

Perhaps the clearest case that illustrates the important role of organized cell structure is the utilization of the common precursor, carbamyl phosphate (CP), in the biosynthesis of the pyrimidines and of arginine in *Neurospora* (figure 1). Davis (1972, 1974) and his associates have found that *Neurospora* possesses two carbamyl phosphate synthetases, one serving the pyrimidine

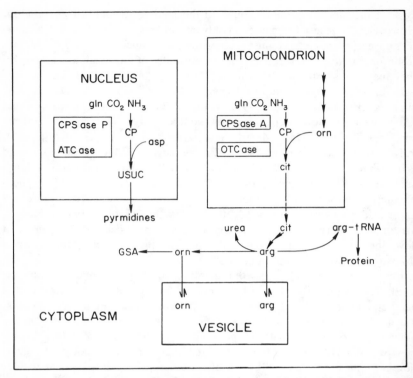

Fig. 1. Diagram of cellular structure and biochemical steps involved in arginine and pyrimidine metabolism in *Neurospora*. The vesicle is a cytoplasmic body that differs from mitochondria and serves as a storage vesicle for some amino acids. Abbreviations: gln, glutamine; CP, carbamyl phosphate; asp, aspartate; USUC, ureidosuccinate; ATCase, aspartate transcarbamylase; CPSase A, carbamyl phosphate synthetaste A; CPSase P, carbamyl phosphate synthetase P; OTCase, ornithine transcarbamylase; cit, citrulline; orn, ornithine; arg, arginine; gsa, glutamic semialdehyde.

synthetic pathway (CPSase P) and one specific for arginine biosynthesis (CPSase A). CPSase P is found exclusively within the nucleus, where it exists aggregated with aspartate transcarbamylase, the next enzyme of the pathway. Because of this bifunctional enzyme complex, carbamyl phosphate destined for pyrimidine synthesis is not released but remains as an enzyme-bound intermediate. This feature permits efficient catalysis with low carbamyl phosphate concentrations and also restricts this CP for exclusive use in pyrimidine synthesis. CPSase P is feedback inhibited by UTP, and, due to the location of the enzyme aggregate in the nucleus, it is directly exposed to a most significant biosynthetic pool—that of pyrimidine triphosphates. Thus control of CPSase P activity appears to be facilitated by its cellular location.

Five enzymes involved in the early steps of arginine synthesis are localized within mitochondria, namely, CPSase A, ornithine transcarbamylase (OTCase), and the three enzymes required for ornithine synthesis (Weiss and Davis, 1973). The final two enzymes of arginine synthesis are situated in the cytoplasm. Citrulline, the product of the OTCase reaction, exits from the mitochondria, and in two steps gives rise to arginine. The carbamyl phosphate pool destined for arginine biosynthesis is confined to the mitochondria so that loss to the potentially competing aspartate transcarbamylase reaction of pyrimidine synthesis is prevented. The five early enzymes for arginine synthesis are all repressible by arginine, although CPSase A is unusual because it is the only one that is fully repressible, the others all having high basal levels.

Even when growing on minimal medium, *Neurospora* cells contain relatively high concentrations of arginine and ornithine. Two rather puzzling questions arise in this context. Why is CPSase A not fully repressed in view of the high content of arginine, which is known to cause repression of this enzyme? Secondly, since the enzymes responsible for metabolism of arginine and ornithine (arginase and ornithine transaminase, respectively) are present, what prevents the continuous, wasteful catabolism of these amino acids? Weiss (1973) found that most of the intracellular arginine and ornithine is contained as a storage pool within an osmotically sensitive organelle, designated the "vesicle." The vesicle serves to segregate the storage forms of arginine, ornithine, lysine, histidine, and perhaps other amino acids from the smaller dynamic pools involved in their synthesis, utilization, and regulation. It was shown that when a small amount of highly radioactive arginine was added to the cells, it was preferentially utilized for protein synthesis and was not diluted by mixing with the storage pool (Subraminian, Weiss, and Davis, 1973). The arginine in this reservoir pool is not normally used for biosynthetic purposes (nor is it metabolized), but it is available as a storage form whenever a deficiency occurs in the biosynthetic pool. The vesicle not only confines a storage pool but also maintains a relatively constant cytoplasmic concentration of arginine. The cytoplasmic concentration so maintained is sufficient to permit protein synthesis but is too low for arginine catabolism by arginase, which has a high K_m for its substrate. Arginine will be catabolized only when it is present in the external medium and is entering the cell so rapidly that the cytoplasmic concentration rises because the vesicles are temporarily flooded. Thus the vesicle plays an important role by permitting storage and consequent metabolic stability but in such a way that it does not interfere with the usual control mechanisms or permit wasteful catabolism. The importance of internal cell structure and storage pools and their consequences for regulatory systems seems well established in the case of arginine biosynthesis and utilization in *Neurospora* and closely related organisms. This example underlines the need to carefully consider the possible role of internal cell structure and compartmentation when studying regulation in fungi, or, indeed in any eukaryotic organism.

AROMATIC AMINO ACID METABOLISM

It has been of considerable interest to determine whether the genes that specify the related enzymes of a single pathway in eukaryotes are clustered together and controlled as a unit as is so familiar in bacteria. The conclusion of many studies with *Neurospora* and yeast is that related structural genes are generally not found in an operon-type arrangement but, in most instances, are widely scattered throughout the genome. Although widely separated from one another, related genes are usually controlled in a parallel manner by common metabolic and genetic regulatory signals (see below). However, there are at least several well-documented cases of the existence of a cluster of two or more structural genes in fungi. We should ask whether these exceptional cases do indeed represent an operon-type of gene arrangement.

The pathway for the biosynthesis of the aromatic amino acids and that for the degradation of quinic acid and related compounds have been studied in *N. crassa* by Giles, Case, and their colleagues. The biosynthetic enzymes were reported to be aggregated in a multienzyme complex (mol. wt. 230,000) containing five different proteins. These five proteins were believed to be encoded by the *arom* gene cluster (*arom*-2, -9, -1, -5, and -4) consisting of five adjacent structural genes. Mutations that map within a specific *arom* gene may affect only individual enzymes or may cause loss of two or more of the activities of the complex. Some of these pleiotropic mutants were thought to represent nonsense mutations that presumably exert polar effects on the translation of a single polycistronic mRNA encoded by the *arom* cluster (Case and Giles, 1968; 1971).

However, recent results from two laboratories convincingly demonstrate that the *arom* cluster is instead a single large structural gene that encodes a single polypeptide chain (Coggins, unpublished results; Gaertner, unpublished results). This large polypeptide (mol. wt. 115,000) is pentafunctional, possessing all five biosynthetic activities. The native enzyme is apparently a homodimer, containing two such identical subunits. The earlier reports of five separate enzymes is readily explained as an artifact that arises during purification, since the enzyme is extremely sensitive to an endogenous alkaline protease, whose action generates enzyme fragments that possess the individual activities. Thus, this case of an apparent clustering of related structural genes, with the attendant expectations for their common control, instead clearly represents the evolutionary fusion of five separate genes into a single one.

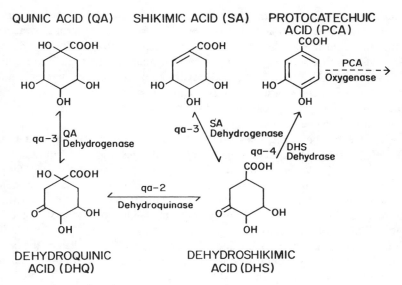

Fig. 2. Quinic acid metabolism in *Neurospora crassa*.

Although the biosynthetic and catabolic pathways for the aromatic amino acids share two intermediates, metabolic flow occurs in such a way that the pathways do not seriously compete with each other. The multifunctional enzyme confines intermediates of the biosynthetic pathway so that they cannot escape to any extent and enter the degradative pathway. Furthermore, the catabolic enzymes are only synthesized when suitable inducers are present.

Even though not all of the criteria necessary to establish the presence of an operon have been met, the genes encoding the enzymes for quinate metabolism in *Neurospora* may well occur in such a regulated unit. The first three enzymes for catabolism of quinic acid (QA) and shikimic acid (SA) are encoded by three tightly linked structural genes (Chaleff, 1974a). Both quinate dehydrogenase and shikimate dehydrogenase activities reside in the same enzyme, which is encoded by the *qa-3* gene. The inducible dehydroquinase and dehydroshikimate dehydrase are coded for by the *qa-2* and *qa-4* genes, respectively (see figure 2). These structural genes are tightly linked and adjacent to a fourth gene, *qa-1*, which apparently encodes a regulatory protein that acts in a positive manner to activate transcription of the structural genes of the cluster.

The three catabolic enzymes are not aggregated and are only synthesized in response to induction, the most effective inducer being quinic acid. Strong induction was achieved with quinic acid in the *qa-3* mutant, which is incapable of further metabolism of this compound, thus providing strong evidence that quinic acid itself is a genuine inducer (Chaleff, 1974b). This system is very sensitive to low concentrations of inducer, half maximal induction being achieved at 5×10^{-6} M quinic acid. Dehydroquinic acid and dehydroshikimic acid are less-effective inducers, and shikimic acid is inactive in this regard. Induction of the *qa* enzymes requires protein synthesis and is completely inhibited by cycloheximide.

All three catabolic enzymes are synthesized coordinately in wild type (Chaleff, 1974b). This fact and the linkage of the *qa* genes in a tight cluster, controlled by the common *qa-1* regulatory gene, suggests that the *qa* genes may constitute an operon. More evidence is needed to settle this issue; identification of a polycitronic mRNA and isolation and study of cis-acting operator- or initiator-type regulatory mutants would constitute strong evidence in favor of the operon concept.

Giles, Case, and their colleagues have made extensive studies of the *qa-1* regulatory gene. Mutants of the *qa-1* locus are pleiotropic and non-inducible for all three enzyme activities, and they complement mutants of each of the other *qa* genes. Several studies have shown that *qa-1* mutants can be divided into two discrete groups, namely *qa-1*ᔆ (slow) and *qa-1*ᶠ (fast), on the basis of how rapidly they complement with other *qa* mutants, e.g., *qa-2*. Several lines of evidence indicate that the *qa-1* regulatory product is a multimeric protein. The isolation of temperature-sensitive *qa-1* alleles (*qa-1*ᶠ mutants) that produce low levels of the *qa* enzymes at 25°C but cannot be induced at 35°C suggests that the *qa-1* product is a protein, since at least most temperature-sensitive mutants produce a thermolabile protein. Intragenic complementation clearly occurs between certain pairs of *qa-1*ᔆ and *qa-1*ᶠ alleles and presumably occurs by the association of subunits into a multimeric protein. The occur-

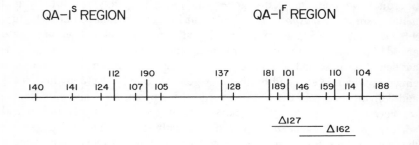

Fig. 3.   Genetic fine structure of the *qa-1* locus. *QA-1*ˢ and *QA-1*ᶠ refer to slow- and fast-complementing *ga-1* alleles, respectively. The vertical lines indicate individual point mutations; Δ 127 and Δ 162 are small deletions.

rence of non-complementing *qa-1* point mutations implies that both *qa-1*^{S} and *qa-1*^{F} mutational alterations occur within a single functional gene despite their different phenotypic characteristics and their distinct distributions on the *qa-1* map (figure 3).

Giles, Case, and Jacobson (1974) have suggested that the *qa-1* coded regulatory protein may function by binding at a specific DNA sequence adjacent to the *qa* structural genes (a promoter or initiator sequence) and thereby activate transcription of these genes (figure 4). The active conformation of the *qa-1* protein is postulated to exist only after it binds an appropriate inducer such as QA. The most plausible mode of action of the *qa-1* protein is to aid RNA polymerase in melting a particular DNA sequence next to the structural genes, which permits initiation of their transcription. If this model for *qa-1* action is correct, several consequences may be predicted. Constitutive *qa-1* alleles (*qa-1*^{C}) may be found that produce a regulatory protein that is active in the absence of inducer. Furthermore, alterations in the postulated DNA recognition sequence for the *qa-1*$^+$ protein should result in initiator-type constitutive mutants (I^c) similar to those found in the *ara* operon of *E. coli*. A relatively large number of mutants constitutive for the quinate catabolic enzymes have been obtained, and all appear to be of the expected *qa-1*^{c} type, i.e., alterations that affect the regulatory protein. Such *qa-1*^{c} constitutive mutants can be isolated in two ways. They occur as revertants of *qa-1*^{S} mutants, and can also be directly isolated from the wild-type strain (Partridge, Case, and Giles, 1972).

According to the model presented above, the *qa-1* locus encodes a diffusible regulatory protein. Consequently, in dominance studies, *qa-1*$^+$ should act both cis and trans and should be dominant (or at least semi-dominant) to *qa-1* mutants. These expected results are obtained (Case and Giles, 1975). The behavior within heterokaryons of various pairwise combinations of *qa-1* alleles—wild type (WT), *qa-1*^{c}, *qa-1*^{S}, and *qa-1*^{F}—indicates that the *qa-1*

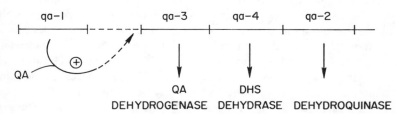

Fig. 4. Proposed mechanism for regulation of the *qa* cluster of structural genes. The *qa-1*$^+$ gene is believed to encode a positive-acting regulatory protein required for transcription of a polycistronic messenger RNA. Function of the *qa-1*$^+$ gene product requires that it first bind the inducer, quinic acid (QA).

product is diffusible. In general, *qa-1* mutants are recessive to WT, which is consistent with the notion that the *qa-1*$^+$ gene produces a regulatory protein that exerts positive control over the synthesis of the enzymes encoded in the *qa* cluster. As expected, certain *qa-1*^{C} mutants are dominant (or semi-dominant) to WT. Yet, when heterokaryons with a suitable set of mutants are examined, it is clear that the *qa-1*^{C} gene product is far more effective in initiating the synthesis of *qa* enzymes within its own nucleus than in other nuclei contained in a common cytoplasm (Case and Giles, 1975). These results appear to be similar to, but not as extreme as those found with, the "nucleus limited" product of the *scon*^{c} gene (see below).

Extensive genetic analysis has shown a clear segmentation of the *qa-1*$^+$ gene in that *qa-1*^{S} and *qa-1*^{F} mutant sites occur in discrete, non-overlapping regions (figure 3). The *qa-1*$^+$ regulatory protein may possess two discrete functional regions—one that interacts with the inducer and a second site that recognizes and binds to a specific DNA sequence essential for transcription of the adjacent *qa* structural genes (Case and Giles, 1975). The inducer-binding and DNA-binding regions of the regulatory protein may be coded for by the *qa-1*^{F} and *qa-1*^{S} segments of the gene, respectively. The *qa-1*^{S} mutants apparently exhibit negative complementation, most likely through the formation of hybrid multimeric regulatory proteins, which are defective for DNA binding or transcription initiation. The regulatory protein produced by *qa-1*^{F} mutants may be faulty in its binding of inducer and thus unable to assume a conformation that can bind to the initiator DNA sequence. Finally, *qa-1*^{C} mutants can readily be explained as producing a *qa-1* protein that exists in an active form (even without inducer) for binding to the initiator DNA sequence.

Further support for this model of regulation of *qa* gene transcription is needed before it can be considered as established. The identification of initiator constitutive (I^c) mutants that would define the DNA binding region would be particularly valuable. Since mutation in even a single base pair of DNA can dramatically alter its local melting characteristics, it seems likely that some I^c mutants would display constitutive synthesis of the *qa* enzymes even in the absence of any *qa-1* gene product. Such I^c mutants could possibly be isolated as constitutive revertants of *qa-1* deletions. Direct biochemical isolation of the postulated *qa-1* regulatory protein and a study of its behavior, when derived from wild type and mutants, would also be very helpful. Since it appears that this protein has a very high affinity for the inducer, quinic acid, techniques that detect QA-binding proteins may be productive. Although we must wait for additional details, it is already clear that the structural genes of the *qa* cluster of *Neurospora* are subject to positive control and in a way reminiscent of several bacterial control systems.

The three enzymes of galactose metabolism in *Saccharomyces cerevisiae*, galactokinase, galactose-1-phosphate uridyl transferase, and UDP-galactose epimerase, are specified by a cluster of three tightly linked structural genes, *gal-1, gal-7,* and *gal-10.* Expression of the *gal* structural genes is controlled by at least two regulatory loci, *gal i* and *gal-4.* The *gal-4* mutants lack galactose permease and the three enzymes of galactose catabolism, which led Douglas and Hawthorne (1964, 1972) to propose that *gal-4*$^+$ specifies a regulatory product that exerts positive control on the unlinked cluster of *gal* structural genes. Klar and Halvorson (1974) have recently shown that a temperature-sensitive allele of *gal-4* affects the synthesis of the *gal* enzymes but does not qualitatively alter them in thermolability or temperature optima from that of wild type. This result argues that *gal-4*$^+$ does not encode a subunit that is shared by the *gal* enzymes and supports the earlier suggestion that the *gal-4*$^+$ product is a positive-acting regulatory protein. Mutants of the *gal i* gene are constitutive and recessive to *gal i*$^+$, suggesting that the *i*$^+$ product acts as a repressor. Starting with a diploid strain to screen out recessive regulatory mutants of the *i*$^-$ type, Douglas and Hawthorne (1966) attempted to isolate cis dominant O^c-like mutants to identify an operator site adjacent to the *gal-1, -7, -10* cluster. However, they instead found dominant constitutive mutants, C, that mapped at or very near the *gal-4* locus. Since C is cis dominant to *gal-4,* it appears that C is formally an O^c mutant and identifies a regulatory region that controls *gal-4* expression. The available evidence suggests a sequential control mechanism in which the *i*$^+$ gene product acts as a repressor of *gal-4* function by binding at an operator site defined by the C mutant. Upon induction the *gal-4*$^+$ regulatory product is made and in turn "turns on" the expression of the unlinked *gal* structural genes and the separate gene for galactose permease. Thus the cluster of *gal* structural genes appears to be organized like a positively controlled operon. Additional evidence is needed to support this concept; particularly valuable would be recovery of initiator-constitutive (I^c) mutants closely linked, and cis-dominant, to the structural genes, which would equally affect the synthesis of all three *gal* enzymes. Although additional instances of operon-like gene clusters exist in fungi, the quinate system in *Neurospora* and the *gal* system of yeast are more than sufficient to point out that the general types of regulatory systems observed in bacteria are also found in eukaryotes, at least the lower eukaryotes, although they may be more complicated than is now evident. Also noteworthy is the prominence of positive control in fungal regulation.

SULFUR-CONTROLLED ENZYMES AND NUCLEUS RESTRICTED CONTROL

In *N. crassa* a family of related enzymes that function in the acquisition of sulfur from the environment are subject to an intricate set of genetic and metabolic controls. A metabolite, probably cysteine, derived from favored sulfur sources such as methionine, represses this set of enzymes, which include aryl sulfatase, choline sulfatase, choline-O-sulfate permease, an aromatic sulfate permease, a specific methionine permease, γ-cystathionase, an extracellular protease, and two permeases for inorganic sulfate (Metzenberg and Parson, 1966; Marzluf, 1970a; Marzluf, 1972a; Hanson and Marzluf, 1973; Pall, 1971). This effect on enzyme synthesis can be considered to result from sulfur catabolite repression, analogous to the more familiar carbon catabolite repression. This entire group of enzymes is also controlled by two unlinked regulatory genes of opposite effect, designated *cys-3* and *scon*.

The *cys-3* gene is believed to encode a positive regulatory product that is required for the synthesis of these enzymes (Marzluf and Metzenberg, 1968). Accordingly, *cys-3* mutants display a pleiotropic loss of all these activities and cannot grow on minimal medium because of the complete loss of sulfate transport activity. Temperature-conditional alleles and revertants of *cys-3* have been studied. They synthesize aryl sulfatase (of normal heat stability) and its congeners at 25°C but fail to do so at 37°C. This result argues that the *cys-3* gene specifies a macromolecule, presumably a protein, that is required to "turn on" the structural genes for the various sulfur enzymes. The structural gene (*ars*) for aryl sulfatase has been identified by mutants that result in an altered electrophoretic mobility of the enzyme (Metzenberg, Chen, and Ahlgren, 1971; Metzenberg and Ahlgren, 1971). The putative structural genes for the distinct sulfate transport systems have also been located (Marzluf, 1970b). The *cys-13* locus encodes sulfate permease I, a form that has a high K_m for sulfate and that predominates in the conidial stage. Sulfate permease II, which has a low K_m for sulfate and is found only in the mycelial phase, is encoded by the *cys-14* gene. These three structural loci (*ars, cys-13,* and *cys-14*) are unlinked to each other and to the separate regulatory genes, *cys-3* and *scon*. Structural genes for the remainder of the sulfur-controlled enzymes have not yet been identified, but they presumably are also unlinked. Although each of the separate structural genes must recognize the *cys-3*$^+$ product, they are not equally sensitive to this positive regulatory signal. This is apparent because different partial revertants of the *cys-3* mutant display completely disproportionate levels of sulfate permease I, sulfate permease II, aryl sulfatase, and choline sulfatase (Marzluf, 1975). This differential response presumably occurs because receptor sites, perhaps within a promoter region, adjacent to each of the structural genes have somewhat different affinities for the common *cys-3* regulatory signal. Mutations in such cis-acting regions might occur that would permit expression of the particular gene in the absence of any *cys-3* product, i.e., I^c-type constitutive mutants. Such I^c mutants should arise during isolation of *cys-3* revertants; and yet a large number of revertants (selected for restoration of sulfate permease activity) have been examined, and all result from alterations within the *cys-3* locus itself (Marzluf, 1975). It appears that the occurrence of I^c mutations may be relatively rare, and special selective procedures may be required for their isolation, if indeed they can be obtained at all in some cases. The use of deletions of the respective positive control gene, when available, should greatly facilitate recovery of I^c-type mutants.

As expected in cases in which a regulatory gene encodes a diffusible product with a positive action, the wild-type allele ($cys-3^+$) is dominant to the $cys-3$ mutant in heterokaryons. An interesting question arises in this regard, namely, can a $cys-3^+$ gene "turn on" expression of structural genes contained in different nuclei of a heterokaryon, or can it only control those genes within its own nucleus? This problem was analyzed by the use of heterokaryons in which $cys-3^+$ and $cys-3$ nuclei carried particular *ars* genes that encode aryl sulfatase with different electrophoretic mobilities (Metzenberg and Ahlgren, 1971). The $cys-3^+$ gene very clearly activated synthesis of both forms of the enzyme regardless of nuclear ratio and thus can act trans-nuclearly. One obvious interpretation of this outcome is that the $cys-3^+$ encodes a macromolecule that is actually synthesized within the common cytoplasm and then enters nuclei (of both types), where it exerts its positive control function. Alternatively, it is entirely possible that this regulatory product acts at the translational level.

An identical type of test was conducted with $scon^c$, a mutant of a second unlinked regulatory locus that results in the constitutive synthesis of the entire group of sulfur-related enzymes (Burton and Metzenberg, 1972). By the use of suitably designed heterokaryons (e.g., $scon^c ars^F + scon^+ ars^S$), $scon^c$ was shown to be codominant with $scon^+$, and the action of each is restricted to just the nucleus in which it resides. Thus, during repressing conditions achieved with excess sulfate or methionine, only the aryl sulfatase species encoded in the $scon^c$ nuclear type is synthesized, whereas both forms are produced during sulfur limitation. Nevertheless, it must be recalled that *scon* regulates the activity of several unlinked structural genes. The results suggest a situation in which the *scon* gene specifies a regulatory product that is freely diffusible within its nucleus but whose activity is confined to the same nucleus, or at least to the immediate vicinity of that nucleus. The product encoded by the *scon* locus might be synthesized within, and confined to, its nucleus or could be synthesized on the outer surface of the nucleus and immediately transported into, and restricted to, that nucleus. Alternatively, the *scon* product might only be limited to the vicinity of its own nucleus. In any case, the dominance test for $scon^c$ and $scon^+$ is meaningless in heterokaryons since the control is nucleus-limited, and there is, consequently, no clear basis to decide whether this locus acts in positive or negative control (partial diploids for the *scon* region of the genome have not yet been tested). One cannot help but wonder whether the *scon* product is a nuclear protein, some type of regulatory RNA species, or perhaps even an activity involved in the maturation or export from the nucleus of a specific class of mRNAs that encode sulfur-related enzymes. Finally, assuming for the moment that both *cys-3*[+] and *scon*[c] act at the level of transcription, it seems possible that these two regulatory genes are sequential in action, with *scon* sensing the sulfur status of the cell and inhibiting or repressing the *cys-3* gene product, which is responsible for "turning on" the entire group of sulfur-related genes. In agreement with this possibility is the finding that *scorn*[c] is hypostatic to *cys-3* since *scorn*[c] *cys-3* double mutants inevitably have the "null" phenotype identified with *cys-3* (Dietrich and Metzenberg, 1973).

The two distinct species of sulfate permease, one encoded by the *cys-13* locus and the second by *cys-14*, are primarily found in different cell types. The pattern of differential synthesis of these sulfate permease isozymes during particular stages indicates that an additional set of developmental controls is somehow superimposed upon the genetic and metabolic controls described above (Marzluf, 1972b). It is not clear whether the developmental regulation somehow interacts with the *scon-cys-3* system or acts independently. The synthesis of both choline sulfatase and aryl sulfatase during spore germination is also subject to developmental control (McGuire and Marzluf, 1974). The mechanism responsible for the developmental regulation of these enzymes and of others in similar situations is unknown, but this is clearly an intriguing area for potential study of developmentally related control elements. It can be hoped that such systems will also be susceptible to genetic disection, perhaps with the aid of mutants that either permit enzyme synthesis at developmentally incorrect times or else eliminate a specific phase of enzyme synthesis that normally occurs at two or more developmental times.

CONTROL OF PHOSPHORUS METABOLISM—SEQUENTIAL GENE ACTION

In *N. crassa* the synthesis of a number of enzymes involved in phosphorus metabolism is repressed as a group by high levels of inorganic phosphate or any similar favored source of phosphate. These include an alkaline phosphatase, an acid phosphatase, a high-affinity phosphate permease, O-phosphorylethanolamine permease, one or more nucleases, and likely additional related enzymes (Lehman et al., 1973; Nyc, 1967; Hasunuma, 1973; Lowendorf, Bazinet, and Slayman, 1975; Littlewood, Chia, and Metzenberg, 1975). At least three distinct regulatory genes control the synthesis of this entire family of phosphorus-related enzymes. Two separate mutants, *pcon*[c] and *preg*[c], lead to the constitutive synthesis of these enzymes, i.e., they are not repressible by high levels of phosphate. Two other mutants, *nuc-1* and *nuc-2*, are designated as "null" and are incapable of producing these same enzymes under any conditions. The *pcon^c* and *nuc-2* mutations actually lie within the same cistron but result in opposite phenotypes.

This wealth of regulatory mutants virtually assures the presence of a complex regulatory system and simultaneously foretells that any analysis of the system will be complicated and difficult. Metzenberg and his colleagues have, nevertheless, gained considerable insight concerning the control mechanism (Lehman et al., 1973; Metzenberg, Gleason, and Littlewood, 1974; Littlewood, Chia, and Metzenberg, 1975) which is summarized by the model presented in figure 5. The most unusual feature of this phosphorus-control system is the series of three sequential steps that necessarily precede the activation of the various structural genes. In this model the *nuc-1*⁺ gene, the final one of the regulatory series, specifies a product that has a positive role in "turning on" the various unlinked structural genes for alkaline phosphatase and its congeners. The *preg*⁺ product is postulated to act negatively to either inactivate or repress the synthesis of the *nuc-1*⁺ product. The *nuc-2*⁺ product likewise acts to inactivate or repress the *preg*⁺ product. The role of phosphate as a corepressor is most adequately explained if it converts the *nuc-2*⁺ product into an inactive form. Thus in the absence of repressing levels of phosphate, the *nuc-2*⁺ product interferes with *preg*⁺ action that permits synthesis of the *nuc-1*⁺ gene product that in turn activates the various structural genes. It is interesting to note that in this proposed system a control gene (*nuc-2*) with a negative action is, nevertheless, required for enzyme synthesis because of its position in the sequential series of regulatory steps.

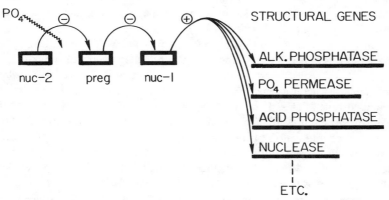

Fig. 5. Model of the sequential regulatory system that controls synthesis of phosphorus-related enzymes in *Neurospora*. The various structural genes that specify phosphorus-related enzymes are "turned on" by the *nuc-1* product. Synthesis or activity of the *nuc-1* product is controlled in a negative manner by the *preg* gene, which itself is controlled in a negative fashion by *nuc-2*. The *nuc-2* product is inactivated by phosphate.

Part of the evidence that supports this model of sequential gene action was obtained by studying the epistatic relationships that occur when two or more mutant genes are placed together in various combinations. For example, if the $nuc-1^+$ product acts in the final step and is indispensible for the expression of the structural genes, then the $nuc-1$ (null) mutant should be epistatic to all alleles of the *preg* locus and the $nuc-2$ locus. This is exactly what is found; the double mutant strains, $preg^c nuc-1$, $nuc-2 nuc-1$, and $pcon^c nuc-1$ as well as $nuc-2 preg^c nuc-1$, all show the "null" phenotype characteristic of $nuc-1$. In contrast, $nuc-2 preg^c$ displays the constitutive phenotype as expected if activity of the $nuc-2$ locus precedes and controls action of the *preg* cistron.

Additional evidence that supports the proposed model was obtained by studying the dominance relationships of the regulatory genes in heterokaryons and in partial diploids. A word here concerning the use of partial diploids in *Neurospora* is in order. The dominance or recessiveness of regulatory gene mutants (such as the "null" and constitutive mutants described here) is nearly always examined in heterokaryons that contain the mutant and wild-type alleles in separate nuclei. Any interpretation of such dominance studies is subject to serious reservations for at least two reasons. In the first place, the proportion of the two types of nuclei present within the heterokaryon can vary widely, and the different nuclei may even be largely segregated from each other. Second, any gene product that is not freely diffusible between nuclei can act only within its own nucleus. This difficulty can be used to advantage to reveal regulatory products that are normally confined to the nucleus (see above) but complicates dominance studies. To circumvent this problem, Metzenberg et al. (1974) made use of partial diploids obtained by crossing normal sequence strains with other strains carrying specific translocations of desired regions of the genome (Perkins, 1972).

$Nuc-1$ mutations ("null") are recessive to the wild-type allele in both heterokaryons and in partial diploids, which lends support to the conclusion that the $nuc-1^+$ gene encodes a diffusible product that is required to "turn on" the relevant structural genes. Similarly, both $nuc-2$ and $preg^c$ are recessive to their wild-type alleles. In contrast, $pcon^c$, whose phenotype is indistinguishable from $preg^c$, is dominant. All of these results are exactly as expected from the sequence and action of the regulatory genes as proposed in the model.

We should inquire into possible types of molecular interactions that might occur within this system of cascading control signals. The available evidence is best interpreted to suggest that the wild-type allele of the $nuc-1$, *preg*, and $nuc-2$ genes all specify a regulatory product that is freely diffusible, at least within its own nucleus. It has not been possible to critically test whether any of these control genes display nucleus-restricted activity because of the lack of electrophoretic or other suitable variants of any of the phosphorus-related enzymes. In each case it seems most plausible that the regulatory product is a macromolecule, likely either a protein or nucleic acid. The isolation of temperature-sensitive *nuc-2* mutants (Toh-E and Ishikawa, 1971; Littlewood et al., 1975) supports the notion that *nuc-2*$^+$ encodes a macromolecule.

It would be valuable to know the nature of the recognition sites for each of the postulated regulatory products. It would also be instructive to know the location of the structural genes that are regulated by this series of control elements. Mutants, designated *pho-2*, that completely lack the repressible alkaline phosphatase but have no other known effects have been isolated and mapped (Gleason and Metzenberg, 1974). The *pho-2* locus is probably the structural gene for the alkaline phosphatase; it is unlinked to any of the control genes described above. Since none of these *pho-2* mutants, or any revertants of them, specify a qualitatively altered enzyme, it is possible, but not likely, that they too are regulatory mutants. One mutant (MKG-2) that maps at the *pho-2* locus is particularly interesting since it makes a reduced amount (approximately 1%) of alkaline phosphatase that is very similar, or identical, to the wild-type enzyme. Alkaline phosphatase from the MKG-2 mutant strain is catalytically as active as the wild-type enzyme as judged by titration with specific antibody. The MKG-2 mutant (and even the "null" alleles) may represent a lesion in a regulatory region immediately adjacent to the *pho* structural gene and could possibly identify the receptor site for the positive control product elaborated by *nuc-1*$^+$. It would be interesting to know whether the low level of alkaline phosphatase synthesis that occurs in MKG-2 would still be found in the presence of a *nuc-1* mutation, i.e., could the former mutant in fact be a low-level initiator constitutive type.

One important lesson to be derived from the analysis of the phosphorus control system is the extreme importance of exhaustive attempts to isolate all of the possible types of regulatory mutants involved in a control system before using them to analyze the nature of the system. Furthermore, the familiar rule that mutational loss of function of a negative control gene results in constitutive enzyme synthesis but a similar lesion in a positive control gene causes a pleiotropic loss of the regulated enzymes cannot be safely applied when two or more regulatory genes are integrated into a sequential series. Here, *nuc-2* mutants are believed to occur in a negative control gene and yet cause a multiple loss of enzymes. Mutation in the first of two negatively acting genes ordered in a series could be easily misinterpreted as a positive control element.

Although it is not yet possible to specify the exact set of interactions that occurs between the phosphorous control genes, it seems likely that each specifies a regulatory product that acts in a definite sequential manner. One cannot help but wonder (and speculate) about the advantages to the cell in possessing such a complex system of cascading regulatory genes. What possible selective pressure would perfect and maintain such an involved regulatory system when, at face value, it would appear that the very same end could be achieved by a single control gene? Perhaps what we are observing is only the "tip" of a very intricate and highly complex regulatory system. One very speculative suggestion is that the regulatory system does not consist of a single series of sequential steps from *nuc-2* to *preg* to *nuc-1*, but instead involves a hierarchy of regulatory genes and a highly branched sequence of control steps. According to this suggestion, *nuc-2*, the "master" control gene of the sequence, may govern the activity of *preg* and several other similar intermediate-level regulatory genes; *preg*, in turn, may control not just *nuc-1* but a group of "final stage" positive regulatory genes, each of which activates a particular set of structural genes. Specific interactions with regulatory products at any level could modulate the control activity of any particular branch of the system. This model suggests that *nuc-2* mutants might be deficient in a multitude of phosphorus-related and perhaps even other types of enzymes (the enzymes could not be essential since *nuc-2* mutants have no nutritional requirements). Although such a complicated system seems unlikely in the case of the phosphorus-related enzymes, it is worth emphasizing that sequential gene action can be the basis of highly branched regulatory systems that could certainly yield many distinct patterns of enzyme synthesis, such as those characteristic of differentiated cell populations. Other possible cellular strategies for sequential control steps include the potential for specific timing of gene expression such as during the cell cycle or during different developmental stages. Other regulatory systems of fungi have also been reported to include sequential regulatory steps with combinations of positive and negative signals. These include those for acid phosphatase (Toh-E et al., 1973), arginase (Dubois, Grenson, and Wiame, 1974) and galactose metabolism in yeast (Douglas and Hawthorne, 1972; Klar and Halvorson, 1974). The presence of such complex regulatory systems in primitive eukaryotes certainly implies that we can anticipate in higher organisms highly intricate, multi-component control systems, such as those proposed by Britten and Davidson (1969).

INTEGRATED REGULATORY SYSTEMS: CONTROL OF
BRANCHED-CHAIN AMINO ACID SYNTHESIS

Gross and his coworkers have studied in much detail the biochemical genetics of leucine synthesis in *Neurospora* and interactions with the synthesis of isoleucine and valine. The regulatory mechanisms that serve to coordinate the synthesis of the branched chain amino acids appear to be a relatively

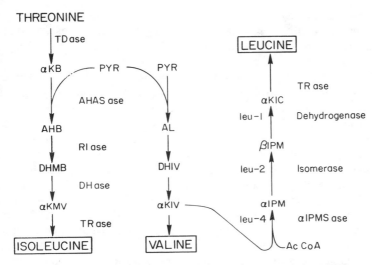

Fig. 6. Pathway of branched-chain amino acid biosynthesis. Abbreviations: PYR, pyruvate; αKB, α-ketobutyrate; DHMB, dihydroxymethylbutyrate; αKMV, α-ketomethylvalerate; AL, acetolactate; DHIV, dihydroxyisovalerate; αKIV, α-ketoisovalerate; AcCoA, acetyl Coenzyme A; αIPM, βIPM, α- and β-isopropylmalate; αKIC, α-ketoisocaproate; TDase, threonine deaminase; AHASase, acetohydroxyacid synthase; RIase, reductoisomerase; DHase, dehydratse; TRase, transaminase(s); α-IPMSase, α-isopropylmalate synthase. The enzymes of leucine synthesis specified by *leu-1, leu-2,* and *leu-4* are indicated.

simple, but nevertheless sophisticated, instance of regulation between related pathways. The pathways and corresponding structural genes involved in the synthesis of these three amino acids are shown in figure 6. Threonine deaminase, the first enzyme in the synthesis of isoleucine, converts threonine into α-ketobutyrate. It is a cytoplasmic enzyme and is inhibited by isoleucine. Four enzymatic steps are required in the conversion of α-KB into isoleucine. These very same four enzymes perform essentially identical reactions in the formation of valine from pyruvate. The last intermediate in the synthesis of valine, α-ketoisovalerate (α-KIV), is also the precursor for leucine biosynthesis.

The four enzymes common to the synthesis of isoleucine and valine are coded by nuclear genes but are located in the mitochondrial matrix, perhaps in an aggregate (Cassady et al., 1972). The individual enzymes, when isolated, have substantial activity, suggesting that the aggregate may not be absolutely essential for synthesis of the amino acid products (Altmiller and Wagner, 1970; Leiter et al., 1971). The enzyme aggregate may be quite important, however, for regulatory interactions and for metabolic channeling. The enzyme acetohydroxyacid synthase (AHASase) can be studied in intact mitochondria, in which it is inhibited by valine. Upon solubilization its valine sensitivity is rapidly lost and several other properties change, suggesting that normal regulation and function of AHASase require that it be integrated within the enzyme complex.

At least two different regulatory signals are involved in modulating the synthesis of the leucine biosynthetic enzymes of *Neurospora* (Gross, 1965). Synthesis of the first enzyme unique to leucine production (α-IPM synthetase) is controlled in a negative manner, being repressed by leucine or, more likely, a repressor complex containing leucine. It appears that leucyl-tRNA is not involved in repression since temperature-sensitive mutants of the leucyl-tRNA synthetase (*leu-5* gene) display normal control of the leucine biosynthetic enzymes at all temperatures. Little else is known concerning this negative signal and in particular neither operator-type (O^c) mutants nor mutants that encode an aporepressor have been identified. Activity of the first enzyme is controlled by feedback inhibition by leucine, limiting synthesis of α-IPM, the inducer of enzymes 2 and 3.

The *leu-3* cistron has been found to be a positive regulatory gene that controls the synthesis of all three enzymes specific for leucine formation. The *leu-3* product plus the positive effector, α-isopropylmalate (α-IPM), are required for expression of the *leu-1* and *leu-2* genes that encode, respectively, β-IPM dehydrogenase and α-IPM isomerase. In addition, the *leu-3* product is required to attain maximum derepression of the first enzyme, α-IPM synthetase, which is specified by *leu-4* and of a branched-chain amino acid permease (Polacco and Gross, 1973). The *leu-1, leu-2,* and *leu-4* genes are unlinked, and *leu-3* is only distantly linked to *leu-4*. Yet, the *leu-3* gene product clearly controls in a parallel (usually coordinated) manner the enzymes encoded by the *leu* structural genes.

The *leu-3*$^+$ gene product (plus α-IPM) may act at the transcriptional level by binding adjacent to each of the structural gene loci to activate their expression. Very recent studies (Reichenberger, Fischer, and Gross, 1975) using cycloheximide and proflavin to inhibit protein and RNA synthesis, respectively, indicate that both messenger RNA and protein synthesis are required for induction of the leucine biosynthetic enzymes. Furthermore, the mRNA for the isomerase has a half life of only a few minutes, whereas the enzyme itself is fully stable. Polacco and Gross (1973) have argued that the *leu-3*$^+$ product must have at least three distinct functional regions, namely, (1) a site for recognition of DNA sequences adjacent to *leu-1*, and similar cistrons, (2) a binding site for the inducer, α-IPM, and (3) a binding site for branched-chain amino acids (see below). If, as has been suggested, the *leu-3* product exists in a multimeric state, a fourth region responsible for subunit association might also be postulated. It is difficult to conceive that any macromolecule other than a protein could possess so many functional sites. However, there is as yet no direct, or even indirect, evidence which argues that the regulatory product is a protein. No temperature-sensitive *leu-3* auxotrophs or *leu-3* revertants have been found in spite of a major effort to identify such mutants (Polacco and Gross, 1973). Furthermore, intragenic complementation has not been found with *leu-3* mutants nor have any suppressible nonsense mutants of the *leu-3* cistron been obtained.

Convincing evidence exists to support the concept that the *leu-3*[+] product binds the inducer, α-IPM, to form an active regulatory complex. A group of intracistronic (or very closely linked) partial revertants of *leu-3*, designated *leu-3*[cc] (see below), were found to be constitutive for the *leu-1* and *leu-2* coded enzymes. The *leu-3*[cc] strains have intermediate levels of the isomerase and the dehydrogenase, but unlike wild type, do not require the inducer α-IMP for synthesis of these enzymes. The inducer, α-IMP, is not transported by *Neurospora;* however, by the use of mutant strains with widely varying levels of endogenous α-IPM, it was demonstrated that *leu-3*[cc] alleles were insensitive to the inducer. Quite recently, Reichenberger, Fischer, and Gross (1975) have used the *leu-4* strain to isolate a secondary mutant that can utilize α-IPM to fulfill its leucine requirement. This new mutant transports α-IPM, permitting a direct demonstration that exogenously supplied α-IPM does induce synthesis of the isomerase.

The amount of the isomerase and dehydrogenase enzymes present in the *leu-3*[cc] mutants could not be elevated any further even in the presence of an excess of α-IPM. This result indicates that the regulatory product specified by *leu-3*[cc] is active without inducer, which implies that the *leu-3*[+] product has a binding site for α-IPM. The *leu-3*[cc] strains are not simply constitutive but require the presence of isoleucine and valine for growth and for the synthesis of *leu-1* and *leu-2* enzymes and therefore were designated *leu-3*[cc] (for conditional constitutive mutants). These findings suggest that the *leu-3*[+] product may have a binding site for branched-chain amino acids although it is difficult to assess whether the wild-type product is active or inactive when this site is occupied.

Olshan and Gross (1974) have found that the *leu-3* product and the positive effector are also involved in regulating the synthesis of the isoleucine and valine biosynthetic enzymes. Even when severely restricted for relevant products, both *leu-3* and *leu-4* mutants fail to display elevated levels of the isoleucine and valine enzymes, which instead remain at the basal level found in wild type during full end-product repression. It is postulated that the *leu-3* product–α-IPM regulatory complex can recognize and bind to regulatory sequences, perhaps within a promoter region, adjacent to each of the pertinent structural genes. This binding may facilitate transcription of this set of genes.

The 7 to 8 individual structural genes are widely scattered in the genome and include the cistrons for isoleucine and valine synthesis, those for leucine synthesis, plus one for a branched chain amino acid permease. Each structural gene may have a similar but possibly different sequence for recognition of the *leu-3* product, similar to the "address" sites suggested by Paul (1972). Thus it appears that the *leu-3* product plays an important role in coordinating the synthesis of the biosynthetic enzymes for all of the branched-chain amino acids. Quite obviously, mutational identification of one or more of the postulated individual *cis*-acting recognition sequences (e.g., as I^c constitutive mutants) would greatly facilitate analysis of this system. Isolation and study of the molecular mechanism of action of the *leu-3*$^+$ product and its various mutant forms will also be of considerable interest. The binding of α-IPM by the *leu-3*$^+$ regulatory product should provide a convenient means for assay and purification of this element. A fine-structure genetic analysis of the *leu-3* cistron might be also instructive in assigning a specific genetic region to a particular regulatory site of the gene product.

In contrast to the situation just described in *Neurospora,* in *S. cerevisiae* the enzyme threonine deaminase has been suggested to have a dual role. In addition to its catalytic function it may also serve as a positive regulatory protein for the synthesis of all of the branched-chain amino acid biosynthetic enzymes. Mutants (*ilv-1*) lacking or having an altered form of threonine deaminase were unable to derepress the *ilv* biosynthetic enzymes when starved for the end-product amino acids (Bollon and Magee, 1973). Bollon (1974) analyzed the fine structure of the *ilv-1* cistron and was able to identify certain segments of the gene related to catalytic, regulatory, and allosteric functions.

CROSS-PATHWAY REGULATION

In bacteria, starvation for an amino acid usually leads to derepression of the biosynthetic enzymes for that particular amino acid. In contrast, in *N. crassa* and *S. cerevisiae,* starvation for a single amino acid may cause derepression of the biosynthetic enzymes for other amino acids as well as those of the deficient amino acid. This phenomenon, known as cross-pathway regulation, has been studied with the histidine, tryptophan, and arginine pathways (Carsiotis et al., 1970). The effect is totally reciprocal, since starvation for any one of these three amino acids derepresses the synthesis of all three sets of biosynthetic enzymes (Carsiotis and Jones, 1974; Carsiotis, Jones, and Wesseling, 1974). The amount of derepression achieved due to the effect of cross-pathway control is approximately the same as obtained when the specific amino acid is limited.

One possible explanation for this effect is that starvation for a specific amino acid, e.g., tryptophan, might also lead to a decreased intracellular concentration of related amino acids and, consequently, to derepression of their respective biosynthetic enzymes. Carsiotis and Jones (1974) found that upon starving a tryptophan auxotroph of *Neurospora* for tryptophan, the enzymes for histidine and arginine synthesis were dramatically elevated even though the cellular content of these amino acids was actually higher than in control (non-starved) cells. Furthermore, the addition of exogenous histidine to tryptophan-starved cells did not prevent derepression of the *his* biosynthetic enzymes, although the histidine pool was elevated 15-fold. However, these results are not completely conclusive since it is known that *Neurospora* possesses at least two distinct intracellular pools of arginine and tryptophan. Thus it is possible that starvation for a specific amino acid somehow causes a redistribution of other amino acids between functionally distinct pools (e.g., pools for protein synthesis, regulation, storage, and catabolism), leading to a lower concentration in the pool that functions in repression. Such an indirect mechanism could serve to coordinate the synthesis of these amino acids, yielding the tripartite regulatory pattern. Transfer RNA species may be involved in cross-pathway regulation. A *Neurospora* mutant with a defective tryptophanyl-tRNA synthetase has elevated levels not only of the *trp* biosynthetic enzymes but also those for histidine and arginine biosynthesis (Carsiotis, 1973). Possibly the cellular pool of specific-charged tRNAs are instrumental in cross-pathway control. Direct studies of the nature and responses of the separate cellular pools of amino acids may provide insight into this phenomenon.

Another possible mechanism for cross-pathway regulation suggests the involvement of a multivalent regulatory signal such that the formation of an active repressor (or activator) complex requires the presence of each of the individual amino acids, perhaps charged to their cognate tRNAs, plus an aporepressor. Such a repressor complex could act at the transcriptional or translational level to provide a coordinated control of all three sets of biosynthetic enzymes, perhaps in a manner similar to that suggested for the coordinated regulation of the branched-chain amino acids (see above). It is significant in this regard that no clustering of the structural genes for the histidine, tryptophan, or arginine enzymes occurs in *Neurospora*. The postulated aporepressor might even be an indispensible macromolecule with multiple functions, e.g., an enzyme such as glutamine synthetase, which has been demonstrated to play a regulatory role in nitrogen metabolism in *Salmonella typhimurium* (Tyler, Deleo, and Magasanik, 1974). In this context it is interesting that glutamine serves as a precursor for the synthesis of arginine, histidine, tryptophan, and also lysine, which has recently been shown to be involved in this same cross-pathway regulatory system. Synthesis of other aromatic and aliphatic amino acids has not been so implicated. Mutations of control genes that alter cross-pathway regulation or affect the synthesis of specific sets of biosynthetic enzymes would greatly facilitate further analysis of this phenomenon.

Some pertinent studies have been accomplished in *S. cerevisiae* (Schurch, Miozzari, and Hutter, 1974; Greer and Fink, 1975). A mutant, designated as *aas,* that fails to display cross-pathway regulation has been isolated as well as another mutant (*tra-3*) that is constitutive for these sets of enzymes. The double mutant strain, *aas tra-3,* displays the *tra-3* phenotype, synthesizing the biosynthetic enzymes in a constitutive fashion. This result suggests that the wild-type *tra*$^+$ gene encodes an aporepressor for negative control of the enzymes. It is most interesting that the *tra-3* mutants are temperature-conditional lethals and thus may play a broader role in regulatory interactions or have other critical functions. The role of the wild-type allele of the *aas* cistron is more difficult to specify, although it has been speculated to work by inactivating the *tra-3*$^+$ product during conditions of amino acid limitation. This postulated sequence of two negative steps could have been easily mistaken for simple positive control if only *aas* mutants were known.

Although cross-pathway regulation is not ordinarily found in bacteria, it has been demonstrated in *N. crassa, S. cerevisiae,* and *Euglena gracilis,* which suggests that this type of control may be widespread in eukaryotic organisms (Carsiotis and Jones, 1974). It remains to be seen whether other patterns for coordinated regulation of different sets of amino acid biosynthetic enzymes may also exist. In what other pathways may there be hidden interdependent regulatory systems that serve to integrate metabolism—perhaps on a much grander scale than we can now envisage?

NITROGEN REGULATION IN FUNGI

A wealth of studies concerning nitrogen metabolism and its control in fungi have been reported recently, particularly in *A. nidulans* and *S. cerevisiae,* and to a lesser extent in *Neurospora.* Nitrogen catabolite repression, often referred to as ammonium repression, governs the synthesis of many enzyme systems involved in the catabolism of various nitrogen sources.

It now seems certain in *Aspergillus* that the synthesis of many nitrogen-related enzymes, such as nitrate reductase, uricase, xanthine dehydrogenase, and extracellular protease requires that two conditions be met. First, there must be a lifting of nitrogen catabolite repression (by growth in very low concentrations of ammonium or in some less-favored nitrogen source). Second, in many cases, specific induction of the enzymes of a particular catabolic pathway by a substrate or intermediate of that pathway must also occur. Distinct regulatory genes appear to mediate the separate steps of repression and induction.

A regulatory gene of *Aspergillus,* which is central to nitrogen catabolite repression, has been identified and designated *areA* (for ammonium repression). Many mutants that appear to be leisions in *areA* have been isolated and display a variety of phenotypic effects (Hynes, 1972; Hynes and Pateman, 1970; Cohen, 1972; Arst and Cove, 1973). One type, designated *areA*^{r} (for repressed) results in the inability to utilize a wide variety of nitrogen sources, such as purines, amino acids, amides, nitrate, and nitrite. Furthermore, the *areA*^{r} mutants cannot be derepressed in the synthesis of certain nitrogen-related enzymes and thus seem analogous to the "null" alleles of regulatory genes described earlier (*nuc-1, cys-3, qa-1*^{F}, *leu-3,* etc.). However, a rather unusual property of *areA* mutants has been found. Different alleles of the *areA* type each show individual patterns of partial or complete loss of enzymes and of nitrogen source utilization and may or may not have temperature sensitivities. One allele, *areA*^{r}-*217,* which was actually isolated from a parental strain already carrying an *areA* mutant (*areA-102*), grows very poorly on all nitrogen sources except NH_4^+. Still others grow even better than wild type on some N sources (e.g., acetamide) but fail to use certain other N-sources, e.g., uric acid.

The second type of mutants, *areA*^{d} (for derepressed), lead to the loss of ammonium repression for certain nitrogen-related enzymes. One of these, which was originally called *xprD-1* but now appears to be an *areA*^{d} mutant, cannot be repressed by NH_4^+ for the synthesis of many enzymes, including nitrate reductase, xanthine dehydrogenase, uricase, and extracellular protease, (Cohen, 1972) acetamidase (Hynes, 1972), and separate permeases for glutamate and for urea (Pateman et al., 1973). All of these enzymes still require induction, however, indicating that the *areA* gene is concerned only with nitrogen catabolite repression. The distinction between *areA*^{r} and *areA*^{d} alleles is far from absolute since a particular *areA* mutant may be derepressed for one ammonium-repressible activity, be normally repressible for another, and lead to abnormally low levels for a third. Consequently each *areA* mutant really has its own highly specific phenotype. It is rather unusual, furthermore, that *areA* mutants cannot only eliminate ammonium repression (or derepression) but can also increase the maximum level of enzyme(s) above that achieved in wild type. For example, *areA-102* can utilize acrylamide and acetamide much better than wild type and has an enhanced level of acetamidase (Hynes and Pateman, 1970) but simultaneously lower than normal levels of nitrate reductase and uric/xanthine permease. These characteristics suggest a functional overlap between the promoter and a binding site for the *areA* regulatory product.

It is believed that the *areA* locus encodes a protein that serves as a positive control element and is essential for the synthesis of the various nitrogen-related enzymes. It is presumably rendered nonfunctional in the presence of ammonium. The heterogeneity of phenotypes exhibited by different *areA* alleles strongly supports the suggestion that this locus encodes a macromolecule, likely a protein, rather than specifying an enzyme responsible for the synthesis of a small molecule involved in derepression. It is not yet clear whether the *areA* product acts at the transcriptional, translational, or yet another level. The *areA* product might also exert some negative effect in addition to its positive role, the latter of which seems clearly established. Dominance studies with *areA* alleles support a positive mode of action; the *areA*^{r} alleles (repressed phenotype) are all recessive to wild type while *areA*^{d} are semi-dominant to *areA*$^+$. A fine-structure analysis of the *areA* locus is badly needed to help understand the relationship of the various types of alleles to each other and, indeed, to ensure that all occur within a single gene.

Upon release from nitrogen catabolite repression, the synthesis of many of the nitrogen-related enzymes in *Aspergillus* requires induction by a substrate or intermediate of the particular catabolic pathway. Regulatory genes whose actions are specific for particular enzymes or pathways intervene in the inductive process, and have been identified by the use of mutants in several instances. The induction by nitrate of nitrate and nitrite reductases requires the activity of a gene designated *nirA*$^+$, for which both "null" (*nirA*$^-$) and constitutive (*nirA*^{c}) alleles are known. Similarly, acetamidase induction depends upon a regulatory gene *amdR,* and both "null" and constitutive mutants of it exist. A gene, *ua-Y,* that controls the induction of the enzymes for purine catabolism has also been identified. In each case the properties of the mutants strongly suggest that the wild-type form of the control gene is required for induction and acts in a positive way to "turn on" enzyme synthesis.

What is the relationship of the specific control genes responsible for induction and the *areA* product? It now seems that their control functions are exerted independently of one another. If the *areA* product is indispensable for the synthesis of the various nitrogen enzymes, *areA*^{r} ("null") should be epistatic to constitutive alleles of the various pathway specific genes, as *nirA*^{c}, *amdR*^{c}, and *ua-Y*^{c}, when present with one of them in a double mutant. This result is obtained, namely the relevant enzymes for nitrate reduction cannot be derepressed in *areA*^{r} *nirA*^{c} under any condition. In an analogous way, *nirA*$^-$ (not inducible) is epistatic to *areA*^{d} (derepressed) and the relevant enzymes cannot be induced in the double mutant. This outcome favors a model in which the regulatory product of both the $areA^+$ gene and the $nirA^+$ gene are independently required to "turn on" the structural genes or at some other step preceding or accompanying enzyme synthesis. Their activities could work at the same step or at entirely separate levels, e.g., one, activating transcription, and a second, translation. Sequential gene action in which these lie in series is virtually excluded since constitutive mutants of the final one should be epistatic to any alleles of the other gene.

CARBON CATABOLITE REPRESSION

The mechanism of carbon catabolite repression in bacteria has been largely elucidated, but the manner in which glucose and other favored carbon sources prevent the synthesis of many enzymes relevant to carbon metabolism in eukaryotes is not yet understood. Bailey and Arst (1975) have isolated mutants in *Aspergillus* named $creA^d$, which are defective in carbon catabolite repression, by selecting for activity of specific catabolite-repressible enzymes in the presence of high levels of glucose. The four, independently isolated, mutants obtained so far all map at the same genetic locus and, interestingly, lead to a compact colony morphology. Synthesis of certain enzymes are relieved of catabolite repression while other enzymes are still subject to its effects in $creA^d$ mutants. The $creA^d$-1 mutant was shown not to alter glucose transport, thus eliminating the possible trivial explanation of exclusion of carbon catabolite-repressing compounds.

Very similar results have been found with yeast mutants that are altered in catabolite repression, including the presence of morphological abnormalities (Ghosh, Montenecourt, and Lampen, 1973). A similar locus has apparently not yet been found in *Neurospora*, although the colonial mutant known as *frost* has a reduced cAMP level and an altered adenyl cyclase (Scott, Mishra, and Tatum, 1973).

Arst and MacDonald (1975) have suggested that carbon catabolite repression might be mediated by a negative control mechanism in *A. nidulans* on the basis of recessive behavior of $creA^d$ mutants, which result in the loss of sensitivity to catabolite repression (see above). Furthermore, extensive attempts to obtain single mutants defective in the use of several carbon sources have failed, which is consistent with the expected rarity of super-repressed phenotype. They also reported that neither cyclic AMP nor its dibutyryl derivative seem to reverse the effects of catabolite repression in *Aspergillus*, although there is no evidence that these possible effectors actually gain entrance into the cells. In contrast, cyclic-3', 5'-AMP and 8-bromo-cAMP, but not 5' AMP, 3' AMP, or 2,3-cAMP, induce the synthesis of tyrosinase in

Neurospora (Feldman and Thayer, 1974). It was also found that caffeine and theophylline, potent inhibitors of cyclic AMP phosphodiesterase, cause highly elevated levels of tyrosinase. This result suggests that tyrosinase is subject to carbon catabolite repression and that cAMP may indeed be an effector molecule in *Neurospora*. This organism clearly possesses adenyl cylase, cAMP, and cAMP phosphodiesterase.

Enzymes for the utilization of compounds that contain carbon but not nitrogen (e.g., acetate) might be expected to be under carbon catabolite repression and subject to control by the *creA* locus. Similarly, enzymes for the use of compounds containing just nitrogen (e.g., nitrate) should only be controlled by ammonium repression (*areA* gene). However, the metabolism of compounds that can be used as both nitrogen and carbon source (e.g., acetamide or proline) may well be subject to both N and C regulation. This suggestion implies that the structural genes encoding certain enzymes may be subject to multiple control signals; the mechanism by which such complex control is exerted is of great current interest. The evidence available at present is quite limited but suggests that C and N regulation are exerted by independent mechanisms, although some degree of interaction between them may occur.

Such considerations suggest that some structural genes coding for enzymes in eukaryotes may be served by a relatively large adjacent region containing one or more recognition sites involved in their regulation. Several interesting genetic studies attempting to define such regions have recently been reported. Two putative structural genes (in *Aspergillus*) that specify activities involved in proline catabolism were found to be very tightly linked to each other (Arst and MacDonald, 1975). The *prnA* locus is thought to encode a protein subunit common to proline oxidase and pyrroline-5-carboxylate dehydrogenase while *prnB* apparently codes for a proline permease. Proline oxidase is subject to both N- and C-catabolite repression whereas proline transport is only regulated by C-catabolite repression in *Aspergillus*. A regulatory mutant, *prn*[d], which acts only *cis* and results in the derepression of these proline metabolic enzymes, was found to map between the *prnA* and *prnB* loci, both of which it apparently controls (*prn*[d] was isolated as a suppressor of an *areA*[r] mutant and uniquely permits utilization of proline as a nitrogen source). Arst and Mac-Donald (1975) favor a model in which the two structural genes have a divergent orientation but are served by a common internal control region. This is an obvious way in which to organize two or more clustered genes that share at least one common control element but also have one (or more) control elements that are not shared. The two *prn* genes (*prnA* and *prnB*) appear to share two regulatory signals, one for induction and one for carbon-catabolite repression. An alteration of the receptor element for carbon repression seems to explain the derepressed phenotype of the *prn*ᵈ mutant. The *prnA* gene alone is also subject to ammonium repression and thus should have an adjacent recognition region for the *areA* positive regulatory product; this recognition site quite possibly also lies between *prnA* and *prnB* but it so situated that it can only activate transcription of the *prnB* locus.

In another study (Arst and Scazzocchio, 1975) with *Aspergillus* designed to detect regulatory elements next to structural genes, revertants of an *areA*ʳ mutant were selected for restoration of a xanthine/uric acid permease. One revertant (*uap-100*) occurred as a rare cis-dominant mutation that mapped immediately adjacent to the putative structure gene (*uapA*) of the permease while the original *areA*ʳ mutant was unchanged. This new mutant resulted in constitutive synthesis of the permease while all other activities missing in *areA-102* were still absent, as expected. Furthermore, *uap-100* displays an "up-promoter" effect since the maximum level of permease is 2.5 times higher than found in wild type. This strain still requires induction, mediated by another positive control gene, *uaY*⁺. The characteristics of *uap-100* are best interpreted to indicate that it is an initiator constitutive mutant which is altered in such a way that, unlike the usual sequence, it can recognize the mutant *areA* product specified by *areA-102*. The concomitant "up-promoter" effect further suggests a functional overlap of the control sites for reception of positive signals (for induction and derepression) with the promoter region.

In a remarkably similar manner, Hynes (1975) isolated a *cis*-dominant Iᶜ-type mutation termed *amdI9* in *Aspergillus* that resulted in derepressed synthesis of acetamidase without affecting the synthesis of other nitrogen-related enzymes. This mutant mapped at the structural gene (*amdS*) which encodes acetamidase, an enzyme whose synthesis requires induction and is subject to both nitrogen and carbon-catabolite repression. The *amd 19* lesion also appears to have an "up-promoter" effect since it results in unusually high levels of acetamidase, which is indistinguishable from the wild-type enzyme by several sensitive criteria (electrophoretic mobility, thermolability, and substrate specificity). These several studies have apparently identified regulatory regions that serve as address sites for particular structural genes. There is a genuine need to isolate and characterize similar cis-acting control mutants in many other fungal regulatory systems and to better understand the regulatory sequences that they identify.

GLUTAMATE DEHYDROGENASE — A REGULATORY PROTEIN?

A new concept that has emerged in recent years in several bacterial systems is that some enzymes serve a significant regulatory function in addition to their familiar catalytic role (Goldberger, 1974; Goldberger and Deeley, this volume). It appears that in both *S. cerevisiae* and *A. nidulans* the enzyme NADP-linked glutamic dehydrogenase (NADP-GDH) may, quite independently of its catalytic function, be a regulatory protein having a major role in the control of nitrogen-related enzymes. Mutations in *gdhA,* the structural locus for NADP-GDH in both of these organisms, relieve the usual ammonium repression of many enzymes, including nitrate reductase, xanthine dehydrogenase, allantoicase, and general amino acid transport (Grenson et al., 1974; Dubois et al., 1973; Pateman et al., 1973). The regulatory defect of the *gdhA* mutants could not be accounted for by a deficiency of glutamate or by an accumulation of the enzyme substrates. Thus NADP-GDH may play a direct role in nitrogen catabolite repression in these fungi, perhaps much in the same way that glutamine synthetase functions in *Salmonella typhimurium* (Tyler, DeLeo, and Magasanik, 1974). Pateman et al. (1973) observed that the level of a permease for ammonium was regulated by the intracellular NH_4^+ concentration, while the synthesis of other N-related enzymes including nitrate reductase and xanthine dehydrogenase was instead controlled by the extracellular concentration of NH_4^+. Because both types of ammonium repression were eliminated by *gdhA* mutants, they suspect that NADP-GDH mediates both effects, and have proposed a mechanism to explain the diverse results. They suggested that NADP-glutamate dehydrogenase located in the cell membrane can sense extracellular ammonium and assume a conformation that represses nitrate reductase, xanthine dehydrogenase, and so on, whereas NADP-GDH contained in the cytoplasm can bind intracellular NH_4^+ and form a different regulatory complex that determines the level of ammonium uptake (by repression or inhibition).

The role of NADP-GDH has been questioned by Arst and Cove (1973), who argue that it probably acts in a more indirect manner such as affecting the intracellular distribution of ammonium. Along with other evidence, they point out that *areA^r-1* mutant is epistatic to *gdh-10* (the double mutant lacks the relevant enzymes rather than being derepressed for them), which implies that the *areA* product plays a later and more direct role in N-regulation than the *gdhA* product. Whatever its exact mechanism of action, it seems well established that NADP-GDH is intimately involved in nitrogen catabolite repression, and additional studies of its role should be illuminating. Both detailed protein chemistry and genetic studies of NADP-glutamate dehydrogenase of *N. crassa* have been accomplished. It is unfortunate and surprising that any possible role that it has in nitrogen catabolite repression has yet to be established. The wealth of *am* mutants, which includes complementing and noncomplementing alleles and nonsense mutants containing only a fragment of the enzyme protein, should provide excellent subjects to investigate the regulatory role, if any, of NADP-GDH in *Neurospora.*

NITRATE REDUCTASE AND AUTOGENOUS REGULATION

The regulation of the pathway for nitrate reduction has been studied in *A. nidulans* and in *N. crassa* and several unusual phenomena have been revealed. In *A. nidulans,* synthesis of nitrate reductase and nitrite reductase is controlled by both induction and ammonium repression. The product of a regulatory gene, *nirA*+, is believed to mediate induction and is required for the production of both of these enzymes. Furthermore, nitrate reductase has been postulated to play a regulatory role in its own synthesis. It has been suggested that the positive acting form of the *nirA*+ product is achieved or stabilized by interaction with nitrate reductase in the presence of nitrate (Cove and Pateman, 1969). Conversely, when complexed with ammonium, nitrate reductase is postulated to convert the *nirA*+ product into a repressor for these same enzymes. These effects could be exerted at the transcriptional, translational, or even other levels. The key observation that suggests this model is that many mutants that lack nitrate reductase result in the constitutive synthesis of the other enzymes of the same pathway. The auto-regulatory role postulated for nitrate reductase is clearly quite speculative, but it should provide a valuable focal point for further investigation. It seems difficult to conceive that the large number of elements that have been implicated in the regulation of nitrate reductase could all be directly involved in the control system. At first glance, there simply seems to be too many control elements, namely, the *areA* product, the *nirA* product, possibly glutamate dehydrogenase, plus nitrate reductase itself. On the other hand, these elements could act at several different levels and provide a more sophisticated and integrated control system than might presently be imagined.

Mutations at five separate loci result in a lack of nitrate reductase activity in *N. crassa,* but the genetic basis of its structure and regulation is still not well understood. *Nit-1* mutants are deficient in a small molecular weight (less than 1,000 daltons) molybdenum cofactor that is also an essential component of xanthine dehydrogenase. Consequently, *nit-1* mutants cannot use nitrate or hypoxanthine as a N-source, but grow normally on later intermediates of either pathway. The *nit-3* locus is the only one for which there is convincing evidence that it encodes an essential polypeptide of nitrate reductase. It seems quite possible that as yet unidentified structural genes may specify other subunits of the enzyme. Mutants of *nit-2, nit-4,* and *nit-5* loci lack both nitrate and nitrite reductases and seem likely to be regulatory genes. Indeed, *nit-2* has recently been shown to be a major regulatory gene that controls the synthesis of many N-related enzymes (Reinert and Marzluf, 1975a).

It was long suspected that the synthesis of nitrate reductase in *N. crassa* required induction by nitrate, most easily interpreted as occurring at the transcriptional level. Sorger and his associates (Subramanian and Sorger, 1972, a, b; Sorger and Davies, 1973; Sorger, Debanne, and Davies, 1974) have used actinomycin D and cycloheximide to analyze the effects of nitrate, ammonia, and nitrogen starvation upon the events of transcription and translation. The rather unexpected results indicate that nitrate is not required for transcription or stability of the mRNA. Rather, nitrate stabilizes nitrate reductase, which in its absence undergoes rapid inactivation. Ammonia represses transcription of the mRNA and also interferes with either the synthesis or stability of the enzyme. It is noteworthy that control of nitrate reductase may be exerted at many levels, transcription, translation, and in the functional half lives of the respective products. Although it is difficult to accept results obtained with the use of inhibitors without some reservations, the complicated picture revealed for control of nitrate reductase is likely to be generally correct and should serve as a warning not to interpret experimental results too simply, nor to assume that regulation will occur solely at the transcriptional level.

PURINE CATABOLISM IN FUNGI

Allantoin can serve as the sole nitrogen source in *S. cerevisiae,* and its catabolism requires five enzymes, at least four of which are induced by allophanic acid, the last intermediate of the pathway. The pertinent structural genes are located in two unlinked clusters, each with two cistrons (Lawther et al., 1974). The enzymes urea carboxylase and allophanate hydrolase form a multienzyme complex and are encoded by contiguous genes in one cluster. The structural genes of the other cluster encode allantoinase and allantoicase, which, however, seem to exist as separate enzymes (Lawther et al., 1974). These four enzymes are induced in a parallel manner by allophanate.

Lawther and Cooper (1973) noted that allophanic hydrolase enzyme activity increased within 3 minutes upon the addition of inducer to a culture. The capacity for enzyme synthesis, i.e., the messenger RNA, also decayed very rapidly with a functional half-life of only 3 minutes. Other yeast enzymes required about 10 minutes for induction, and their mRNAs had a half-life of 20 minutes. These observations suggested the possibility that allophanic hydrolase (and, presumably, the other three related enzymes) is controlled at a post-transcriptional step. To examine this possibility in detail, Lawther and Cooper (1975) used lomofungin and cycloheximide to specifically interfere with transcription and translation, respectively. Lomofungin apparently acts by chelating the divalent metal cations required by RNA polymerase (Lawther, Phillips, and Cooper, 1975). These studies revealed that: (1) induction of the hydrolase begins immediately upon adding the inducer; (2) induction of the capacity to make the enzyme (i.e., presumably its mRNA) occurs in the absence of protein synthesis; (3) half-life of the mRNA increases when protein synthesis is blocked; and (4) the enzyme itself is not degraded in the absence of inducer. They concluded that the addition of inducer had two effects. First, it immediately increased hydrolase mRNA synthesis, and second, it also influenced the rate of messenger translation. Thus in this case it appears that both induction and repression do act at the transcriptional level, but that the inducer also controls the rate of enzyme synthesis.

Both *N. crassa* and *A. nidulans* can utilize various purine bases such as xanthine or uric acid as their sole nitrogen source, and control of this pathway is very similar in these two organisms (Scazzocchio and Darlington, 1968). In *N. crassa,* Reinert and Marzluf (1975a) have isolated putative structural gene mutants for most of the catabolic enzymes. Two types of mutants lack xanthine dehydrogenase activity. The first mutant, *nit-1,* is deficient in both nitrate reductase and xanthine dehydrogenase because it lacks a molybdenum cofactor shared by these two enzymes. The second type of mutant, *xdh,* lacks only xanthine dehydrogenase and may be the structural gene for this enzyme. Allantoinase and allantoicase are apparently encoded by the genes *aln* and *alc.* None of these genes are linked to each other or to a common regulatory gene. The last two enzymes of the pathway, urease and ureidoglycolate hydrolase, are constitutive, whereas synthesis of the earlier enzymes requires both induction and nitrogen-derepression. By the use of mutant strains blocked at specific steps in the degradative pathway, it was concluded that uric acid is the genuine inducer of these enzymes (Reinert and Marzluf, 1975 a, b). Hypoxanthine can be metabolized to yield the inducer but is not itself an inducer of the purine enzymes. Both uricase and allantoinase are stable enzymes, whereas allantoinase is quite labile both *in vivo* and *in vitro,* with a half-life *in vivo* of approximately 20 minutes in the presence of cycloheximide. It is not clear whether allantoinase turnover contributes to the control of flow along this pathway.

The regulated purine enzymes are all present in only basal levels in mutants of a control gene designated *amr* (for ammonium regulation). The *amr* gene appears to play a major role in the control of nitrogen metabolism in *Neurospora* and may be similar to the *areA* gene of *Aspergillus.* Mutation at the *amr* (also called *nit-2*) locus confers a pleiotropic loss in the ability of *Neurospora* to utilize a large number of nitrogen sources, including nitrate, nitrite, purines, many amino acids, and exogenous proteins. It appears that the *amr* product is required for "turning on" the expression of many genes subject to nitrogen catabolite repression. The *amr* mutants are deficient in many enzymes, including nitrate reductase, nitrite reductase, the purine catabolic enzymes, an extracellular protease, amino acid transport, uric acid and xanthine transport, and probably numerous other activities (Reinert and Marzluf, 1975 a, b; Facklam and Marzluf, 1975; Tsao and Marzluf, unpublished results). For example, the general amino acid transport system of wild type is derepressed approximately 10-fold when cells are grown on less-favored nitrogen sources. In contrast, although the *amr* mutant has the same basal level of transport as found in the wild type during growth with excess NH_4^+, it cannot be derepressed during nitrogen limitation. On the other hand, some enzymes of nitrogen metabolism do not appear to be regulated by *amr* or subject to ammonium repression. Currently, it would appear that enzymes of nitrogen metabolism in *Neurospora* occur in at least four groups in relation to their control, namely, (1) constitutive enzymes (e.g., urease); (2) enzymes that require induction but are not subject to ammonium repression, as arginase and ornithine transaminase; (3) enzymes controlled only by ammonium repression, as the general amino acid permease; and (4) enzymes that require both induction and N-catabolite derepression, as uricase and allantoicase. The *amr* gene appears to be a major control gene that regulates synthesis, in a positive manner, of those enzymes controlled by N-repression.

CONCURRENT REGULATION OF COMPETING PATHWAYS

Competing biosynthetic and degradative pathways offer a typical case of concurrent pathways that must be regulated in an opposite manner. One can visualize two separate and independent systems for regulation of biosynthetic and catabolic enzymes, as appears to be the case for histidine synthesis and utilization in *Salmonella typhimurium* (Tyler, Deleo, and Magasanik, 1974). Alternatively a common system might control both groups of concurrent activities. This integrated type of regulation for arginine synthesis and catabolism in *S. cerevisiae* has been revealed by the interesting work of Wiame and his collaborators (Wiame, 1971; Dubois, Grenson, and Wiame, 1974; Ramos et al., 1970). A number of compounds, including arginine and ornithine, repress synthesis of the arginine biosynthetic enzymes in *S. cerevisiae*. Without exception these same compounds induce synthesis of the catabolic enzymes. Three unlinked regulatory mutations, *argRI, argRII,* and *argRIII* have similar phenotypes. In each case five biosynthetic enzymes (e.g., ornithine transcarbamylase) are rendered constitutive while simultaneously the arginine catabolic enzymes (arginase and ornithine transaminase) are missing. This phenotype suggests that a common control system or element exerts negative control over the biosynthetic enzymes and positive control over catabolic enzymes (figure 7). Wiame (1971) suggested that the three unlinked *argR* genes contribute subunits to a heteromultimeric regulatory protein that controls the expression of the various unlinked structural genes. A cis-dominant mutant was found that specifically elevates uninduced ornithine transaminase levels about 100-fold but has no effect on arginase. A similar O^c-type mutant was recovered that renders arginase constitutive with no change in OTAse. These cis-dominant mutants were interpreted to be operator constitutive (O^c) types, which would imply that the catabolic enzymes are also under negative control.

Thus Wiame (1971) proposed a model whereby the multimeric regulatory protein acted negatively to repress the activity of the structural genes for the biosynthetic enzymes and to also repress or inhibit an additional postulated control gene (R2) which itself acted negatively to repress the genes for the catabolic enzymes (figure 7). However, this model would predict the existence of an important class of R2 mutants, constitutive for all of the catabolic enzymes but unaffected for biosynthetic enzymes. This type of mutant has apparently not been found. Alternatively, it would seem that the cis-dominant mutants with O^c behavior could be I^c mutants. There appears to be no ready

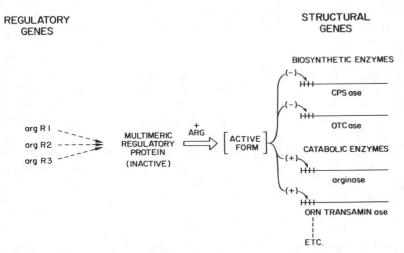

Fig. 7. Modified scheme for the concurrent regulation of arginine anabolic and catabolic enzymes in *Saccharomyces cerevisiae*. The three unlinked *argR* genes specify subunits of a multimeric regulatory protein, which is converted into its active form upon binding arginine. The active *argR* regulatory product is proposed to "turn on," in a positive manner, synthesis of arginine catabolic enzymes and also to repress activity of structural genes for the arginine biosynthetic enzymes. According to the model as proposed by Wiame (1972) the *argR* product actually controls the synthesis (or activity) of a second repressor that, in turn, represses synthesis of the biosynthetic enzymes.

criteria to distinguish between such cis-acting constitutive mutants. Thus the multimeric regulatory product specified by *argRI, argRII,* and *argRIII* genes may act directly in a dual manner, activating expression of the genes encoding the catabolic enzymes and repressing activity of the related biosynthetic genes. Whatever the exact mechanism, control of the concurrent pathways for metabolism is clearly intricately controlled by a common system and is worthy of much more detailed study.

Although different conformational forms of the *araC* protein have been demonstrated to act as an activator and repressor of the *ara* operon in *E. coli* (Wilcox et al., 1974), no case where a single active form of a regulatory product can act both positively and negatively has yet been documented.

An additional unusual control device for arginine metabolism was uncovered in *S. cerevisiae.* Ornithine transcarbamylase (OTCase) activity very rapidly declines in whole cells upon the addition of arginine. This rapid loss of OTCase activity results from a direct binding with arginase synthesized under these conditions—in the presence of both arginine and ornithine as effectors (Wiame, 1971). When examined *in vitro,* a strong binding between arginase and OTCase is observed when both arginine and ornithine are present. Although the activity of OTCase is severely inhibited, no reciprocal effect on arginase activity occurs, nor does arginase affect any of the other biosynthetic enzymes. The inhibitory effect of arginase does not require its catalytic activity since an arginase-less mutant (*ag-1*) has been found that possesses a defective enzyme that retains the ability to inhibit OTCase. Other *ag* mutants eliminate both activities. Interestingly, mutation in the OTCase structural gene can render the enzyme insensitive to the arginase-mediated inhibition. Wild-type OTCase can likewise be desensitized to this inhibition by chemical modification, also implying separate catalytic and regulatory sites (Wiame, 1971).

This unusual behavior may permit rapid responses to changing metabolic conditions. Thus, in the presence of exogenous arginine, the catabolic enzyme, arginase, is rapidly synthesized and forms an aggregate with any preexisting OTCase, whose activity is immediately inhibited. This arrangement leaves the cells with a potential capacity for rapid arginine synthesis if the effectors, especially arginine, should become depleted, thus avoiding a prolonged lag before growth can resume.

CONVERGENCE OF DISTINCT REGULATORY CIRCUITS

A recently developed concept with both bacterial and fungal systems is the importance of multiple control circuits converging upon, and regulating expression of, one or more structural genes. The synthesis of a number of inducible enzymes in *E. coli* requires not only their specific inducer but also a lifting of catabolite repression as signaled by cyclic AMP and its receptor protein (Pastan and Perlman, 1970). Even more intricately controlled are the two histidine utilization (*hut*) opersons of *Salmonella* (Tyler, Deleo, and Magasanik, 1974). Transcription of these operons has been demonstrated to require specific induction plus either a positive regulatory signal related to carbon or to nitrogen catabolite repression. Tyler et al. (1974) convincingly demonstrated that the nonadenylylated form of the enzyme glutamine synthetase is also a regulatory macromolecule and that it signals a lifting of nitrogen catabolite repression.

A clear case of multiple control is found in *N. crassa,* where it has been demonstrated that an extracellular protease is synthesized in response to an exogenous protein and a limitation for either sulfur, nitrogen, or carbon (Matile, 1965; Drucker, 1972; Hanson and Marzluf, 1973). Production of the protease is not simply a general response to starvation conditions as shown by its absence during starvation for other metabolites, such as individual amino acids or phosphate. Hanson and Marzluf (1975) demonstrated that the very

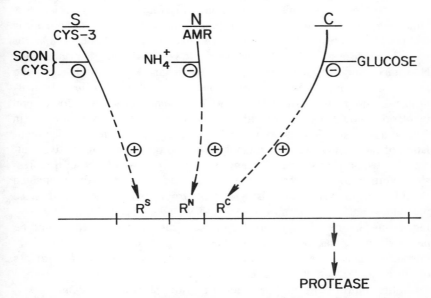

Fig. 8. Proposed model for the complex regulation of an extracellular protease in *Neurospora*. S and N represent the *cys-3* and *amr* positive regulatory genes, respectively. R^S, R^N, and R^C are the receptor sites postulated to exist in a promoter region adjacent to *prt,* the structural gene for the enzyme. These sequences are predicted to be specific binding regions for the distinct control signals of the sulfur, nitrogen, and carbon regulatory circuits.

same alkaline protease is synthesized and secreted in response to a limitation of S, N, or C. The extracellular protease synthesized under each of these three different conditions is identical by a number of biochemical criteria, which include gel filtration, ion exchange chromatography, thermal inactivation, electrophoresis, catalytic activity, and immunochemical cross reaction. Genetic analysis with electrophoretic variants of the protease indicated the presence of only a single structural locus. Thus it has been postulated that a single structural gene is served by a complex adjacent regulatory region that contains a promoter and three separate receptor sites for positive regulatory signals, one each for the sulfur, nitrogen, and carbon status of the cell (figure 8). Unlinked to the structural gene and to each other are postulated to be at least three positive regulatory genes, each of whose respective products has affinity for one of the specific receptor sites, as well as individual sensitivity to the pertinent metabolite that reflects the S, N, or C status of the cell. Apparently, a regulatory macromolecule from any one of the three different control circuits would bind at its specific receptor in the promoter region and would be sufficient to activate expression of the structural gene (*prt*). The *cys-3*[+] regulatory gene, which controls the synthesis of a number of enzymes of sulfur metabolism (see above), mediates the S-control over protease synthesis, *cys-3* mutants being unable to make this enzyme during S-limitation, although it is still produced in response to either N or C starvation. Similarly, the *amr* (or *nit-2*) locus discussed earlier, which seems to be a major regulatory gene for N metabolism in *Neurospora,* appears to signal a lifting of N-catabolite repression to many N-related structural genes, one of which is *prt*. By analogy, regulatory mutants similar to *cys-3* and *amr* but specific for carbon regulation should also exist, although none have yet been identified (in *Neurospora*). Additional work is needed to exactly define the complex regulation of this system. Particularly helpful would be I^c-type constitutive mutants that would alter the requirement for signals related to C, N, or S repression. Furthermore, cis-acting I^- types (inactivating one of the postulated specific receptors) should be distinguishable from "null" gene mutants since it would be predicted that enzyme synthesis would not occur during limitation for one metabolite (as S) but that protease identical to wild type would be produced during starvation for the other two (as N or C). Indeed, such I^- mutants might arise more frequently than I^c types, since they only require loss of function. Such mutants have been observed in the system for carbon catabolite control in *E. coli* and often are associated with the promoter.

A very similar situation was described by Cohen (1973) who found that in *Aspergillus* the synthesis of several extracellular protease species is regulated by C, N, and S repression. Furthermore, it was shown that an activation step required for activity of the beta intracellular protease is inhibited by the presence of carbon, nitrogen, sulfur, and phosphorus compounds. The synthesis of several additional enzyme systems in *Aspergillus* are also controlled by two or more converging signals that indicate the lifting of catabolite repression for C, N, S, or P; e.g., Bartnik and Weglenski (1973) found that both arginase and ornithine transaminase are subject to C and N repression, as was also observed in the case of proline oxidase (Arst and MacDonald, 1975).

The presence of such complex regulatory circuits in fungi in which the expression of a single gene can be "turned on" by several different control signals certainly argues that higher eukaryotes may possess very sophisticated and complicated regulatory systems. A regulatory system in which a number of independent circuits can control the expression of an entire set of structural genes, each of which may be served by a distinctive pattern of address sites for the regulatory signals, could clearly be a basic feature underlying the complicated processes of differentiation and morphogenesis.

REGULATION OF DEVELOPMENT

Fungi may be ideally suited as experimental organisms with which to study basic relationships between gene expression, morphogenesis, and development. *Neurospora* has been employed to advantage to investigate the genetic and biochemical basis of morphological abnormalities and simple developmental sequences (Brody and Tatum, 1966; Brody and Tatum, 1967; Scott, Mishra, and Tatum, 1973; Scott and Solomon, 1975). The very exciting area of the biochemical genetics of abnormal colonial morphology has been recently reviewed (Scott, Mishra, and Tatum, 1973) and will not be covered here. Other fungi such as the mushroom *Laccaria laccata* may be useful for examining more complex developmental patterns.

N. crassa has several well-defined stages, vegetative hyphae, aerial hyphae, and macroconidia in the asexual life cycle. Each stage consists of but a single cell type, and changes in the developmental stage can be quickly and specifically elicited by proper environmental signals (Matsuyama, Nelson, and Siegel, 1974). Siegel and his colleagues have searched for phase-specific genes, in particular, genes that function only in the differentiation of asexual spores (conidia), while Brody and his associates have looked for genes active only during spore germination. By proper manipulations, aerial hyphae can be obtained in a synchronized fashion and soon give rise to lateral branches, which form the conidiophores and conidia. Aerial hyphae themselves never directly yield conidia and thus are clearly distinct from the lateral branches.

Conidiogenesis occurs in at least five fairly discrete steps: (1) conidiophore formation; (2) nuclear migration into the conidiophore tips; (3) swelling of the coniophore; (4) conidiophore budding, which results in a chain of presumptive conidia; and (5) septation, which yields the individual spores. At least seven different mutants that interrupt conidiogenesis, but have no other detectable effect, have been studied (Matsuyama et al., 1974). These genes are scattered throughout the genome and are located on six different chromosomes. Each mutant gene seems to interrupt conidiogenesis at a certain point in the developmental sequence, e.g., the mutant aconidial-2 (acon-2) completes steps 1 and 2, but rarely reaches the third step in conidia formation. Similarly, the csp-1 and csp-2 (conidial separation) mutants complete stage 5, but the conidia fail to separate from each other (Selitrennikoff, Nelson, and Siegel, 1974). These genes seem to function only in the production of an autolytic activity that is required for the conversion of proconidial chains into free spores. By the use of temperature-sensitive mutants and temperature-shift experiments, a distinction can be made between the time of gene action and the period when prior activity becomes critical for development. The various genes that have a role in conidiogenesis can be ordered into a sequence in terms of the timing of their respective activities, e.g., acon-2, acon-3, fl, and csp-1 act in that order. One principle that seems clear from this work is that certain genes are highly phase-specific and may act only during a limited part of the life cycle. Much work remains to be done, however, and many important questions have yet even to be framed. What are the particular regulatory signals that "turn on" these specific genes for conidiogenesis? How are they "turned on" in a sequential fashion? What, in fact, determines whether conidia formation will proceed? It can be anticipated that many important new concepts will be derived by additional research in this and related areas, including the events that occur during spore germination and outgrowth.

NEEDED RESEARCH AND POSSIBLE FUTURE DIRECTIONS

There is an urgent need to develop cell-free transcriptional and translational systems with which to study fungal mRNA synthesis, protein synthesis, and the functions of various regulatory elements. It is likewise most important to develop the capability to identify and assay specific mRNAs, most likely by the use of DNA probes with which particular RNA sequences can be detected by hybridization techniques. Such systems should be invaluable for the detection, purification, and detailed study of various regulatory products, which so far have only been identified by mutational studies. Careful studies of the nuclear proteins of fungi also need to be undertaken. One cannot help but wonder whether any of the positive-acting regulatory products such as those specified by the qa-1, leu-3, cys-3, areA, and nuc-1 genes may be non-histone chromosomal proteins, which have been postulated to effect gene control in mammalian cells. Chromatin reconstitution studies with any of these positive control systems could be very exciting and illuminating. The fact that regulatory proteins may be expected to occur in only very low concentrations argues against the possibility that they are the acidic nuclear proteins that can be visualized by staining following their separation by zone electrophoresis. The authentic regulatory proteins might instead be present as minor species in preparations of nuclear proteins.

Work is needed to study the structure of chromatin and DNA sequences in fungi and the nature of primary RNA transcripts and messenger processing and secretion. Further studies need to be accomplished with the multiple RNA polymerases found in fungi, including their ability to utilize native and reconstituted fungal chromatin as a template. Conditional mutants that affect the RNA polymerases, elements of the protein synthesis apparatus, and the processes of messenger maturation and secretion would be of great use. There is a genuine need for a specific inhibitor of RNA synthesis in fungi that is readily permeable, effective at low concentrations, and easily reversed. Although actinomycin D, proflavin, and lomofungin have all been used to inhibit transcription, none of them are ideal for this role. In short, additional insight into regulation in fungi seems to depend primarily upon the development of techniques and systems for studies at the molecular level. With their emergence great progress in our understanding of regulation in eukaryotes should follow. Another area in which considerable work is needed is the biochemical genetics of developmentally regulated events such as conidiogenesis, spore germination, colonial morphology, and differentiated patterns of enzyme synthesis.

CLOSING REMARKS

Our present understanding of regulation of gene expression in fungi is encouraging and suggests that considerable progress at the molecular level can now be anticipated. It seems clear that fungi possess regulatory systems similar to those found in bacteria and that operons do exist in fungi, but are relatively infrequent. The more usual situation in the fungi finds related structural genes widely scattered from each other but, nevertheless, controlled as a group. Present knowledge suggests that in most cases structural genes are "turned on" by a positive-acting regulatory product (such as the products of *qa-1, leu-3, cys-3, areA,* and *nuc-1* genes) although some instances of negative control may also occur. In some instances regulatory proteins may be strictly confined to the nucleus that encodes them whereas, in others, they may have at least a transient existence in the cytoplasm.

An understanding of regulation in fungi requires a knowledge of the highly organized cell structure and of the presence of various pools of metabolities, including storage pools, as well as the confinement of certain enzymes or pathways to specific cell organelles. We must be alert for both transcriptional and translation controls as well as possibilities for controlling enzyme levels by dynamic turnover or by reversible modification. A striking feature of control in fungi is the prevalence of very complex regulatory systems. A definite sequential action of a series of regulatory loci that necessarily precede the final step of positive activation of structural loci has been identified in several cases. Highly integrated systems are apparent in the control of nitrogen metabolism, branched-chain amino acid biosynthesis, cross-pathway control, and the concurrent regulation of competing pathways. The regulatory signal may itself be quite complex and may be an aggregate of regulatory products, each of which is required for proper function of the whole. Regulatory signals that arise from distinct control circuits may converge upon, and independently activate, a single structural gene, which, accordingly, is probably served by a complex adjacent control region containing separate sites for recognition of the various signals. Finally, in some instances, fungal enzymes seem to play a regulatory role in addition to their catalytic function and may control the synthesis of many other enzymes as well as their own synthesis.

ACKNOWLEDGMENTS

I wish to thank Dr. Lloyd Wolfinbarger, Dr. Robert Metzenberg, and Dr. Tom Byers for careful reading of the manuscript. Research in the author's laboratory is supported by Public Health Service Grant 1-RO1 GM 18642 from the National Institutes of Health. G.A.M. is supported by a P.H.S. Career Development Award K4-GM-00052.

[1]From *Alice's Adventures in Wonderland.*

REFERENCES

Adman, R., L. Schultz, and B. D. Hall. 1972. Transcription in yeast: Separation and properties of multiple RNA polymerases. Proc. Nat. Acad. Sci. USA 69:1702–6.

Altmiller, D. H., and R. P. Wagner. 1970. Purification and properties of dihydroxyacid dehydratase from soluble and mitrochondrial fractions of *Neurospora crassa.* Arch. Biochem. Biophys. 138:160–70.

Arst, H. N., Jr., and D. J. Cove. 1973. Nitrogen metabolite repression in *Aspergillus nidulans.* Molec. Gen. Genet. 126:111–42.

Arst, H. N., Jr., and D. W. MacDonald. 1975. A gene cluster in *Aspergillus nidulans* with an internally located cis-acting regulatory region. Nature 254:26–31.

Arst, H. N., Jr., and C. Scazzocchio. 1975. Initiator constitutive "up-promoter" effect in *Aspergillus nidulans*. Nature 254:31–34.

Bailey, C., and H. N. Arst, Jr. 1975. Carbon catabolite repression in *Aspergillus nidulans*. Eur. J. Biochem. 51:573–77.

Bartnik, E., and P. Weglenski. 1973. Ammonium and glucose repression of the arginine catabolic enzymes in *Aspergillus nidulans*. Mol. Gen. Genet. 126:75–84.

Bollon, A. P. 1974. Fine structure analysis of eukaryotic multifunctional gene. Nature 250:630–34.

Bollon, A. P., and P. T. Magee. 1973. Involvement of threonine deaminase in repression of the isoleucine-valine and leucine pathways in *Saccharomyces cerevisiae*. J. Bacteriol. 113:1333–44.

Britten, R. J., and E. H. Davison. 1969. Gene regulation for higher cells: A theory. Science 165:349–57.

Brody, S., and E. L. Tatum. 1966. The primary biochemical effect of a morphological mutation in *Neurospora crassa*. Proc. Nat. Acad. Sci. USA 56:1290–97.

Brody, S., and E. L. Tatum. 1967. Phosphoglucomutase mutants and morphological changes in *Neurospora crassa*. Proc. Nat. Acad. Sci. USA 58:923–30.

Brooks, R. R., and P. C. Huang. 1972. Redundant DNA of *Neurospora crassa*. Biochem. Genet. 6:41–49.

Burton, E. G., and R. L. Metzenberg. 1972. Novel mutation causing repression of several enzymes of sulfur metabolism in *Neurospora crassa*. J. Bacteriol. 109:140–51.

Carsiotis, M. 1973. Tryptophan-mediated control of histidine and arginine biosynthetic enzymes in *Neurospora crassa*. Abstr. Ann. Meeting Am. Soc. Microbiol. P 70, p. 152.

Carsiotis, M., and R. F. Jones. 1974. Cross-pathway regulation: Tryptophan-mediated control of histidine and arginine biosynthetic enzymes in *Neurospora crassa*. J. Bacteriol. 119:889-92.

Carsiotis, M., R. F. Jones, A. M. Lacy, T. J. Cleary, and D. B. Fankhauser. 1970. Histidine-mediated control of tryptophan biosynthetic enzymes in *Neurospora crassa*. J. Bacteriol. 104:98–106.

Carsiotis, M., R. F. Jones, and A. C. Wesseling. 1974. Cross-pathway regulation: Histine-mediated control of histidine, tryptophan, and arginine biosynthetic enzymes in *Neurospora Crassa*. J. Bacteriol. 119:893–98.

Case, M. E., and N. H. Giles. 1968. Evidence for nonsense mutations in the arom gene cluster of *Neurospora crassa*. Genetics 60:49–58.

Case, M. E., and N. H. Giles. 1971. Partial enzyme aggregates formed by pleiotropic mutants in the arom gene cluster of *Neurospora crassa*. Proc. Nat. Acad. Sci. USA 68:58–62.

Case, M.E., and N. H. Giles. 1975. Genetic evidence on the organization and action of the *qa-1* gene product: A protein regulating the induction of three enzymes in quinate catabolism in *Neurospora crassa*. Proc. Natl. Acad. Sci. USA 72:553–57.

Cassady, W. E., E. H. Leiter, A. Bergquist, and R. P. Wagner. 1972. Separation of mitochondrial membranes of *Neurospora crassa*. II. Submitochondrial localization of the isoleucine-valine biosynthetic pathway. J. Cell. Biol. 53:66–72.

Chaleff, R. S. 1974a. The inducible quinate-shikimate catabolic pathway in *Neurospora crassa*: Genetic organization. J. Gen. Microbiol. 81:337–55.

Chaleff, R. S. 1974b. The inducible quinate-shikimate catabolic pathway in *Neurospora crassa:* Induction and regulation of enzyme synthesis. J. Gen. Microbiol. 81:357–72.

Cohen, B. L. 1972. Ammonium repression of extracellular protease in *Aspergillus nidulans.* J. Gen. Microbiol. 71:293–99.

Cohen, B. L. 1973. Regulation of intracellular and extracellular neutral and alkaline proteases in *Aspergillus nidulans.* J. Gen. Microbiol. 79:311–20.

Cove, D. J., and J. A. Pateman. 1969. Autoregulation of nitrate reduction in *Aspergillus nidulans.* J. Bacteriol. 97:1374–78.

Davis, R. H. 1972. Metabolite distribution in cells. Science 178:835–40.

Davis, R. H. 1974. Metabolic organization in Neurospora. Stadler Sympos. 6:61–74.

Dietrich, P. S., and R. L. Metzenberg. 1973. Metabolic suppressors of a regulatory mutant in Neurospora. Biochem. Genet. 8:73–84.

Douglas, H. C., and D. C. Hawthorne. 1964. Enzymatic expression and genetic linkage of genes controlling galactose utilization in *Saccharomyces.* Genetics 49:837–44.

Douglas, H. C., and D. C. Hawthorne. 1966. Regulation of genes controlling synthesis of the galactose pathway enzymes in years. Genetics 54:911–16.

Douglas, H. C., and D. C. Hawthorne. 1972. Uninducible mutants in the gal i locus of *Saccharomyces cerevisiae.* J. Bacteriol. 109:1139–43.

Drucker, H. 1972. Regulation of exocellular proteases in *Neurospora crassa:* Induction and repression of enzyme synthesis. J. Bacteriol. 110:1041–49.

Dubois, E., M. Grenson, and J. M. Wiame. 1973. Release of the "ammonia effect" on three catabolic enzymes by NADP-specific glutamate dehydrogenaseless mutations in *Saccharomyces cerevisiae.* Biochem. Biophys. Res. Comm. 50:967–72.

Dubois, E., M. Grenson, and J. M. Wiame, 1974. The participation of the anabolic glutamate dehydrogenase in the nitrogen catabolite repression of arginase in *Saccharomyces cerevisiae.* Eur. J. Biochem. 48:603–16.

Dutta, S. K. 1974. Repeated DNA sequences in fungi. Nucleic Acids Res. 1:1411–19.

Facklam, T., and G. A. Marzluf. 1975. Nitrogen regulation of amino acid metabolism in *Neurospora crassa.* Genetics 80:s29.

Feldman, J. R., and J. P. Thayer. 1974. Cyclic AMP induced tryosimase synthesis in *Neurospora crassa.* Biochem. Biophys. Res. Comm. 61:977–82.

Flawia, M. M., and H. N. Torres. 1972. Adenylate cyclase activity in lubrol-treated membranes from *Neurospora crassa.* Biochim. Biophys. Acta 289:428–32.

Ghosh, B. K., B. Montenecourt, and O. J. Lampen. 1973. Abnormal cell envelope ultrastructure of a *Saccharomyces* mutant with invertase formation resistant to hexoses. J. Bacteriol. 116:1412–20.

Giles, N. H., M. E. Case, and J. W. Jacobson. 1974. Genetic regulation of quinate-shikimate catabolism in *Neurospora crassa. In* B. A. Hamkalo and J. Papaconstantinous (eds.). Molecular cytogenetics. Pp. 309–14. Plenum Publishing, New York.

Gleason, M. K., and R. L. Metzenberg. 1974. Regulation of phosphate metabolism in *Neurospora crassa:* Isolation of mutants deficient in the repressible alkaline phosphatase. Genetics 78:645–59.

Goldberger, R. F. 1974. Autogenous regulation of gene expression. Science 183:810–16.

Greer, J., and G. R. Fink. 1975. Isolation of regulatory mutants in *Saccharomyces cerevisiae. In* D. M. Prescott (ed.). Methods in cell biology, vol. 11: Yeast cells. Academic Press, New York.

Grenson, M., E. Dubois, M. Piotrowska, R. Drillien, and M. Aigle. 1974. Ammonia assimilation in *Saccharomyces cerevisiae* as mediated by the two glutamate dehydrogenases. Evidence for a gdhA locus being a structural gene for the NADP-dependent glutamate dehydrogenase. Mol. Gen. Genet. 128:73–85.

Gross, S. R. 1965. The regulation of synthesis of leucine biosynthetic enzymes in *Neurospora.* Proc. Nat. Acad. Sci. USA 54:1538–46.

Hanson, M. A., and G. A. Marzluf. 1973. Regulation of sulfur-controlled protease in *Neurospora crassa.* J. Bacteriol. 116:785–89.

Hanson, M. A., and G. A. Marzluf. 1975. Control of the synthesis of a single enzyme by multiple regulatory circuits in *Neurospora crassa.* Proc. Nat. Acad. Sci. USA 72:1240–44.

Hasunuma, K. 1973. Repressible extracellular nucleases in *Neurospora crassa.* Biochim. Biophys. Acta 319:288–93.

Hsiang, M. W., and R. D. Cole. 1973. The isolation of histone from *Neurospora crassa.* J. Biol. Chem. 248:2007–13.

Hynes, M. J. 1973. Mutants with altered glucose repression of amidase enzymes in *Aspergillus nidulans.* J. Bacteriol. 111:717–22.

Hynes, M. J. 1975. A cis-dominant regulatory mutation affecting enzyme induction in the eukaryote *Aspergillus nidulans.* Nature 253:210–12.

Hynes, M. J., and J. A. Pateman. 1970. The genetic analysis of regulation of amidase synthesis in *Aspergillus nidulans.* I. Mutants able to utilize acrylamide. Molec. Gen. Genet. 108:97–106.

Klar, A. J., and H. O. Halvorson. 1974. Studies on the positive regulatory gene, *Gal 4,* in regulation and galactose catabolic enzymes in *Saccharomyces cerevisiae.* Molec. Gen. Genet. 135:203–12.

Lawther, R. P., and T. G. Cooper. 1973. Effects of inducer addition and removal upon the level of allophanate hydrolase in *Saccharomyces cerevisiae.* Biochem. Biophys. Res. Comm. 55:1100–1104.

Lawther, R. P., and T. G. Cooper. 1975. Kinetics of induced and repressed enzyme synthesis in *Saccharomyces cerevisiae.* J. Bacteriol. 121:1064–73.

Lawther, R. P., S. L. Phillips, and T. G. Cooper. 1975. Lomofungin inhibition of allophanate hydrolase synthesis in *Saccharomyces cerevisiae.* Molec. Gen. Genet. 137:89–99.

Lawther, R. P., E. Riemer, B. Chojnacki, and T. G. Cooper. 1974. Clustering of the genes for allantoin degradation in *Saccharomyces cerevisiae.* J. Bacteriol. 119:461–68.

Lehman, J. F., M. K. Gleason, S. K. Ahlgren, and R. L. Metzenberg. 1973. Regulation of phosphate metabolism in *Neurospora crassa.* Characterization of regulatory mutants. Genetics 75:61–73.

Leiter, E. H., D. A. La Brier, A. Bergquist, and R. P. Wagner. 1971. *In vitro* mitochondrial complementation in *Neurospora crassa.* Biochem. Genetics. 5:549–61.

Littlewood, B. S., W. Chia, and R. L. Metzenberg. 1975. Genetic control of phosphate-metabolizing enzymes in *Neurospora crassa:* Relationships among regulatory mutations. Genetics 79:419–34.

Lowendorf, H. S., G. F. Bazinet, Jr., and C. W. Slayman. 1975. Phosphate transport in *Neurospora.* Derepression of a high-affinity transport system during phosphorus starvation. Biochim. Biophys. Acta 389:541–49.

Marzluf, G. A. 1970a. Genetic and biochemical studies of distinct sulfate permease species in different developmental stages of *Neurospora crassa.* Arch. Biochem. Biophys. 138:254–63.

Marzluf, G. A. 1970b. Genetic and metabolic controls for sulfate metabolism in *Neurospora crassa:* Isolation and study of chromate resistant and sulfate transport-negative mutants. J. Bacteriol. 102:716–21.

Marzluf, G. A. 1972a. Genetic and metabolic control of sulfate metabolism in *Neurospora crassa:* A specific permease for choline-O-sulfate. Biochem. Genet. 7:219–33.

Marzluf, G. A. 1972b. Control of the synthesis, activity, and turnover of enzymes of sulfur metabolism in *Neurospora crassa.* Arch. Biochem. Biophys. 150:714–24.

Marzluf, G. A. 1975. Genetic and developmental regulation of distinct sulfate permease species in *Neurospora crassa. In* C. L. Markert (ed.). *Isozymes III Developmental Biology.* Pp. 239–52. Academic Press, New York.

Marzluf, G. A. and R. L. Metzenberg. 1968. Positive control by the *cys-3* locus in regulation of sulfur metabolism in *Neurospora.* J. Mol. Biol. 33:423–37.

Matile, P. 1965. Intracellular location of proteolytic enzymes of *Neurospora crassa.* Z. Zellforsch. 65: 884–96.

Matsuyama, S., R. Nelson, and R. W. Siegel. 1974. Mutations specifically blocking differentiation of macroconidia in *Neurospora crassa.* Developmental Biology 41:278–87.

McGuire, W. G., and G. A. Marzluf. 1974. Developmental regulation of choline sulfatase and aryl sulfatase in *Neurospora crassa.* Arch. Biochem. Biophys. 161:360–68.

Metzenberg, R. L., and S. K. Ahlgren. 1971. Structural and regulatory control of aryl sulfatase in *Neurospora:* The use of interspecific differences in structural genes. Genetics 68:369–81.

Metzenberg, R. L., G. S. Chen, and S. K. Ahlgren. 1971. Reversion of aryl sulfataseless mutants of *Neurospora.* Genetics 68:359–68.

Metzenberg, R. L., M. K. Gleason, and B. S. Littlewood. 1974. Genetic control of alkaline phosphatase synthesis in *Neurospora:* The use of partial diploids in dominance studies. Genetics 77:25–43.

Metzenberg, R. L., and J. W. Parson. 1966. Altered repression of some enzymes of sulfur utilization in a temperature-conditional lethal mutant of *Neurospora.* Proc. Nat. Acad. Sci. USA 55:629–35.

Nyc, J. R. 1967. A repressible acid phosphatase in *Neurospora crassa.* Biochem. Biophys. Res. Commun. 27:183–88.

Olshan, A. R., and S. R. Gross. 1974. Role of the *leu-3* cistron in regulation of the synthesis of isoleucine and valine biosynthetic enzymes of *Neurospora.* J. Bacteriol. 118:374–84.

Pall, M. L. 1971. Amino acid transport in *Neurospora crassa.* IV. Properties and regulation of a methionine transport system. Biochim. Biophys. Acta 233:201–14.

Partridge, C. W. H., M. E. Case, and N. H. Giles. 1972. Direct isolation in wild type *Neurospora crassa* of mutants *(qa-1ᶜ)* constitutive for the catabolism of quinate and shikimate. Genetics 72:411–17.

Pastan, I., and R. Perlman. 1970. Cyclic adenosine monophosphate in bacteria. Science 169:339–44.

Pateman, J. A., J. R. Kinghorn, E. Dunn, and E. Forbes. 1973. Ammonium regulation in *Aspergillus nidulans.* J. Bacteriol. 114:943–50.

Paul, J. 1972. General theory of chromosome structure and gene activation in eukaryotes. Nature 238:444–46.

Perkins, D. D. 1972. An insertional translocation in *Neurospora* that generates duplications heterozygous for mating type. Genetics 71:25–51.

Polacco, J. C., and S. R. Gross, 1973. The product of the *leu-3* cistron as a regulatory element for the production of the leucine biosynthetic enzymes of *Neurospora*. Genetics 74:443–59.

Ramos, R. P. Thuriaux, J. M. Wiame, and J. Bechet. 1970. The participation of ornithine and citrulline in the regulation of arginine metabolism in *Saccharomyces cerevisiae*. Eur. J. Biochem. 12:40–47.

Reed, J., and E. Wintersberger. 1973. Adenylic acid-rich sequences in messenger RNA from yeast polysomes. FEBS Lett. 32:213–17.

Reichenbecher, V. E., M. Fischer, and S. R. Gross. 1975. A mutant of *Neurospora* which allows utilization of exogenous a-isopropylmalate. Genetics 80:s67.

Reinert, W. R., and G. A. Marzluf. 1975. Genetic and metabolic control of the purine catabolic enzymes of *Neurospora crassa*. Mol. Gen. Genet. 139:39–55.

Reinert, W. R., and G. A. Marzluf. 1975. Regulation of the purine catabolic enzymes in *Neurospora crassa*. Arch. Biochem. Biophys. 166:565–74.

Scazzocchio, C., and A. J. Darlington. 1968. The induction and repression of the enzymes of purine breakdown in *Aspergillus nidulans*. Biochim. Biophys. Acta 166:557–68.

Schurch, A., J. Miozzari, and R. Hutter. 1974. Regulation of tryptophan biosynthesis in *Saccharomyces cerevisiae*: Mode of action of 5-methyl-tryptophan and 5-methyl-tryptophan sensitive mutants. J. Bacteriol. 117:1131–40.

Scott, W. A., N. C. Mishra, and E. L. Tatum. 1973. Biochemical genetics of morphogenesis in *Neurospora*. Brookhaven Symp. Biol. 25:1–18.

Scott, W. A., and B. Solomon. 1973. Cyclic 3′, 5′-AMP phosphodiesterase of *Neurospora crassa*. Biochem. Biophys. Res. Comm. 53:1024–30.

Scott, W. A., and B. Solomon. 1975. Adenosine 3′, 5′-cyclic monophosphate and morphology in *Neurospora crassa*: Drug induced alterations. J. Bacteriol. 122:454–63.

Selitrennikoff, C., R. Nelson, and R. W. Siegel. 1974. Phase-specific genes for macroconidiation in *Neurospora crassa*. Genetics 78:679–90.

Sorger, G. J., and J. Davies. 1973. Regulation of nitrate reductase of *Neurospora crassa* at the level of transcription and translation. Biochem. J. 134:673–85.

Sorger, G. J., Debanne, M. T., and J. Davies. 1974. Effects of nitrate on the synthesis and decay of nitrate reductase of *Neurospora crassa*. Biochem. J. 140:395–403.

Subramanian, K. N., and G. J. Sorger. 1972a. Regulation of nitrate reductase in *Neurospora crassa*: Stability in vivo. J. Bacteriol. 110:538–46.

Subramanian, K. N., and G. J. Sorger. 1972b. Regulation of nitrate reductase in *Neurospora crassa*: Regulation of translation and transcription. J. Bacteriol. 110:547–53.

Subramanian, K. N., R. L. Weiss, and R. H. Davis. 1973. Use of external, biosynthetic, and organellar arginine by *Neurospora*. J. Bacteriol. 115:284–90.

Timberlake, W. E., and G. Turian. 1974. Multiple DNA-dependent RNA polymerases of *Neurospora*. Experientia 30:1236–38.

ToH-E, A., and T. Ishikawa. 1971. Genetic control of the synthesis of repressible phosphatase in *Neurospora crassa*. Genetics 69:339–51.

ToH-E, A., Y. Ueda, and Y. Oshima. 1973. Genetic regulatory system for acid phosphatase formation in *Saccharomyces*. Genetics 74:s277.

Tyler, B., A. Deleo, and B. Magasanik. 1974. Activation of transcription of *hut* DNA by glutamine synthetase. Proc. Nat. Acad. Sci. USA 71:225–29.

Weiss, R. L. 1973. Intracellular localization of ornithine and arginine pools in *Neurospora*. J. Biol. Chem. 248:5409–13.

Weiss, R. L., and R. H. Davis. 1973. Intracellular localization of enzymes of arginine metabolism in *Neurospora*. J. Biol. Chem. 248:5403–8.

Wiame, J. M. 1971. Regulation of arginine metabolism in *Saccharomyces cerevisiae*. Current Topics in Cellular Regulation. 4:1–38.

Wilcox, G., K. Clemetson, P. Cleary, and E. Englesberg. 1974. Interaction of the regulatory gene product with the operator site in the L-arabinose operon of *Escherichia coli*. J. Mol. Biol. 85:589–602.

ERIK ZEUTHEN

Studies on the Cell Cycle

7

Each functional step in the cell cycle is the end of a sequence extending from transcription, through translation and assembly, to physiological function. Thus to account for the cells' progression in the cycle, we must account for a series of interlocked and mutually controlled functions. In yeast and perhaps in all cells, the progression through the cell cycle is governed by sequential gene action and related to complex physiological gene expression during the cycle (Hartwell et al., 1974).

For one who examines cell populations with the microscope and aims at inducing the cells to divide together, problems of cell cycle controls tend to unfold themselves at the physiological level. It is only when one has the proper synchronized system that one is tempted to ask questions about prior gene transcription and translation. As will be evident in this review, I continue to see these problem from the viewpoint of a cellular physiologist.

This paper contains two parts. The first deals with synchrony induction in *Tetrahymena* and in *Schizosaccharomyces* populations by use of heat shocks, and with problems that arose upon analysis of the first synchronized *Tetrahymena* system. These problems relate to the dissociation of DNA synthesis from phenomena coupled to processes that occur during G_2 and division, and later with the same processes, some of which permit the cells to complete G_2, D, and S, and others that do not. These studies led to new synchronization procedures.

The second part deals with precise microgasometric measurements of unperturbed and of synchronized cells during the cell cycle. Together with part

Biological Institute of the Carlsberg Foundation, 16 Tagensvej, 2200 Copenhagen N, Denmark.

one they will indicate that heat shock-synchronized systems behave rather normally, and further, that the growth potential of normal cells doubles at or during division.

CELL CYCLE CONTROLS IN *TETRAHYMENA*

Tetrahymena pyriformis, the amicronucleate strain GL, was grown exponentially under standard conditions (protease peptone, liver, salts, 28°C) with 150–170 min. doubling time, or synchronously after treatment with temperature shocks. The normal cell cycle of this organism as shown in figure 1A can be divided into G_1, S, G_2, and D (Cameron and Nachtwey, 1967). Nilsson (1970), in comparable experiments, studied morphological changes through

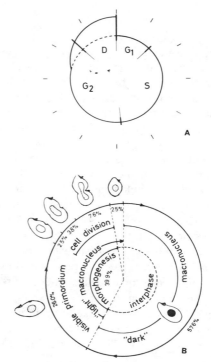

Fig. 1. (A) Cell cycle of *Tetrahymena pyriformis,* amicronucleate strain GL, the strain used throughout these studies. The diagram shows how the cycle time (in this study, 150 minutes) is divided between G_1, S, G_2, and D. The "transition point" is around 9:30 o'clock (data from Cameron and Nachtwey, 1967). (B) Morphological changes through the cell cycle of strain GL. The cells grew exponentially with a generation time of 170 minutes. The fraction of the cell cycle time that is spent in the indicated stages of oral morphogenesis, cell division, and "interphase" are shown, the latter defined as the stage with dispersed chromatin. (From Nilsson, 1970).

the cell cycle of strain GL (figure 1B). The polyploid macronucleus (henceforth, nucleus) stands out as "dark" in the phase contrast microscope for slightly more than half of the cycle and appears "light" for a slightly shorter time. It is darker from well before to well after the S-period and appears "light" prior and during division. Parallel examination in the electron microscope showed that "dark" chromatin is dispersed and "light" chromatin is granulated. Nilsson refers to the phase with dispersed chromatin as "interphase." By inference the phase with a visible primordium for the new oral apparatus (cf. fig. 1B) would be prophase or pre-prophase, terminologies not agreed on for *Tetrahymena* but well known for mitotic cells. Thus chromatin condensation goes hand in hand with the assembly of structures in the cytoplasmic cortex, e.g., the oral primordium and apparatus, and undoubtedly the contractile ring. It will be seen that oral morphogenesis begins with the appearance of the primordium and continues through division. Comparison of figures 1A and B shows that the chromatin of *Tetrahymena* loosens quickly in G_1, and that it again condenses in G_2—well before it gets partitioned to the daughter nuclei. In these respects the "amitotic" *Tetrahymena* behaves as a mitotic cell equipped with regular chromosomes.

The Use of Heat Shocks to Control the Cell Cycle: Dissociation and Association of Cell Division and DNA Replication

Using temperature shocks, Scherbaum and Zeuthen (1954), Zeuthen and Scherbaum (1954), and Hotchkiss (1954) independently phased animal cells (*Tetrahymena*) and bacteria (*Pneumococcus*) for cell cycle functions. Heat-shock synchronized cells look quite healthy, and in all probability the heat shocks act by putting normal cell cycle control mechanisms under stress. This technique permits study of the cell cycle control mechanisms and can also aid in the development of additional steps to improve cell synchrony. Furthermore, it was hoped that with time these procedures could be applied to synchronization of other cell types. This has been partly accomplished, as will be discussed later.

Age-dependent division delays. Cells of a ciliate protozoan, a yeast, a bacterium, and a mammalian cell, grown at or near the optimum temperature, all show similar age-dependent responses to a temperature shock defined as short-term chilling or heating. This response appears to be widespread for fast growing cells and is illustrated in figure 2, which displays early experiments by Thormar (1959). These studies were performed to shed light on the mechanisms of the heat shock synchronization of *Tetrahymena* populations. Curve A_1 shows the duration of a cell generation as a function of age when the cells were heat-shocked. Age is measured as the time elapsed since the cell di-

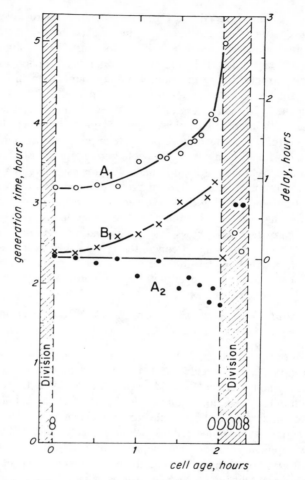

Fig. 2. *Tetrahymena pyriformis:* curves A_1 and A_2: cells grown at 28.5°C were exposed to 34.1°C for 15 minutes at the various ages shown on the abscissa. The duration of the treated generation (A_1) and of the first untreated generation (A_2) is shown on the left ordinate. Curve B_1: as A_1, but exposure is to 31.1°C for 20 minutes. (From Thormar, 1959.)

vided. The heat shock extends the treated cell generation time considerably over normal, always by more than the duration of the shock, and up to that characteristic of "old" cells. The later the shock is initiated, the more pronounced the effect. Thormar found such potentiation of effect with cell age also using a lower temperature (31.1°C, figure 2, curve B_1). Increase in cellular response with increase in cell age can be traced through G_1 and S (first

1¼ hour), and reaches its maximum during G_2 (last hour). Just prior to cell division (seen best in figure 2, curve B_1), at what we later termed the "transition point" (Rasmussen and Zeuthen, 1962), there is an abrupt transition to insensitivity to the heat shock. One can thus visualize periodic repeats of this curve during subsequent cell cycles showing increasing sensitivity to heat-shock prior to each transition point and a steep decline afterward. Curves resembling the one just described for normal cells were later observed for temperature-shocked synchronized *Tetrahymena* cells (Frankel, 1962; Zeuthen, 1964) and also for quite unrelated cells: normal and synchronized *Escherichia coli* (Smith and Pardee, 1970), synchronized *Schizosaccharomyces pombe* (Kramhøft and Zeuthen, 1971), and with normal mouse L-cells (Miyamoto et al., 1973). With normal and synchronized *Tetrahymena* cells, response patterns essentially similar to those seen in figure 2 can also be obtained with cold shocks (Thormar, 1959; Frankel, 1962; Zeuthen, 1964).

The transition point marks a time when the cell moves from a reversible to an irreversible commitment for a forthcoming division. As described, the transition point can be characterized by temperature shocks. However, *Tetrahymena* exhibits similar response patterns to anaerobiosis (Rasmussen, 1963) and to inhibitors of glycolysis, respiration, and oxidative phosphorylation (Hamburger, 1962) as well as to the addition of amino acid analogues (Rasmussen and Zeuthen, 1962; Frankel, 1962), or inhibitors of protein synthesis (Rasmussen and Zeuthen, 1962; Frankel, 1967). The transition point splits G_2 into two parts. The second part is the one that leads to cell division, D (see figure 1A). The first part is sensitive to inhibitors of various sorts, but the second is largely insensitive. Although a cell cycle is normally measured from the end of one division to the end of the next, it can also be conveniently measured from one transition point to the next, i.e., from the point in one cell generation when division is irreversibly triggered, to the corresponding point in the next generation. This is illustrated in figure 7, and will be further discussed later in different connections.

Recovery from temperature shock is a function of cell age in the cycle. This recovery occurs in a way that suggests that the shock causes loss of investments made for the forthcoming division, during a period that began even before the preceding division. The time required for recovery could reflect a loss of stored material or loss in accumulated structural organization or even an alteration in the genetic program, as has been discussed (Byfield and Scherbaum, 1967; Byfield and Lee, 1970). In fact, distinct loss of structural organization can be observed in *Tetrahymena*. This ciliate protozoan carries a structural marker that defines its position in the cell cycle (the developing oral primordium and apparatus), and it behaves as if it represented some part of the prior investment for division. This structure dissociates in response to a temperature shock given prior to a particular time late in the cell cycle. "Structural stabilization" of the oral primordium (Frankel, 1962, 1967) occurs at a time point coincident with the "transition time point" for cell division.

We are ignorant as to whether proteins used for constructing an oral structure or a division apparatus are synthesized constitutively or in a regulated manner during the cell cycle. Microscopic observation reveals that structures are assembled discontinuously; we propose that the response curves to pulse heating (or chilling) of cells proceeding through the cycle reflect changes from low to high, and from invisible to visible, levels of organized aggregation of macromolecules into cellular structures that have some relevance to cell division.

Synchrony induction of cell division by use of heat shocks. The patterns of differential delay of cell division account for the observation that *Tetrahymena, Schizosaccharomyces,* and *Escherichia coli* can be induced to divide in synchrony after exposure to a single, or to a series of, temperature shocks. Because cells of different ages are differently delayed with respect to the forthcoming division, they tend to be collected in a common phase. Cells

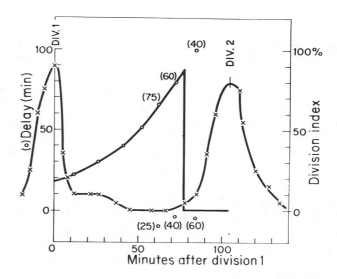

Fig. 3. *Tetrahymena* synchronized with a succession of closely spaced heat shocks, essentially according to the "old method" of Scherbaum and Zeuthen (1954). The crosses show percentage of dividing cells, and the circles, delay of the second division in response to a new heat shock (34°, 1/3 hour) at the times indicated by the circles. The first division maximum comes 85 minutes after the last shock has been terminated. (From Zeuthen, 1964.) About the time of the transition point some cells are maximally, others minimally, delayed. The percentage distributions between the extremes are indicated in parantheses. Curves are drawn through means.

thus synchronized show much the same pattern of response to temperature shocks as do normal cells.

Generally a sequence of well-chosen and well-administered temperature shocks gives better division synchrony than a single shock. Multiple shocks collect more cells more closely than does a single shock. With respect to *division synchrony,* it matters little if one spaces the temperature shocks one-half hour apart (figure 3), which blocks the division cycle for the duration of the shocks (Scherbaum and Zeuthen, 1954), or if the shocks are administered a cell generation apart (figure 7) so as to allow each cell precisely one division between consecutive shocks (Zeuthen, 1971). However, the results do differ with respect to *replication synchrony.* We shall deal first with the "old system" in which shocks are spaced one-half hour apart. With this sytem replication is only parasynchronous: between the two synchronous divisions from 50 to 80% of the cells initiate replication (Hjelm and Zeuthen, 1967a, b), and little more than 50% (Andersen, Brunk, and Zeuthen, 1970) to 70% (Hardin, Einem, and Lindsay, 1967) of the DNA is replicated. The synchrony of cell division is better than the synchrony of DNA replication, which indicates that heat shocks must have dissociated the two processes in some of the cells.

Such dissociation is very apparent in *E. coli.* A single heat shock delays cell division, the effect being greater the farther the cells are in the division cycle. However, rounds of replication are not much affected by the shock (Smith and Pardee, 1970).

Synchrony induction of cell division and of DNA replication by use of heat shocks in Tetrahymena. From the previous discussion it can be concluded that the dissociation of cell division from replication (which is affected by single or by closely spaced heat shocks) is either not recovered (*E. coli*) or not fully reverted (*Tetrahymena*) after a single cell division. We shall later discuss the reassociation of these two processes, and here only state that in *Tetrahymena* not one but several divisions are required to reassociate cell division and DNA replication in all cells of a population. In the "old" system reassociation occurs several divisions after synchrony induction with heat shocks. These divisions are free-running (no heat shocks between them), and they result in *asynchrony* of both cell division and DNA replication. We wanted to achieve *synchrony* of both processes as they occur in the normal cell cycle. Development of the "new" system was based on a lesson learned from analysis of the "old" one: heat shocks synchronize cell divisions, and endogenous signals coupled to cell division, in turn, phase DNA replication. To obtain full synchrony of division *and* of DNA replication, not one or two but a sequence of well-synchronized cell divisions must be achieved at more or less normal intervals. Thus when temperature shocks are the inducers of synchrony, good

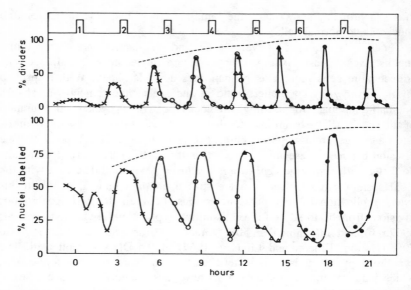

Fig. 4. *Tetrahymena:* synchrony induction using the "new procedure." Heat shocks (34°C, 1/2 hour) are spaced normal cell generations (160 minutes) apart. Otherwise, growth is at the optimum temperature (28°C). After 6 shocks the system is nicely phased, for oral morphogenesis in G_2 (not shown), for cell division (upper curve shows percentage of dividers) and for DNA replication (lower curve shows percentage of cells in nuclear DNA replication after 15 minute pulses with ^{14}C-thymidine). (From Zeuthen, 1971.)

"repetitive division synchrony" may be a prerequisite of "repetitive replication synchrony."

The "new" synchronization procedure takes these principles into account. With this method shocks are spaced normal cell generations apart so that each cell divides one time between consecutive shocks. Division occurs in better synchrony after each new shock and in fine synchrony after 5–7 shocks (fig. 4). It will be seen that the early heat shocks lead to considerable disturbance of the order in which cells engage in DNA synthesis, but after 5–6 shocks the desired relationship is eatablished: there is cyclic repeat of a sequence in which the large majority of cells perform G_2-morphogenesis, divide and replicate, all in excellent synchrony. This result was not obtained earlier because spacing of the temperature shocks (155 ± 5 min) is more critical than was expected (Zeuthen, 1971).

Figure 5 illustrates features of the repetitive synchrony obtained with *Tetrahymena*. Protein and RNA increase logarithmically through two cycles without perturbation due to the temperature shocks. However, analysis at higher resolution than obtainable with chemical analyses reveals such pertur-

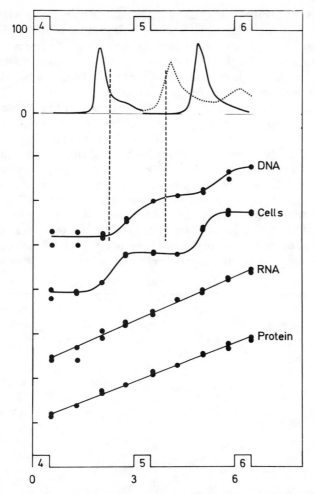

Fig. 5. *Tetrahymena:* repetitive synchrony of cell division and DNA replication. The heat shock program is indicated on top and bottom of the figure. The upper left ordinate shows percentage of dividing cells (had heat shock 5 been omitted, the dotted curve should have been followed). The lower left ordinate is logarithmic. Units show doublings, and the curves are placed arbitrarily on the ordinate. (From Zeuthen, 1971.)

bations. Nucleic acid metabolism in this system was recently reviewed (Andersen, Rasmussen, and Zeuthen, in press). DNA doubles by normal replication one time per cycle, but the replication order is random between successive S-periods (Andersen and Zeuthen, 1971). *Tetrahymena* has numerous

(500–1,000) nucleoli, which harbor the ribosomal genes. This rDNA replicates at the very beginning of the S-period, just after the nuclei have separated and, in some cells, perhaps before the daughter cells have come apart (Andersen and Engberg, 1975). Figure 6 shows these reuslts. This sharp doubling of gene dose should double the cell's capacity for synthesis of ribosomal RNA, though not necessarily for assembling ribosomes. The latter question relates to what will be discussed in part two, but it is relevant here to mention that ribosomal proteins are synthesized one cell generation ahead of the ribosomal RNA (Plesner, 1971). Thus ribosomal RNA, including 5S RNA, are better candidates than the ribosomal proteins for limiting ribosome production.

Figures 4 and 5 illustrate heat-shock controlled repetitive synchrony in *Tetrahymena;* figure 7 shows the same system running free after 6 shocks. Synchrony of cell division decays in the same way as in the "old" system (cf. figure 3), and a subsequent division, the first, second, or third after the shocks have been terminated, suffers increasing delay in response to a heat shock administered up to the time of the transition point. Figure 7 also illustrates a point made earlier concerning normal cells: the cell cycle can be conveniently

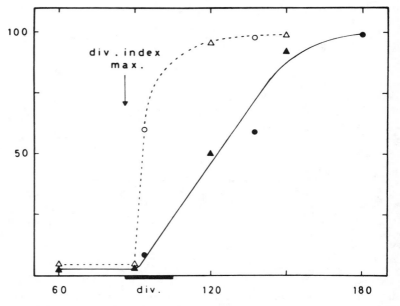

Fig. 6. *Tetrahymena:* open symbols demonstrate that the replication of the ribosomal genes (rDNA) takes place in a short time interval at the time of the initiation of the macronuclear S period, following immediately after the cellular division. The solid symbols show that total macronuclear DNA replicates in 70–80 minutes. (Results from Andersen and Engberg, 1975.)

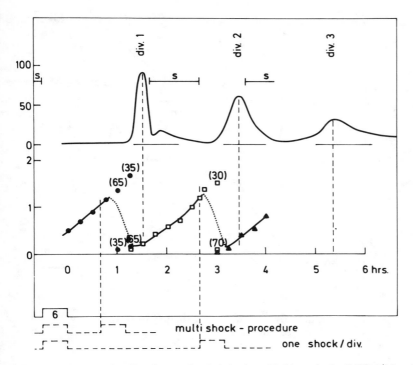

Fig. 7. *Tetrahymena* running free after synchrony induction with 6 heat shocks (34°C, 1/2 hour) spaced normal generation times apart. The upper curve shows percentage of dividing cells after the shocks are terminated; the S-periods are indicated. The lower curve shows how division 1 (solid circle), division 2 (open square), or division 3 (solid triangle) become delayed if a new heat shock is initiated at the different times indicated by the points. Below the frame of the figure is shown when the next heat shock would have come had the shock program been continued, or had we shifted to the multishock procedure. (From Zeuthen, 1971.)

measured from the transition point in consecutive cycles. It also clearly demonstrates both the similarity and the difference between the "old" and the "new" systems. A subsequent division is delayed maximally by exposure to a heat shock when given just prior to a transition point. This timing of heat shocks is what collects the cells in a common phase of oral morphogenesis.

Synchrony induction of cell division and of DNA replication by application of heat shocks to Schizosaccharomyces pombe. It has been rewarding to see that cellular response patterns to temperature changes that account for synchrony induction exist in a variety of quite unrelated cells, including the ciliate *Tetrahymena* in which these patterns were discovered, a yeast, and a bacterium. With *Tetrahymena* we learned that, in response to repeated heat

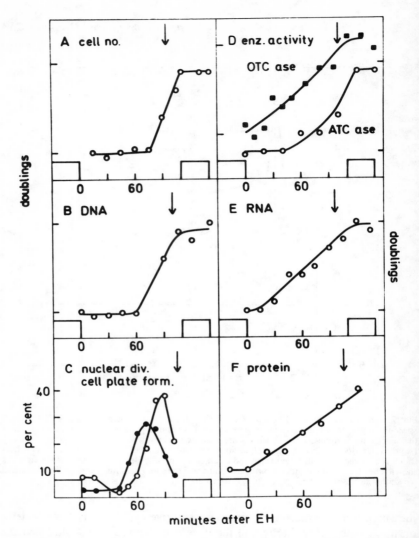

Fig. 8. *Schizosaccharomyces pombe:* repetitive synchrony induced with 5 heat shocks spaced normal cell generations (110) minutes apart. In each of the frames A-F the arrow indicates when 50% of the cells have divided. A synchronized division step is illustrated in frame A. Generally this comes 5–10 minutes before the next heat shock is initiated. The figure illustrates that nuclear and cell division occur sequentially in the last part of the interval between shocks. First the nuclei divide (frame C: solid circles show fraction of cells with stretching, not yet doubled nucleus), then a cell plate forms (frame C: open circles show percentage of cells with cell plate), next DNA (B), and finally the cells (A) double. Protein (F) increases from shock to shock, and there is little synthesis during the shock; however, we cannot safely distinguish this from linear increase (cf. part two). RNA synthesis (E) stops during, and for some time after, the heat shock. When RNA synthesis begins, it occurs rapidly, and doubling of RNA is accomplished before the next shock. Two enzyme activities, ATCase and OTCase (D) nearly double between the shocks. Increase of the latter begins earlier than increase of the former. All measured parameters nearly double between each two shocks, and most of them in distinct steps that follow each other in a regular manner. The separation of daughter cells completes this process. (From Kramhøft and Zeuthen [1975].)

shocks, cells grown at the optimum temperature can shift from an exponential, asynchronous mode of growth and division (normal) to exponential and synchronous growth and division. Periods at the elevated temperature ("shocks") are interspersed with periods at the optimal temperature for precisely the doubling time of a population. Heating is at a temperature that is sufficiently high to block cell division and low enough not to kill the cells even after long exposures. Is this reaction pattern specific for *Tetrahymena,* or is it shared by other cells?

We tested *Schizosaccharomyces pombe,* Mitchison's choice of cell types for cycle studies. With this cell type we obtained the results shown in figure 8, from which we conclude that the ciliate and the yeast respond similarly to these heat treatments. It may be significant that both kinds of synchronized cells are slightly oversized. In *Schizosaccharomyces* the sequence of events between two divisions is the same as those found when this same strain is tudied by selection-synchronization (Mitchison, 1971; Kramhøft and Zeuthen, 1971, 1975), as shown in figure 9.

Miyamoto, Rasmussen, and Zeuthen (1973) later studied murine L-cells in surface culture, but found them not to be readily synchronized with heat shocks. Perhaps the reason we cannot yet synchronize L-cells with heat shocks is because of the considerable spread in response to a heat shock shown by individual cells of equal age. This spread should not totally discourage future attempts to synchronize mammalian cells with temperature shocks.

Tolerance of Cell Cycle Controls: Studies with the System of Scherbaum and Zeuthen

This section deals with studies of *Tetrahymena* cultures in transition from asynchrony to or toward a synchronous mode of DNA replication and cell division. The transition occurs in response to temperature shocks and dissociate processes that normally follow each other sequentially in the cycle. Such troubled cells can be likened to a cell fused from cells representing different stages in the cell cycle.

These studies were aimed at determining the nature and tolerance of *Tetrahymena* cell cycle controls. For example, what is the cell's response to experimentally controlled shifts in the relative timing of the two key events in the cell cycle, DNA replication and cell division? How far in time can the two be separated? How close can they be pushed together? Can these two processes coincide; and if not, when must one wait for the other?

Dissociation and reassociation of cell division and DNA replication. In the "old" system division is blocked during the entire period of 6–8 heat shocks (34°C), each 30 (or 20) minutes in duration and separated from the next one

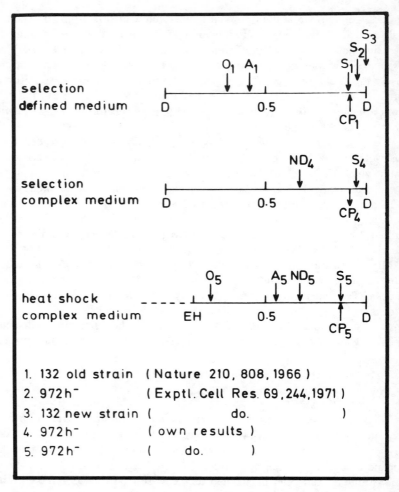

Fig. 9. *Schizosaccharomyces pombe:* cell cycle events in selection-and heat shock-synchronized cells. Numeral indices refer to the strains and authors listed in the figure. (1) from Bostock et al., 1966; (2), (3) from Mitchison and Creanor, 1971; (4), (5) from Kramhøft and Zeuthen, 1975; (D) division; (EH) end of final heat shock; (O) initiation of ornithinetranscarbamylase step (OTCase); (A) initiation of aspartatetranscarbamylase step (ATCase); (ND) midpoint in nuclear division; (CP) midpoint in cell plate formation; (S) midpoint in DNA synthesis. (From Kramhøft and Zeuthen, 1975.)

by 30 (or 40) minutes. However, growth and DNA replication continue during this period. Thus there is dissociation between cell division and DNA replication. Autoradiography with ^{3}H-thymidine (Hjelm and Zeuthen,

1967a), collection of the cells at the entry of S phase using thymidine starvation followed by release for continued DNA synthesis (Zeuthen, 1970), BUdR incorporation studies (Andersen, Brunk, and Zeuthen, 1970) and determination of DNA content per cell (Scherbaum, Louderback, and Jahn, 1959), all indicate that the division-blocked, but growing, cells initiate S-periods asynchronously, much the same as in the original cell population. The S-periods are not extended very much by the temperature cycling, but the time between adjacent S-periods is 4–5 hours. This interval between S-periods in heat-shocked cells is nearly three times greater than the normal interval, which is 97 minutes according to Cameron and Nachtwey (1967). Thus a pathway from S to S stays open in cells that do not divide because of the temperature shocks, but the time interval is long. The time between S phases requires 4–5 temperature cycles, and in this time the cells nearly double their content of protein and RNA. A cell that replicates its DNA early in the period of 6–8 heat shocks will thus replicate again before the treatment is over, and thereby acquire an excess of DNA. Cells that have reached G_2 prior to the heat shocks may even start a third round of DNA replication during the shock treatment and thus have even more DNA.

Because DNA replication stays essentially asynchronous in the population, some cells engage in a first or second round of excess replication so late in the temperature program that this places replication in these cells in conflict with the synchronous division. This conflict arises because replication is biologically timed by the past history of an individual cell, whereas cell division is controlled by the experimenter's heat shock program. However interesting they may be, such conflicts are not easily studied. They are limited to a minor fraction of cells and, furthermore, even differ from cell to cell in this fraction because replication is asynchronous. However, inhibitors of DNA synthesis can be applied during the period of heat shocks to collect the division-blocked cells at or near the point of entry into S. Thus, using a combination of heat shocks and DNA inhibitors, the cells become independently phased for capacity to replicate and for capacity to divide. It becomes possible to individually release the two independently phased processes of the cell cycle to study their interrelationship in time.

Synchronization of DNA Synthesis

Thymidine starvation was used to block DNA synthesis, and subsequent thymidine restoration released the cells for continued and synchronized synthesis. Methotrexate (M) and uridine (U) (Zeuthen, 1968) together affect depletion of the cells' pool of thymidinetriphosphate (Nexø, 1975, Zeuthen, 1974) and thus block DNA synthesis (Villadsen and Zeuthen, 1970). The first

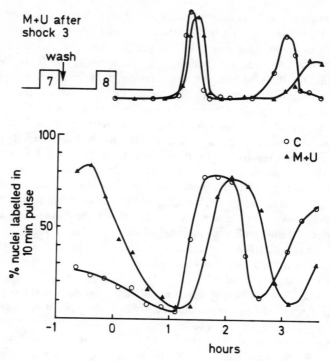

Fig. 10. Synchronization with 8 heat shocks. Two parallel 150 ml cultures, one of which served as a control (open circles). The second received M + U after shock 3 (solid triangles). Aliquots were drawn from both flasks and were pulsed (10 min pulses) with ³H-thymidine. Samples were fixed for autoradiography. Percentage of macronuclei labeled in acid-stable compounds (DNA) were plotted at the end of the incorporation intervals (*lower curves*). *Upper curves* show percentage of dividing cells versus time. The control goes from 0 to 95% in division 1 (visual estimates). (Adapted from Zeuthen, 1970).

agent (M) blocks thymidylate synthesis; the second, U, stops for some time the flow of exogenous thymidine (present in rich medium) into new DNA. In the experiment of figure 10 cells were synchronized with 8 shocks, and M + U was added after shock 3. After shock 7 thymidine was added to release synthesis of DNA, after which 85% of the cells were in S as compared with 25% in the control. Thus M + U trapped 60% of the cells when they were beginning S, and from this state they can be released for DNA synthesis, in replication synchrony. It is far from perfect, but this technique can be used to attempt to overlap DNA replication with cell division.

Cells with conflicting DNA replication and cell division cycles. In normal *Tetrahymena* cells the midpoint in cell division comes 121 minutes after S has

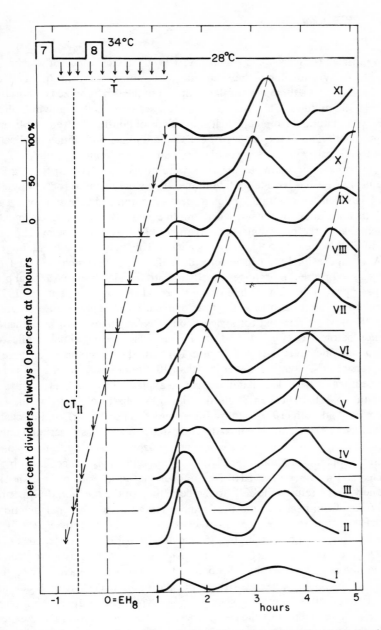

Fig. 11. *Abscissa:* hours; *ordinate:* percentage of dividing cells, always 0% at 0 hrs. Synchronization with 8 heat shocks (visual estimates of division activities). M + U added after shock 3, thymidine (T) at arrows, or not at all (curve I). Ordinate scale for percentage of dividers applies to all curves when 0% is at the level of the horizontal line under a curve. (Adapted from Zeuthen, 1970.)

been initiated (Cameron and Nachtwey, 1967). The technique of synchronizing DNA synthesis has been used to demonstrate that in division-
synchronized cells there is a similar midpoint in the synchronized cell division
cycle at 130 minutes. This time, termed CT_1, separates cells that will replicate
and divide naturally from cells that show signs of conflict between replication
and division. The first category of cells predominate and initiate replication
prior to CT_1, the smaller second class of cells begin replication after CT_1. In
the experiments of figure 11 the cells were collected at (or in) S for a long
time using M + U. By adding thymidine, they were released for new synthesis of DNA at various times prior to heat-synchronized cell division. Apart
from this variation in time when thymidine was added, this experiment is
comparable to the preceding one. Figure 11, I, shows that the synchronous
division is blocked if no thymidine is added. This may be due to shortage of
DNA or, more likely, to incapacity of cells that have embarked on DNA
synthesis to progress morphogenetically toward division before a critical point
has been passed that comes late in the S-period (Buhse and Zeuthen, 1974).
To obtain division furrows at the time dictated by the temperature program,
the cells must be released for synchronous DNA synthesis not later than 40
minutes before EH (fig. 11, II-IV). These cells may not finish replication
until about one hour later (cf. figure 10), but they become insensitive to
inhibitors of DNA synthesis after less than 40 minutes, i.e., at or even before
EH (Zeuthen, 1970). This paradox may be explained by the later-discovered
20 minute overlap between S and functional G_2 phases observed in the new
system by Andersen (1972) and by Buhse and Zeuthen (1974), and discussed
by Zeuthen (1974). Thus we must distinguish between G_2 as describing only a
"gap" and G_2-functions such as oral morphogenesis and build-up of other
structural apparatus required for division. "Functional G_2" exceeds G_2 by 20
minutes and thus begins at EH. This implies that in a series of heat shocks,
each new shock returns the cells to the beginning of the *functional* G_2 period.
"Recovery from heat" would then require repetition of a normal functional
G_2 phase. The normal G_2 is 58 minutes (Cameron and Nachtwey, 1967), or
some 20 minutes shorter than the 85 minutes from EH to synchronous division. Figure 11, IV-XI, also illustrates that the sequence of synchronized S,
G_2 and division, followed by a second cell cycle, can be delayed for up to 2
hours by postponing release of the replication-inhibited system. Block and
release of cell division by heat shocks bring division in conflict with replication in a minor fraction of the cells. There is no evidence from these experiments that the two events can be brought in conflict by manipulation of
replication, although this possibility is not excluded.

   Consideration of the subfractions of the population. In the following we
first (1) consider the major fraction of cells (~80%) that enter a final replica-

tion round before the critical time at EH—40 minutes. Next (2) we turn to the minor fraction of cells (~20%) that engage in DNA synthesis later than this, and in which a conflict between DNA replication and division occurs.

(1) Normally the major fraction, some 80% of the cells, enters a final replication round before the critical time. These cells divide in good synchrony, and most of them synchronously replicate again, skipping G_1. In each of these cells a G_2 interval becomes defined the moment the cell undergoes the synchronous division, but the duration of this G_2 varies greatly from cell to cell, from ~1 (normal) to ~5 hours. This occurs because the heat shocks hold the cells in the first part of G_2, the phase that precedes the transition point (cf. figure 1A). During this time (G_2) a cell can be heat-shocked maximally 4 times. It then divides in the absence of additional shocks or replicates if again heat-shocked. Although time indications are imprecise, the important point is that all the good synchronous dividers have spent at least the normal time in G_2 since they last replicated. Some of these cells even tolerated being blocked in G_2 for several hours. During this extension of the G_2 period the cells grow, but do not seem to be making preparations for the subsequent division. Morphological demonstration of this point has been available for some time when it was observed that the oral structures were held in an early morphogenetic stage (Frankel, 1962, 1964).

Synchrony of cell division in this fraction of cells, following asynchronous replication and highly flexible G_2 time, is an indication that replication and cell division can tolerate great separation in time provided there is an excess of normal G_2 time. Synchrony induction depends on this.

It needs to be pointed out that regardless of the excess amount of DNA per cell already available, engagement in new synthesis commits a cell to a full replication round and a full G_2 period. This new engagement in S may be in response to increased cellular mass, which according to Zeuthen and Rasmussen (1972) doubles in 4–5 hours during heat shocks.

(2) Let us now consider the minor fraction of cells that initiate DNA replication in the interval from 40 minutes before to 40 minutes after the time EH. This interval is between the latest time when the cells can finish DNA replication and take part in the synchronized division, *and* the time when oral morphogenesis and the following division block further engagement in DNA synthesis (Zeuthen, 1971).

Throughout the heat shock program, the cells engage in S at the rate of 17% per hour (Zeuthen, 1970), so the fraction we are dealing with is roughly 22% of all cells. This fraction of cells can be blocked in S (or collected at S) by use of M + U; they then can be released for continued DNA synthesis by the addition of thymidine. Through such procedures, it was found possible to collect those cells that normally replicate in the critical interval here dealt with

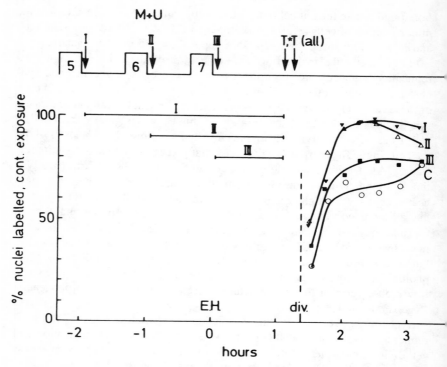

Fig. 12. Synchronization with 7 heat shocks. Three samples (I-III) were treated with M + U as indicated; a fourth served as the control (C). The four samples all received radioactive thymidine (T, *T) as indicated. Subsequently samples were withdrawn at intervals from I-IV for autoradiography. Curves show percentage of cells with labeled macronuclei. Note that 100% nuclei pulse-label after the synchronous division if cells are blocked in, and collect at, S for as long as indicated by II. The collected cells, when released, do not necessarily divide. (Adapted from Zeuthen, 1970.)

and let them continue DNA synthesis *after* the first synchronized division (figure 12). They were found to add to the group of synchronously replicating cells (two-thirds of total), making the sum close to 100%. Thus the cells that fail to replicate between the two synchronized divisions are those that replicate very late before the first synchronized cell division (Zeuthen, 1970). They can also be characterized by their capacity to develop furrows and perhaps to divide two times after EH without new DNA synthesis (Hamburger and Zeuthen, 1957; Lowy and Leick, 1969), 20–30 minutes faster than normal (Zeuthen, 1968).

Thus a minor fraction of the heat-shocked cells may have reversed the normal order between a replication round and a cell division, so that two consecutive rounds of replication are followed by two consecutive cell divisions. I mentioned earlier that a single heat shock of a series can channel a cell away from division and into excess DNA synthesis. The shock commits the cell to a full replication round and a full functional G₂ period before cell division becomes possible again. When this shock occurs very late in the sequence, the cell has insufficient time first to replicate and then undergo the synchronous division. It finds other solutions: division may be delayed or even cancelled ($<^1/_5$ of the cells), or an excess replication round is inserted, so that two consecutive replication rounds may be succeeded by two consecutive divisions as described.

The growth-division cycle of the cytoplasm is matched by a chromatin-condensation, DNA-synthetic cycle of the nucleus. The two are interlocked, probably at several points, but most clearly at division. The initiation of division correlates with chromatin condensation, and its completion is accompanied by chromatin loosening, apparently a condition required for DNA synthesis (cf. figure 1).

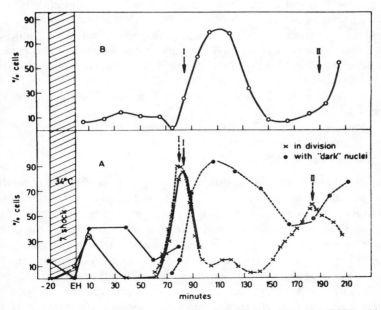

Fig. 13. *Tetrahymena* synchronized according to Scherbaum and Zeuthen (1954) with heat shocks space 1/2 hour apart. (A) Percentage of dividing cells (crosses, 2 exps.). There is some abortive division (circled cross) after the shock (unusual), then the first and second divisions follow normally. Percentage of cells with "dark" nuclei, i.e., with dispersed chromatin, shown by solid circles. (B) Percentage of cells in DNA synthesis shown by open circles (curve from Hjelm and Zeuthen, 1967b). Note the correlation between chromatin dispersal and DNA replication. (Adaped from Nilsson and Zeuthen, 1974.)

Treatment with heat shocks blocks cell division but lets chromatin cycle run asynchronously though slowly, the interval from S to S being extended. As this is the phase with condensed chromatin, the sequence of heat shocks causes visible chromatin condensation. Whenever the shocks are discontinued, some cells should be ready to immediately loosen their chromatin and enter DNA synthesis. Figure 13A illustrates this for the state of the chromatin ("dark" nuclei have dispersed chromatin), and for DNA synthesis (B). It is assumed that the small fraction of cells that replicate within the first hour past EH is contained in the minor fraction of cells that loosen the chromatin at this time and again condense it, presumably when the cell first engages in preparation for division 40 minutes past EH.

Experiment *B* shows fewer nuclei in DNA synthesis before (and more after) division than seen in most other experiments; recall (figure 1) that the chromatin remains loose for considerably more than the S-period itself. I propose that figure 13 demonstrates a clear correlation between structural and functional states of the chromatin, and, further, that the chromatin cycles of condensation and DNA synthesis are similar in normal and synchronized cells.

Deficiencies in synchrony as observed by Scherbaum and Zeuthen (1954) indeed seem to relate to conflict between cytoplasmic and nuclear functions (dissociated by heat shocks) that become evident at the time of reassociation of cellular subcycles. Finally, the synchronized decondensation of chromatin that follows the synchronized cell division as illustrated in figure 13 may represent (or contain) the signal that is required to trigger cells into synchronized DNA replication.

GROWTH THROUGH THE CYCLE: EVIDENCE THAT THE
CELL DOUBLES FUNCTIONALLY AT DIVISION

Mitchison (1971) concluded that cell growth through the cycle is continuous, and follows an exponential, linear, or even some other course. Cell growth is the integrated sum of separate processes making up the cell's many chemical and structural components. I found a linear over-all growth pattern in *Tetrahymena* measuring respiration (Zeuthen, 1953); Kubitchek (1970) found linear growth in bacteria and stressed the generality of this principle. It follows that in growing cells there must exist discontinuities, i.e., discrete doublings of undefined "synthetic centers" once per cycle, or of physiological functions that control cell growth, e.g., capacities for transport of nutrients into the cell. It seems worthwhile to study growth patterns throughout the cell cycle, not simply for synthetic products or selected physiological functions, but for the sum of functions that are reflected by cell size or other properties of the cell. Such integrated functions are heat production, oxygen uptake, and carbon dioxide output (fermenting cells), all measures of the cell's energy metabolism. Another integrated function is the increase in the live cell's dry weight, which will be described below.

Methods

The first Cartesian Diver was introduced and developed by Linderstrøm-Lang (1937, 1943) and his associate Holter (1943). My inspiration stems from my early association with these two men. The Ampulla Diver (Zeuthen, 1953), its construction and operation as a Cartesian Diver, is demonstrated in figure 14. The ampulla diver is an excellent growth chamber for cloned cells.

It can also be used as a non-Cartesian Gradient Diver (Løvlie and Zeuthen, 1962); it will migrate down an aqueous density gradient (figure 15) when the resident cells consume gas, and up the gradient when they produce gas, respectively oxygen and carbon dioxide. Migrations can be followed by automatic photographic recording (Løvlie and Zeuthen, 1962; Hamburger and

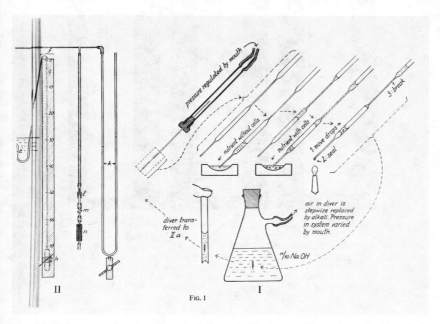

Fig. 14. (I) The *Ampulla Diver* is made from a suitable glass capillary, charged with a single *Tetrahymena* cell, balanced to float, and (II) transferred to a pressure-controlling, pressure-measuring device, "the sensitive manometer," with attached flotation chamber (far left). The sensitive manometer with flotation chamber is hooked over the edge of a regulated water bath under conditions that permit continued microscopic observation of the cell and its progeny. (Adapted from Zeuthen, 1953.)

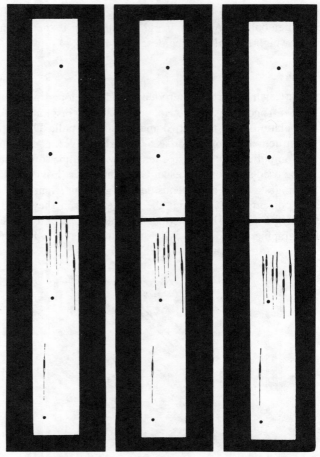

Fig. 15. *Ampulla Gradient Diver*. Three photographs of an aqueous density gradient (Na_2SO_4) taken at intervals of a few hours. Five density standards (small dark spheres) are to be seen, and two control divers (bottom, and upper right). The other 5 divers are each loaded with a single sea urchin egg (*Psammechinus miliaris*). They travel down the gradient because O_2 is consumed and CO_2 is absorbed. The diver's narrow tail (pointing downward) is open for pressure equilibration, so gas consumed in the diver is replaced with gradient fluid. The crossbar is a reference mark on the front of the thermostatic bath. (Adapted from Andersen, Nexφ, Hamburger, and Zeuthen, 1972.)

Zeuthen, 1974; Zeuthen and Hamburger, in press), and a simple equation permits calculation of rates of gaseous exchanges from known diver and gradient specifications and recorded migration rates. We have used diver gasometers to follow cloned cells and their progeny. With these instruments respiration and fermentation rates can be followed with greater precision than is possible with any other vital function.

The Cartesian Diver Balance (Zeuthen, 1948, 1961) floats in biological medium. The equilibrium (flotation) pressure can be adjusted and read on a double-branched water manometer; it differs when the balance pan (open plastic cup attached to the outside of the diver) is empty and when it is loaded, e.g., with a living amoeba, *Chaos chaos* or *Amoeba proteus*. The balance can be calibrated with standard weights made of polystyrene, so the change in equilibrium pressure due to loading of the balance with cells can be interpreted in terms of submerged weight (Reduced Weight, RW) of the live cell. Cell water weighs nothing under water, and this is nearly true also of cell lipids. Thus the RW of a cell can be attributed to its protein, carbohydrates, nucleic acids, and salts (Holter and Zeuthen, 1948). Brzin, Kovic, and Oman (1964), working in my laboratory, developed the Magnetic Diver Balance. In this instrument the air bubble of the Cartesian Diver Balance is replaced with an AlNiCo particle, and this instrument is floated electromagnetically (Brzin, Kovic, and Oman, 1964). The "Magnetic Diver" is a magnetic diver balance that floats an ampulla diver at constant pressure (Brzin and Zeuthen, 1964; Brzin et al., 1965); thus the balance substitutes for a manometer, or a density gradient.

Results.

Mitotic respiratory cycles in cleaving eggs. Single frog eggs show a constant over-all respiration rate during cleavage, but faint waves in rate of

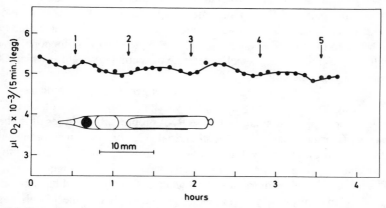

Fig. 16. Rates of oxygen uptake ($\Delta O_2/\Delta t$) in a single egg of *Rana platyrrhina*. Arrows indicate when cleavages 1–5 begin. Insert shows diver used; it floats "egg-down." (Adapted from Zeuthen and Hamburger, 1972.)

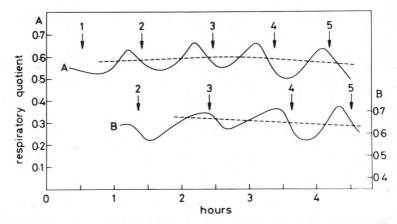

Fig. 17. Respiratory quotients calculated on basis of values for $\Delta O_2/\Delta t$ (fig. 16) and $\Delta CO_2/\Delta t$. Arrows indicate when cleavages 1–5 begin. (Adapted from Zeuthen and Hamburger, 1972.)

oxygen uptake and in carbon dioxide output accompany the cell cycles. For every mitotic cycle a phase with slight increase in rate of O_2 consumption/CO_2 output gives way to a phase with a slight decrease. However, the mitotic waves for O_2 and for CO_2 are phase-shifted almost one-half cycle, and mitotic rate-changes are more pronounced in the case of CO_2 than of O_2. Thus, the respiratory quotient correlates with mitotic cycles (figs. 16, 17).

Oxygen uptake decreases during mitosis and increases during interphase, whereas the opposite holds true for the rate at which the egg liberates CO_2 to the atmosphere. No final interpretation of these observations can be offered without other data, but the findings are compatible with the idea that mitotic chromosome condensation is instrumental in determining the immediate balance between the oxidative energy supply generated by the mitochondria and a multitude of phenomena, which determine the cumulative rate at which CO_2 is liberated from the cell.

It seems reasonable to suggest that messenger RNAs are produced in a pulse during each interphase and quickly disposed of in each mitosis. The limited macromolecular syntheses these RNAs represent might result in these small and transient changes of mitochondrial activity. Such macromolecular syntheses lead to extremely limited over-all growth, but they may serve to control the sequence of mitoses that is characteristic of cleavage.

The sea urchin egg is much smaller than that of the frog, and its respiration rate builds up considerably during cleavage, slowly before the 16-cell stage, then faster (figure 18). This results from activation of a constant population of mitochondria (Gustafson and Lenique, 1952), and such activation can be

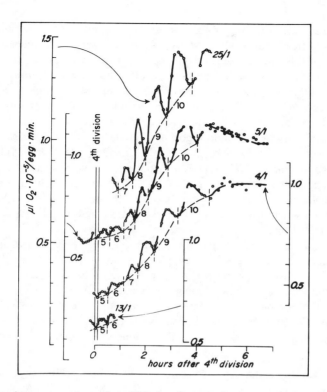

Fig. 18. *Dendraster excentricus:* all available data for rates of oxygen uptake per egg (*ordinate*) plotted against hours of development. The time of division 4 is taken as zero. The respiratory cycles are separated by minima (marked by short vertical lines) presumably around cell division at telophase. The number of a cycle thus precedes the time of the division. The small area from one vertical line to the next, and between curve and smooth auxiliary line is termed the "excess-O₂" of a division cycle. (Adapted from Frydenberg and Zeuthen, 1960.)

obtained with DNP (Immers and Runnström, 1960). During the early mitoses oxygen uptake cycles precisely as in the frog egg. This is true of other marine eggs too (Zeuthen, 1949). Increased O_2 consumption occurs during interphase and decreases during mitosis (Holter and Zeuthen, 1957), as observed with the frog egg. After the 16-cell stage the mitotic rate slows down differentially in the embryo, and this is caused by differential lengthening of the interphases rather than of the mitoses. This is demonstrated in figure 19, which shows nuclear counts (Holter and Zeuthen, 1957). Thus the accelerating over-all increase in respiration rate past the 16-cell stage can be interpreted as the result of increasing interphase activities of the embryonic cells. i.e., as a reflection of growth.

The amplitude of the respiratory waves that accompany the later mitoses in cleaveage differs from study to study, if not from species to species. It may increase considerably as cleavage proceeds as found with *Dendraster* (figure 18 from Frydenberg and Zeuthen, 1960) and *Psammechinus miliaris* (Zeuthen, 1950), or only slightly as in *Psammechinus microtubercultus* (Holter and Zeuthen, 1957). These differences should surprise no one, because as measured, the mitotic respiratory waves accompanying cleavage in populations of embryos or in single embryos (Scholander et al., 1952; Zeuthen, 1955; Scholander, Leivestad, and Sundness, 1958; Zeuthen, 1960; Hamburger and Zeuthen, 1975) represent a balance between steadily increasing rate variations in most of the cells (cf., figure 18) and a damping due to mitotic asynchrony (figure 19) that develops in the population of embryos. The mitotic asynchrony varies with environmental factors and with the quality of the batch of eggs used.

Increase in respiration rate through the cell cycle of Tetrahymena. A *Tetrahymena* cell in the stationary phase is large when culture growth is limited by oxygen such as occurs in an upright test tube. Such large stationary phase cells were individually cloned axenically in ampulla divers (Zeuthen, 1953) with a complex, rich medium (proteose peptone, liver extract). Each cell showed a 2–3 hour lag in respiration rate and then began to grow, initiating division at the same time. Each clone showed stepwise exponential

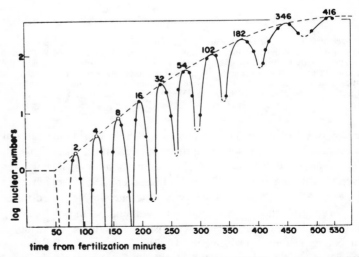

Fig. 19. Mitotic steps in the cleavage of *Psammechinus microtuberculatus* were followed by phase contrast microscopy of samples removed at intervals from the batch. Nuclei with envelopes ("whole") stood out bright in lightly compressed eggs; nuclei in mitosis ("open") did not. The curve gives "whole" nuclei per egg. (Adapted from Holter and Zeuthen, 1957.)

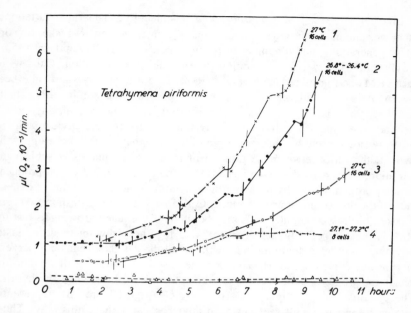

Fig. 20. *Tetrahymena:* four experiments with cloned cells in Cartesian ampulla divers. The respiration rate of the original cell and of its progency is followed concomitantly with observations of cell divisions. The open triangles represent a control showing slight autooxidation of the medium. (Adapted from Zeuthen, 1953.)

growth and multiplication into 16-cells. These events were followed closely, both visually and gasometrically. Finally, the cells were closely inspected and counted. The cloned cells were smaller than the original one.

In figure 20 curves 1 and 2 demonstrate an increase in respiratory rate of cells that grow and divide without environmental restrictions. Once the lag is broken, the respiratory rate increases from division to division and occurs linearly in the first part of each cycle. For some time prior to the beginning of each cytokinetic period, there is little change. This predivisional phase with blocked growth in respiration rate lasts 15–30 minutes. This may reflect reduction of transcriptional activity due to chromatin condensation, which occurs through most of G_2 (Nilsson, 1970) and through cell division (cf. figure 1A). In figure 20 note that when cytokinesis begins, the respiratory rate again increases, in some cases to nearly double the rate exhibited in the previous interphase (table 1). Thus the rate of growth in what may be termed the "respiratory mass" (RM) may double around division, at a time when the chromatin is condensed, and prior to the actual event of separation of the nucleus and the cytoplasm into two cells.

Like cell size, the RM in *Tetrahymena* is subject to considerable variation. In clones and in synchronized populations adjustment to new RM takes one or more generations, and a number of parameters are involved (Zeuthen, 1953, Løvlie, 1963). First, the generation time is subject to variation. Cells with large RM, and large reduced weight (RW), take a relatively short time between divisions, and the converse is true of cells that are initially small (Løvlie, 1963). Large heat-shock-synchronized cells are normal in this sense. Second, the time from division to division can be crudely divided into a post-divisional growth phase and a pre-divisional phase with blocked growth in RM; the ratio between the time spent in these two phases is subject to variation. Thus cells that have large RM at the time of one division produce smaller progeny cells by reduction in generation time and by relative extension of the predivisional growth block. Cells in balanced growth show no such block. Third, two daughter cells may begin their life, each growing as fast in RM as the mother cell (at her birth), and together growing twice as fast; anything less than a doubling in growth rate of the daughters can be observed (figure 20, curves 3 and 4). The extreme case would be that of a clone in which the progeny cells together respire at the rate of the original single cell. The egg in cleavage (figure 16), or early cleavage (figure 18), represents this case, and we shall see that even amoebae can behave this way. Thus what doubles at cell division is the *capacity* of the cell to increase its respiratory rate to double the rate possessed by the mother cell when it originated.

Increase in respiration rate and in reduced weight in amoebae. Ideally, one should follow growth in mass and in respiration through the cycle of the same cell. This has not been done, but I propose to make comparisons between three rather disparate studies with three amoebae.

The first study to be described is by Prescott (1955, 1956) who followed mass growth in *Amoeba proteus*. In this cell type, increases in reduced weight, protein, and in cell volume occur in parallel. They are fastest in newly divided cells, then slow down and come to a complete halt a few hours before the next division. The negative correlation between cell size at division and duration of the forthcoming cycle that was found in *Tetrahymena* was also found by RW measurements in *Amoeba*.

The second study to be discussed was by Hamburger (1975), who grew *Acantamoeba sp.* axenically and followed rates of oxygen uptake with the ampulla diver. From the results (figures 21 and 22) Hamburger concluded that the increase in the respiratory rate from one division to the next may follow at least three patterns. The respiration rate may (1) increase linearly through the cell cycle; it may increase (2) linearly through most of the cell cycle but stop increasing for a short period just before cell division; or it may (3) increase to

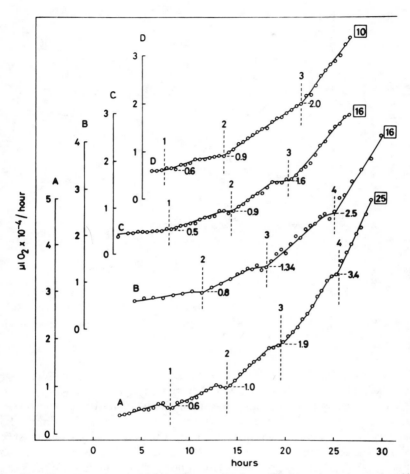

Fig. 21. Automatic recordings of respiration rates using four cells of *Acanthamoeba sp*. cloned in gradient divers. Zero is the time when the single cell was isolated into the diver. The clones were established from cells in exponential growth. The framed values at the extreme right show the final number of cells in the diver. At the level of the horizontal dashed lines is shown the total respiratory rate ($\mu l \times 10^{-4}$), read from the ordinate. (Adapted from Hamburger, 1975.)

a maximum early, and then decrease to a minimum late in the cell cycle. In the last case there is little or no over-all increase of the respiratory rate. Of these patterns the first one may pertain to cells in balanced growth, as will be seen again with *Schizosaccharomyces*. The second pattern is the one most often observed in diver experiments, and it may be characteristic for cells in late exponential growth (50,000–500,000 cells/ml). It is similar to the one found with *Tetrahymena*, and also tends to parallel the growth curves just

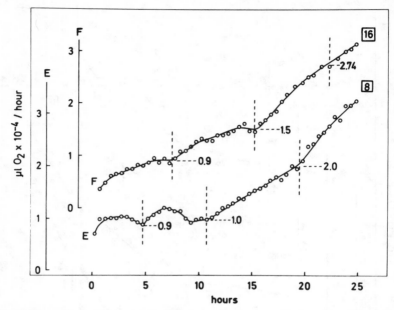

Fig. 22. Rates of oxygen consumption of 2 clones of *Acanthamoeba sp.* established from cells in stationary phase. Zero is the time when automatic recording of the diver position began. (Adapted from Hamburger, 1975.)

described for *Amoeba proteus*. The third pattern was found with very large stationary-phase cells during growth after transfer to fresh medium.

We now ask whether the term "respiratory mass" is justified. Is the respiration rate of single growing cells a reasonably good measure of cell mass? By and large the data answer this question in the affirmative, but caution must be used when considering cells that cease to grow. The large *Acanthamoeba* (figure 22E) cell and its progency show little growth. Through two divisions there is no over-all increase in "respiratory mass." This cell behaves like a cleaving egg, and so do the respiration rate cycles.

When dealing with the egg of frogs and sea urchins, I interpreted the respiratory cycles as reflecting cyclic variations in the rate of macromolecular syntheses (the cells having constant mass). However, with growing cells it is not obvious how to quantitatively split the energy metabolism between growth and maintenance. Nevertheless, the curves for growth (in RW) in *Amoeba proteus* support the notion that in *Acanthamoeba* the predivisional respiratory plateaus and dips in RM (see figures 21 and 22) do reflect predivisional reductions in cellular growth rate; the cell mass stays constant, but the respiration rate decreases. This warns against rigid interpretation of respiration rates as a relative measure of cell mass. On the other hand, the smallness of the respiratory waves that accompany division cycles in eggs, and of the premitotic plateaus and depressions in growing cells, suggests that in practice curves for increase in cell mass and in respiration rate follow each other closely. Thus the term "respiratory mass" can be used with discretion to study fast-growing cells with the high precision offered by diver gasometry.

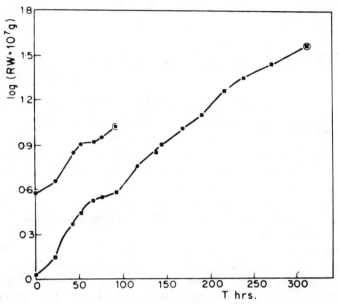

Fig. 23. Growth cycle in *Chaos chaos* followed by increase in reduced weight (RW). The curves are discontinued when the large and the small sister cell (obtained microsurgically) divided, respectively. (Adapted from Satir and Zeuthen, 1961.)

The third study was done by Satir and Zeuthen (1961), who folllowed rates of growth in RW in the large multinucleate amoeba *Chaos chaos;* it shows great natural variation in size even in the same culture. The smallest amoeba (designated B2) was obtained by cutting a cell into two unequal places. Over the first 100 hours the large (B1) and the small piece (B2) showed parallel growth (figure 23). The small cell grew in a cyclic manner to 35 times its original size before it divided; in the process it extended the length of the cell cycle that it first shared with the yet undivided larger sister.

The important observation that arose from these studies is that growth rate over a growth cycle appears to be a function of the surface to volume ratio of the cell at the beginning of a cycle (this is illustrated in figure 24). Said more

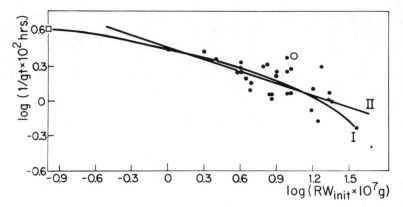

Fig. 24. The relation (solid circle) between growth rate and RW at the initiation of a growth cycle in *Chaos chaos* (open circle, result obtained from Prescott). Curve I is simply fitted to the points. II is calculated with the assumption that growth rate (1/gt) is proportional to $RW_{init}^{-1/3}$. (Adapted from Satir and Zeuthen, 1961.)

directly, change in RW with time (as an index of the rate of synthesis of cytoplasm) is proportional to the surface area of the amoeba. Therefore, the finding in *Chaos chaos* of a synchronized nuclear division cycle (Kudo, 1947) and of a growth cycle resembling the one found in *Amoeba proteus* may be interpreted as before: directly or indirectly, the feeding function of the cell surface is under nuclear control.

Growth followed by measurements of fermentation rate in Schizosaccharomyces. In the yeast *Schizosaccharomyces pombe* grown aerobically in broth, CO_2 output exceeds O_2 uptake 12 times. So what is measured gasometrically (when CO_2 is not absorbed) is essentially CO_2. Furthermore, mitochondrial oxygen consumption is uncoupled from phosphorylation (Heslot, Gafteau, and Louis, 1970). Thus fermentation rates may be indicative of rates of energy production and consumption, and also, when interpreted with caution, of cell mass.

Rates of CO_2 evolution were measured (Kramhøft et al., in press) during the cell cycle of cells naturally synchronized or synchronized by the selection procedure of Mitchison and Vincent (1965) or by the heat-shock procedure of Kramhøft and Zeuthen (1971). The results suggest that in all three cases the fermentation rate increases linearly from division to division and doubles at about the time of division. Growth, as measured by fermentation rate, *appears* to be linear from division to division in all three situations studied; it *definitely deviates* from an exponential course, and toward arithmetic linearity, at least in the two synchronized systems (figures 25 and 26). Although these two systems are essentially similar, they are different with respect to the *extent* of growth in fermentation rate in one generation. This parameter shows

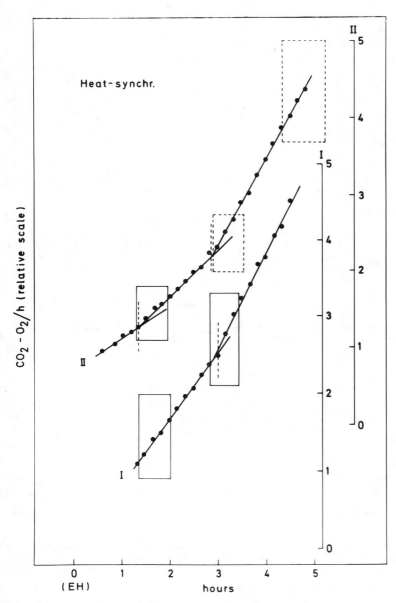

Fig. 25. Gasometry at constant 31°C of two small samples of *Schizosaccharomyces pombe*. Synchrony was induced by 5 heat shocks, ending at zero hours. Cell divisions were followed by inspection of small samples incubated similarly. Division times are framed and with full lines if actually observed. The ordinates are arithmetic and in relative units because the number of cells per diver is unknown. (Adapted from Hamburger et al., in preparation.)

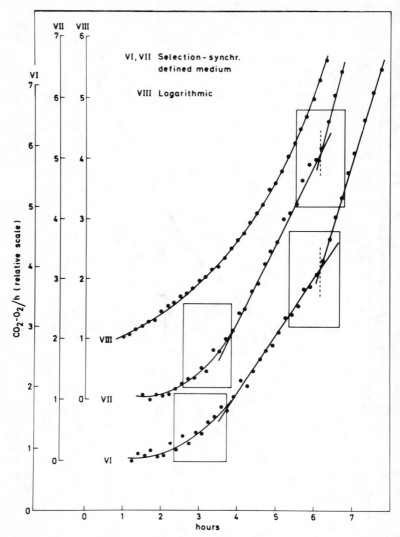

Fig. 26. Gasometry at 31°C of three samples of *Schizosaccharomyces* representing exponentially multiplying and selection-synchronized cells. (Adapted from Hamburger et al., in preparation.)

a doubling in selection-synchronized cells, but somewhat less in heat-synchronized cells. The latter cells were initially slightly oversized because of the temperature treatment, and were studied here while in the process of being reduced to a smaller size.

In conclusion we find that the rate of CO_2 output (glycolysis) increases linearly through the cycle of *Schizosaccharomyces* and doubles at the synchronized cell division. We consider that this reflects a linear increase in energy output to maintain cell mass and to support its linear growth. We suspect that enzymes which control rates of glycolysis are located at ER membranes that are present in several layers in the cortex of this cell. These membranes can peel apart and invaginate, forming mesosome-like structures (Birch-Andersen et al., 1974). *Schizosaccharomyces* has the shape of a rod and grows by elongation only. The growth zone is located at one end of the cell (Johnson, 1965). We often see signs of membrane activity at the end of the cell that might relate to the expected linear accumulation of glycolytic enzymes throughout the cycle. At division a new growth point comes into being (Johnson, 1965) and this could account for the suggested doubling of the glycolytic system. This linear growth, a function of the cell surface, and doubling of glycolytic rate at division might well be under nuclear control, as discussed for *Tetrahymena* and the amoebae.

From the studies reported here, it may be concluded that divers are unusual in offering a combination of high sensitivity with high precision that is necessary for following cleaving eggs and suitably cloned axenically growing cells through a number of cell cycles.

Cleaving eggs show reproducible faint cycles in respiration rate, reflecting a decrease in respiration rate through mitosis and an increase during interphase, beginning with the reconstitution of the daughter nuclei at telophase. In a general way this revitalization of the cells at division appears to be a common feature shared by growing cells, regardless of presence or absence of a pre-divisional or divisional block. Further increase of the measured parameters, Δ O_2/min., Δ CO_2/min., or Δ RW/min. occur after division. These parameters may double in rate at cell division to the rate expressed by the mother cell. Thus what I refer to as "revitalization" of the daughter cells at division also reflects doubling, or possible doubling, of the growth potential, whether or not this is made use of in the next generation. It does not occur in cleaving eggs, nor always in *Tetrahymena,* but in our experiments it always is found in *Schizosaccharomyces.*

This presentation is based on Kubitschek's idea that linear growth through the cell cycle is a basic theme, which cells modulate. Implicit in this concept is the postulate that there is a functional doubling of the cell at some point during the cycle, as documented by the experimental evidence reported here. Support for the concept is not compelling because of uncertainties about how to relate measured gasometric rates to cell mass and cell function. If, however, we assume that maintenance and growth metabolism are distinguishable, it seems clear that changes in growth metabolism are indeed demonstrable through the growth-division cycle, and particularly around the time of cell division. This does not preclude that situations exist in which the cell's shifting synthetic activities are fitted less well in time so that discontinuities appear at the level of respiratory energy supply. In fact, Løvlie (1963) working with *Tetrahymena pyriformis* and Buhse and Hamburger (1974) with *Tetrahymena vorax* have reported cases in which there is respiratory depression about midway in the cycle, probably toward the end of the S period. On the other hand, the mechanical work of cytokinesis is not reflected at the level of respiration in the cleaving frog egg. The cycle shown in figure 16 persisted in a fertilized egg that failed to divide (figure 5A in Zeuthen, 1946).

In the literature we can also find supporting evidence for the view that over-all growth through the cell cycle is basically exponential (Mitchison, 1971), in which case neither replication nor cell division should reflect on clonal growth except by modulation of the basic theme. I have chosen to emphasize the basic pattern of linear growth (and not exponential growth) but without fully committing myself. My choice was determined by the reported results of growth in $\Delta CO_2/t$ through the cycle of *Schizosaccharomyces:* linear without modulations, a simple basic pattern though not necessarily a general one.

To summarize the basic concepts and experimental results presented here, I tentatively conclude that cell cycle controls include mechanisms by which the cell doubles its rate of integrated functions at a discrete point in the cycle. The evidence obtained from studies with *Tetrahymena* and with *Schizosaccharomyces* suggests that this event occurs around the time when the cell splits into two, which agrees with Mitchison's (1971) conclusion that in the lower eukaryotes functional doubling occurs toward the end of the cycle.

REFERENCES

Andersen, H. A. 1972. Requirements for DNA replication preceding cell division in *Tetrahymena pyriformis*. Exptl. Cell Res. 75:89–94.

Andersen, H. A., C. F. Brunk, and E. Zeuthen. 1970. Studies of the DNA replication in heat synchronized *Tetrahymena pyriformis*. C. R. Trav. Lab. Carlsberg 38:123–31.

Andersen, H. A., and J. Engberg. 1975. Timing of the ribosomal gene replication in *Tetrahymena pyriformis*. Exptl. Cell Res. 92:159–63.

Andersen, H. A., and E. Zeuthen. 1971. DNA replication sequence in *Tetrahymena* is not repeated from generation to generation. Exptl. Cell Res. 68:309–14.

Andersen, H. A., L. Rasmussen, and E. Zeuthen. 1975. Cell division and DNA replication in synchronous *Tetrahymena* cultures. *In* Current topics in microbiology and immunology. W. Arber et al. (eds.). Springer Verlag, Berlin.

Birch-Andersen, A., B. Kramhøft, H. Ravn, and E. Zeuthen. 1974. Membranes in the cortical cytoplasm, and mesosome-like structures in the fission yeast *Schizosaccharomyces pombe*. C. R. Trav. Lab. Carlsberg 40:9, 101–6.

Brzin, M., and E. Zeuthen. 1964. Notes on the possible use of the magnetic diver for respiration measurements (error 10^- μl/hour). C. R. Trav. Lab. Carlsberg 39:493–505.

Brzin, M., W. - D. Dettbarn, P. Rosenberg, and D. Nachmansohn. 1965. Cholinesterase activity per unit surface area of conducting membranes. J. Cell Biol. 26:353–64.

Brzin, M., M. Kovič, and S. Oman. 1964. The magnetic diver balance. C. R. Trav. Lab. Carlsberg 34:407–26.

Buhse, H. E., Jr., and K. Hamburger. 1974. Induced macrostome formation in *Tetrahymena vorax* strain V_2: Patterns of respiration. C. R. Trav. Lab. Carlsberg 40:77–89.

Buhse, H. E., Jr., and E. Zeuthen. 1974. Oral morphogenesis in *Tetrahymena* cells synchronized with one heat shock per generation. C. R. Trav. Lab. Carlsberg 39:493–505.

Byfield, J. E., and C. L. Lee. 1970. Do synchronizing temperature shifts inhibit RNA synthesis in *Tetrahymena pyriformis?* J. Protozool. 17:445.

Byfield, J. E., and O. H. Scherbaum. 1967. Temperature dependent decay of DNA and of protein synthesis in a heat-synchronized protozoan. Proc. Natl. Acad. Sci. USA 57:602–6.

Cameron, I. L., and D. S. Nachtwey. 1967. DNA synthesis in relation to cell division in *Tetrahymena pyriformis*. Exptl. Cell Res. 46:385–95.

Frankel, J. 1962. The effects of heat, cold and p-fluorophenylalanine on morphogenesis in synchronized *Tetrahymena pyriformis* GL. C. R. Trav. Lab. Carlsberg 33:1–52.

Frankel, J. 1964. Cortical morphogenesis and synchronization in *Tetrahymena pyriformis* GL. Exptl. Cell Res. 35:349–60.

Frankel, J. 1967. Studies on the maintenance of oral development in *Tetrahymena pyriformis* GL-C. II. The relationship of protein synthesis to cell division and oral organelle development. J. Cell Biol. 34:841–58.

Frydenberg, O., and E. Zeuthen. 1960. Oxygen uptake and carbon dioxide output related to the mitotic rhythm in the cleaving eggs of *Dendraster excentricus* and *Urechis caupo*. C. R. Trav. Lab. Carlsberg 31:423.

Gustafson, T., and P. Lénicque. 1952. Studies on mitochondria in the developing sea urchin eggs. Exptl. Cell Res. 3:251–74.

Hamburger, K. 1975. Respiratory rate through the growth-division cycle of *Acanthamoeba* sp. C. R. Trav. Lab. Carlsberg 40:175–85.

Hamburger, K. 1962. Division delays induced by metabolic inhibitors in synchronized cells of *Tetrahymena pyriformis*. C. R. Trav. Lab. Carlsberg 32:359–70.

Hamburger, K., and E. Zeuthen. 1957. Synchronous division in *Tetrahymena pyriformis* as studied in an inorganic medium. The effect of 2,4-dinitrophenol. Exptl. Cell Res. 13:443–53.

Hamburger, K., and E. Zeuthen. 1974. Recording mitotic cycles in single cleaving frog eggs. Gasometric studies with the gradient diver. C. R. Trav. Lab. Carlsberg 39:415–32.

Hardin, J. A., G. E. Einem, and D. T. Lindsay. 1967. Simultaneous synthesis of histone and DNA in synchronously dividing *Tetrahymena pyriformis*. J. Cell Biol. 32:709–17.

Hartwell, L. H., J. J. Culotti, J. R. Pringle, and B. J. Reid. 1974. Genetic control of the cell division cycle in yeast. Science 183:183–189.

Heslot, H., A. Gafteau, and C. Louis. 1970. Respiratory metabolism of a petite negative yeast. *Schizosaccharomyces pombe* 972 h^{-1}. J. Bact. 104:473–81.

Hjelm, K. K., and E. Zeuthen. 1967a. Synchronous DNA synthesis induced by synchronous cell division in *Tetrahymena*. C. R. Trav. Lab. Carlsberg 36:127–60.

Hjelm, K. K., and E. Zeuthen. 1967b. Synchronous DNA synthesis following heat-synchronized cell division in *Tetrahymena*. Exptl. Cell Res. 48:231–32.

Holter, H. 1943. Technique of the Cartesian diver. C. R. Trav. Lab Carlsberg 24:399–478.

Holter, H., and E. Zeuthen. 1948. Metabolism and reduced weight in starving *Chaos chaos*. C. R. Trav. Lab. Carlsberg 26:277–96.

Holter, H., and E. Zeuthen. 1957. Dynamics of early echinoderm development, as observed by phase contrast microscopy and correlated with respiration measurements. Staz. Zool. Napoli 29:285–306.

Hotchkiss, R. D. 1954. Cyclical behaviour in pneumococcal growth and transformability occasioned by environmental changes. Proc. Nat. Acad. Sci. USA 40:49–55.

Immers, J., and J. Runnström. 1959. Release of respiratory control by 2,4-dinitrophenol in different stages of sea urchin development. Devel. Biol. 2:90–104.

Johnson, B. F. 1965. Autoradiographic analysis of regional cell wall growth of yeasts. Exptl. Cell Res. 39:613–24.

Kramhøft, B., K. Hamburger, S. B. Nissen, and E. Zeuthen. 1975. Rates of gaseous exchanges (CO_2 and O_2) through the synchronized and the normal cell cycle of *Schizosaccharomyces pombe*. Yeast News Letter 24:27.

Kramhøft, B., and E. Zeuthen. 1971. Synchronization of cell divisions in the fission yeast, *Schizosaccharomyces pombe*, using heat shocks. C. R. Trav. Lab. Carlsberg 38:351–68.

Kramhøft, B., and E. Zeuthen. 1975. Synchronization of the fission yeast, *Schizosaccharomyces pombe*, using heat shocks. *In* D. M. Prescott (ed.). Methods in cell biology 12: in press. Academic Press, New York.

Kubitschek, H. E. 1970. Evidence for the generality of linear cell growth. J. Theor. Biol. 28:15–29.

Kudo, R. R. 1947. *Pelomyxa carolinensis* Wilson. II. Nuclear division and plastomy. J. Morphol. 80:93–144.

Linderstrøm-Lang, K. 1937. Principle of the Cartesian diver applied to gasometric technique. Nature 140:108.

Linderstrøm-Lang, K. 1943. On the theory of the Cartesian diver micro respirometer. C. R. Trav. Lab. Carlsberg Ser. Chim. 24:333–98.

Lowy, B., and V. Leick. 1969. The synthesis of DNA in synchronized cultures of *Tetrahymena pyriformis* GL. Exptl. Cell Res. 57:277–88.

Løvlie, A. 1963. Growth in mass and respiration rate during the cell cycle of *Tetrahymena pyriformis*. C. R. Trav. Lab. Carlsberg 33:377–413.

Løvlie, A., and E. Zeuthen. 1962. The gradient diver—a recording instrument for gasometric micro-analysis. C. R. Trav. Lab. Carlsberg 32:513.

Mitchison, J. M. 1971. The biology of the cell cycle. At the University Press, Cambridge, England.

Mitchison, J. M., and W. S. Vincent. 1965. Preparation of synchronized cell cultures by sedimentation. Nature, 205:987–89.

Miyamoto, H., L. Rasmussen, and E. Zeuthen. 1973. Studies of the effect of temperature shocks in preparation for cell division in mouse fibroblast cells (L cells). J. Cell Sci. 13:889–900.

Nexô, B. A. 1975. Ribo- and deoxyribonucleotide triphosphate pools in synchronized populations of *Tetrahymena pyriformis*. Biochim. Biophys. Acta. 378:12–17.

Nexô, B. A., K. Hamburger, and E. Zeuthen. 1972. Simplified microgasometry with gradient divers. C. R. Trav. Lab. Carlsberg 39:33–63.

Nilsson, J. R. 1970. Macronuclear changes in *Tetrahymena pyriformis* GL. during the cell cycle and in response to alterations in environmental conditions. C. R. Trav. Lab. Carlsberg 37:285–300.

Nilsson, J. R., and E. Zeuthen. 1974. Microscopical studies on the macronucleus of heat synchronized *Tetrahymena pyriformis* GL. C. R. Trav. Lab. Carlsberg 40:1–18.

Plesner, P. 1971. Alternative pathways for ribosomal protein. Exptl. Cell Res. 67:255.

Prescott, D. M. 1955. Relations between cell growth and cell division. I. Reduced weight cell volume, protein content, and nuclear volume of *Amoeba proteus* from division to division. Exptl. Cell Res. 9:328–37.

Prescott, D. M. 1956. Relation between cell growth and cell division. II. The effect of cell size on cell growth rate and generation time in *Amoeba proteus*. Exptl. Cell Res. 11:86–98.

Ramussen, L. 1963. Delayed divisions in *Tetrahymena* as induced by short-time exposures to anaerobiosis. C. R. Trav. Lab. Carlsberg 33:53–71.

Rasmussen, L., and E. Zeuthen. 1962. Cell division and protein synthesis in *Tetrahymena* as studied with p-fluorophenylalanine. C. R. Trav. Lab. Carlsberg 32:333–58.

Satir, P., and E. Zeuthen. 1961. Cell cycle and the relationship between growth rate to reduced weight (RW) in the giant amoeba *Chaos chaos*. C. R. Trav. Lab. Carlsberg 32:241–63.

Scherbaum, O. H., A. L. Louderback, and T. L. Jahn. 1959. DNA synthesis phosphate content and growth in mass and volume in synchronously dividing cells. Exptl. Cell Res. 18:150–66.

Scherbaum, O. H., and E. Zeuthen. 1954. Inducation of synchronous cell division in mass cultures of *Tetrahymena pyriformis*. Exptl. Cell Res. 6:221–27.

Scholander, P. F., C. L. Claff, S. L. Sveinsson, and S. J. Scholander. 1952. Respiration of single cells. III. Oxygen consumption during cell division. Biol. Bull. 102:185–99.

Scholander, P. E., H. Leivestad, and G. Sundnes. 1958. Cycling in the oxygen consumption of cleaving eggs. Exptl. Cell Res. 3:505–11.

Smith, H. S., and A. B. Pardee. 1970. Accumulation of a protein required for division during the cell cycle of *Escherichia coli*. J. of Bact. 3:901–9.

Thormar, H. 1959. Delayed division in *Tetrahymena pyriformis* induced by temperature changes. C. R. Trav. Lab. Carlsberg 31:207–25.

Villaden, I., and E. Zeuthen. 1970. Synchronization of DNA synthesis in *Tetrahymena* populations by temporary limitation of access to thymidine compounds. Exptl. Cell Res. 61:302–10.

Zeuthen, E. 1946. Oxygen uptake during mitosis. Experiments on the eggs of the frog. C. R. Trav. Lab. Carlsberg. Sér. Chim. 25:191–228.

Zeuthen, E. 1948. A Cartesian diver balance weighing reduced weights (R.W.) with an accuracy of ± 0.01 γ. C. R. Trav. Lab. Carlsberg. Sér. Chim. 26:243–65.

Zeuthen, E. 1949. Oxygen consumption during mitosis: experiments on fertilized eggs of marine animals. Amer. Nat. 83:303–22.

Zeuthen, E. 1950. Respiration during cell division in the egg of the sea urchin *Psammechinus miliaris*. 98:144–51.

Zeuthen, E. 1953. Growth as related to the cell cycle in single cell cultures of *Tetrahymena pyriformis*, J. Embryol. Exp. Morph. 1:239–49.

Zeuthen, E. 1955. Mitotic respiratory rhythms in single eggs of *Psammechinus miliaris* and of *Ciona intestinalis*. Biol. Bull. 108:366–85.

Zeuthen, E. 1960. Cycling in oxygen consumption in cleaving eggs. Exptl. Cell Res. 19:1–6.

Zeuthen, E. 1961. The cartesian diver balance. General Cytochemical Methods 2:61–92.

Zeuthen, E. 1964. The temperature-induced division synchrony in *Tetrahymena*. In E. Zeuthen (ed). Synchrony in cell division and growth. Pp. 79–158. Interscience Publishers, New York.

Zeuthen, E. 1968. Thymine starvation by inhibition of uptake and synthesis of thymine-compounds in *Tetrahymena*. Exptl. Cell Res. 50:37–46.

Zeuthen, E. 1970. Independent synchronization of DNA synthesis and of cell division in same culture of *Tetrahymena* cells. Exptl. Cell Res. 61:311–25.

Zeuthen, E. 1971. Synchrony in *Tetrahymena* by heat shocks spaced a normal cell generation apart. Exptl. Cell Res. 68:49–60.

Zeuthen, E. 1971. Synchronization of the *Tetrahymena* cell cycle. In D. M. Prescott, L. Goldstein, and E. McConkey (eds.). Advances in cell biology. 2:110–52. Appleton-Century-Crofts, New York.

Zeuthen, E. 1974. A cellular model for respective and free-running synchrony in *Tetrahymena* and *Schizosaccharomyces*. In G. M. Padilla, I. L. Cameron, and A. Zimmerman (eds.). Cell cycle controls. Pp. 1–30. Academic Press, New York.

Zeuthen, E., and K. Hamburger. 1972. Mitotic cycles in oxygen uptake and carbon dioxide output in the cleaving frog egg. Biol. Bull. 143:699–706.

Zeuthen, E., and K. Hamburger. 1977. Microgasometry with single cells using ampulla divers operated in density gradients. In D. Glick and R. M. Rosenbaum (eds.). Techniques of biochemistry and biophysics morphology. 3: in press. Wiley-Interscience, New York.

Zeuthen, E., and L. Rasmussen. 1972. Synchronized cell division in protozoa. In T. T. Chen (ed.). Research in protozoology. 4:11–145. Pergamon Press, Oxford.

Zeuthen, E., and O. H. Scherbaum. 1954. Synchronous division in mass cultures of the ciliate protozoan *Tetrahymena pyriformis*, as induced by temperature changes. In J. A. Kitching (ed.). Recent developments in cell physiology. Pp. 141–56. Butterworth, London.

ROBERT DOTTIN, ALLAN M. WEINER, TOM ALTON,
JEANNE P. MARGOLSKEE, AND HARVEY F. LODISH

Messenger RNA Structure, Synthesis, and Translation in the Cellular Slime Mold *Dictyostelium discoideum*

8

Understanding the molecular details of genetic regulation in eukaryotic cells requires extensive studies of simple systems that are relatively amenable to genetic and biochemical manipulation. The cellular slime mold *Dictyostelium discoideum* offers many advantages for such detailed analysis and is especially attractive for studying the structure of a eukaryotic genome and differentiation in a simple organism. Recent reviews on *Dictyostelium* include Ashworth (1971), Bonner (1971), Newell (1971), Robertson and Cohen (1972), Killick and Wright (1974), Loomis (1975), and Jacobson and Lodish (1975).

Wild-type amoeba can be cultivated in the laboratory only by using bacteria as a food source, but mutants such as AX3 are available that are capable of axenic growth in liquid medium (Sussman and Sussman, 1967; Watts and Ashworth, 1970). The doubling time of cells in axenic medium is 8–12 hours at 22°C with mitosis, G1, S, and G2 lasting about 1.5, 2, 1.5, and 4 hours respectively (Katz and Bourguignon, 1974). When amoebae are starved and placed on a moist surface, they undergo a well-defined series of morphological changes (see fig. 1) leading to the formation of a multicellular fruiting body containing only two major cell types, spore cells and stalk cells (Sussman, 1966). Development of large numbers of fruiting bodies can be made to occur synchronously by harvesting the amoebae, resuspending them in a solution containing only inorganic salts, and depositing them either on Millipore filters, on discs of filter paper resting on absorbent pads, or on non-nutrient agar. Thus the entire developmental sequence can be studied

Department of Biology, Massachusetts Institute of Technology, Cambridge, Massachusetts 02139

THE LIFE CYCLE OF THE CELLULAR SLIME MOLD

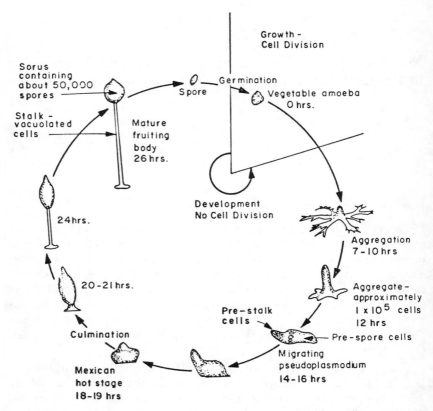

Fig. 1. Life cycle of *Dictyostelium discoideum*. This figure depicts the commonly studied aspects of the slime mold life cycle: vegetative growth of haploid amoebae and formation of fruiting bodies. Not shown here is the formation and germination of macrocysts, which is reviewed by Jacobson and Lodish (1975).

under defined experimental conditions with a sufficient number of cells to permit most conventional analytic procedures. In particular, the biochemical changes that accompany the morphological changes can be well documented.

Morphogenesis occurs only after céll growth, DNA replication, and other biochemical activities characteristic of growing cells have ceased (Katz and Bourguignon, 1974). After an interphase of about six to seven hours, groups of cells stream toward centers and aggregate in mounds containing about 10^5 cells. This aggregation is a chemotactic response to cyclic AMP (Bonner, 1971). The local concentration of cyclic AMP is regulated by a phosphodiesterase that is excreted and that destroys cyclic AMP; moreover, this phosphodiesterase may in turn be inactivated by an inhibitor (Gerisch et al., 1974). The cell membrane contains cyclic AMP binding proteins, phosphodiesterases, carbohydrate binding proteins, and a 5' nucleotidease that also appear to be involved in the aggregation process (Gerisch et al., 1974; Rosen et al., 1974; Rossomando and Sussman, 1973). The aggregating cells of *Dictyostelium* remain as individual uninucleated cells throughout morphogenesis. This is in contrast with the other slime molds, *Myxomycetes,* which aggregate and fuse to form a multinucleate syncytial plasmodium. To avoid confusion, the aggregated *Dictyostelium* cell mass was called a pseudoplasmodium (VanTeghem, 1880). The fingerlike pseudoplasmodium is enclosed in a sheath of cellulose that is continually secreted by the cells (Francis, 1962). The pseudoplasmodium migrates with a distinct polarity so that anterior and posterior ends can be functionally defined (Garrod, 1969). At this stage there is evidence of cell determination in what was initially a homogeneous cell population; microdissection studies have suggested that the cells in the posterior two-thirds of the pseudoplasmodium are committed (albeit reversibly) to differentiate into spore cells (Raper, 1940); these cells contain a characteristic prespore vesicle (Hohl and Hamomoto, 1969). The anterior cells of the pseudoplasmodium appear to be committed to differentiate into stalk cells. The culmination phase of differentiation is favored under conditions of high ionic strength, medium-low humidity, higher temperatures, and overhead light (Newell, Ellingson, and Summer, 1969). The anterior tip of the pseudopolasmodium turns upward and a cellulose-containing ring is formed where the tip joins the cell mass. A tubular stalk sheath is deposited by the pre-stalk cells, and a basal disc is deposited where the stalk sheath contacts the solid support. The cells included in the stalk sheath also vacuolize and expand in volume forming a rigid stalk within the cell mass (Loomis, 1975). The organism now assumes the characteristic Mexican hat appearance. The stalk extends downward as more anterior cells move into the sheath, vacuolize, and secrete cellulose. The peripheral cell mass is raised on the elongating stalk and forms an apical sorus. Culmination is complete in twenty-four hours, and the mature fruiting body consists of a spore mass surmounting a cellulose enclosed stalk of dead cells.

The profound morphological changes observable during development are accompanied by equally striking changes in the specific activities of many enzymes. Among those enzymes that display a considerable increase in specific activity, some maintain the new level of enzyme activity throughout culmination, while the activity of others undergoes a subsequent decline upon further morphogenesis. In theory such changes in specific activity may be due to enzyme activation, *de novo* synthesis of enzyme protein, or the selective sparing of particular proteins from rapid degradation. The one case in which this question has been closely examined, that of uridine diphosphoglucose pyrophosphorylase, remains controversial (Franke and Sussman, 1973; Gustafson, Kong, and Wright, 1973), but increase in enzyme activity does appear to be due to *de novo* enzyme synthesis. Recent studies in which mRNA synthesis is effectively blocked by using a combination of inhibitors have shown that there is only a short lag between synthesis and translation of mRNAs encoding the developmentally regulated enzymes N-acetyl glucosaminidase, uridine diphosphoglucose pyrophosphorylase, and alkaline phosphatase. Thus translational control of the synthesis of these enzymes is unlikely (Firtel, Baxter, and Lodish, 1973). Furthermore, as we will discuss below, changes in the rates of synthesis of specific polypeptides may be detected at discrete stages in the life cycle by labeling with radioactive amino acids and identifying polypeptide "bands" on polyacrylamide gels by autoradiography (Tuchman, Alton, and Lodish, 1974). The specific labeling patterns are qualitatively similar even in very short pulses of amino acids, a result which shows that selective protein turnover is not the mechanism responsible for any gross changes in the synthesis of those polypeptides.

Dictyostelium discoideum is a haploid organism containing seven chromosomes (Sussman, 1961; Brody and Williams, 1974). Mutants blocked at different stages in morphogenesis are easily obtained in large numbers. In addition, mutants are now available that are blocked in the synthesis of specific gene products known to accumulate at particular stages in development. The patterns of morphogenesis and macromolecular synthesis in such mutants can suggest a function for the wild-type gene product in the developmental program (Dimond, Brenner, and Loomis, 1973; Freeze and Loomis, 1974). Sophisticated genetic analysis like that done in prokaryotes is difficult because of the lack of an obligatory sexual phase in the life cycle of this organism. However, *Dictyostelium discoideum* can undergo a parasexual stage involving the rare fusion of two haploid strains to yield diploid progeny from which haploid segregants may be obtained at a low frequency. Genetic exchange occurs during this process (Loomis and Ashworth, 1968). To date, mutations have been localized onto five linkage groups (Kessin, Williams, and Newell, 1972; Katz and Kao, 1974; Williams, Kessin, and Newell, 1974; Gingold and Ashworth, 1974).

Recently it has been shown that when amoebae from different strains of *Dictyostelium discoideum* are incubated together, cells may aggregate in groups of one hundred to form macrocysts (Erdos, Raper, and Vogen, 1973). In the closely related species, *Dictyostelium mucuroides,* meiosis occurs at this stage (MacInnes and Frances, 1974). There is now evidence that the macrocysts of *Dictyostelium discoideum* may also represent a sexual cycle

(Erdos, Raper, and Vogen, 1975), a finding that could enormously facilitate genetic studies in *Dictyostelium discoideum*. As we shall see, some of the mutant types described above are becoming increasingly useful in a biochemical analysis of the developmental program.

Such studies are also facilitated by the relative simplicity of the genome. The nuclear DNA contains about fifty-four million base pairs (Sussman and Bayner, 1971). Fragmented denatured nuclear DNA reanneals in two distinguishable stages One third of the DNA reanneals rapidly at Cot-1/2 of 1 and the remaining two-thirds reanneal at a Cot-1/2 of about 100. This latter fraction represents sequences present only once per genome. The complexity of the unique sequences that presumably code for most structural proteins is about one-fiftieth that of mammalian cells and only seven times greater than that of *E. coli* (Firtel and Bonner, 1972). As we shall discuss, the mode of mRNA synthesis is conservative and involves a much shorter precursor than in mammalian cells (Firtel and Lodish, 1973; Lodish, Firtel, and Jacobson, 1973; Lodish et al., 1974); these properties facilitate labeling and RNA:DNA hybridization studies (Firtel and Lodish, 1973; Firtel, Jacobson, and Lodish, 1972). Such experiments have shown that approximately half of the non-reiterated portion of the genome is transcribed at some stage in the life cycle. Of the RNA transcribed, half appears to be present in cells of all developmental stages, and half can be subdivided into stage-specific classes (Firtel, 1972).

Our own research is directed primarily toward the factors that regulate synthesis and translation of mRNA during differentiation. In this paper we summarize our recent work in these areas.

DICTYOSTELIUM MESSENGER RNA

Dictyostelium messenger RNA has many features in common with mRNA from higher eukaryotes such as HeLa cells (Darnell, Jelinek, and Molloy, 1973). The average *Dictyostelium* mRNA contains about 1,300 nucleotides, large enough to encode a single protein of molecular weight 40,000. The bulk of the mRNA is transcribed from non-reiterated sequences in the DNA; less than 10% of mRNA is complementary to (i.e., derived from) the 30% of nuclear DNA sequences—repetitive DNA—that are present in 100–300 copies per genome (Firtel et al., 1972). At the 3' end of most mRNAs is a sequence of polyadenylic acid about 100 bases long. As in mammalian cells, this sequence is added to the mRNA after it is transcribed from DNA. Each *Dictyostelium* mRNA contains also a second sequence of poly(A), this only 25 bases long. It is located near the 3' end but is separated from the $poly(A)_{100}$ by from 1 to 20 bases (Lodish, Firtel, and Jacobson, 1973; Jacobson, Firtel, and Lodish, 1974a, 1974b).

STRUCTURE AND TRANSCRIPTION OF DICTYOSTELIUM DNA

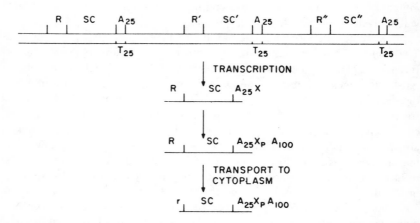

Fig. 2. A model of *Dictyostelium* nuclear DNA. The primary genetic unit in *Dictyostelium* contains a repetitive DNA sequence (R) that averages 300 to 350 nucleotides at the 5′ end; a sequence of nonreiterated or single-copy (SC) DNA of 1,100 to 1,200 nucleotides; and a sequence of 25 adenylic acid residues (A_{25}) at the 3′ end. This unit is transcribed by RNA polymerase, and then poly(A) of 100 to 150 residues is added after transcription. Before transport of the heterogeneous RNA to the cytoplasm, the majority of the 5′ repetitive sequences are removed, leaving a short repetitive sequence. The evidence for the presence of a portion of the repetitive sequence transcript (r) on the majority of mRNA molecules is given in Lodish et al. (1973). Since the poly(A)$_{25}$ and poly(A)$_{100}$ are separable on polyacrylamide gels after digestion with RNase T1 and RNase A, at least one other nucleotide (*x*) must be present between the 3′ end of the short poly(A)$_{25}$ and the 5′ end of the larger poly(A)$_{100}$ (Jacobson, Firtel, and Lodish, 1974).

The poly(A)$_{25}$, in contrast to the poly(A)$_{100}$ sequence, is believed to be transcribed from poly(T)$_{25}$ sequences in the *Dictyostelium* genome (fig. 2); there are about 15,000 poly(dT)$_{25}$ sequences in *Dictyostelium* DNA—about one per gene (Lodish, Firtel, and Jacobson, 1973; Jacobson, Firtel, and Lodish, 1974a, 1974b).

The experiment in figure 3 shows that the poly(A)$_{100}$ sequences are added just before the RNA exits from the nucleus and also supports the notion that the poly(A)$_{25}$ sequences are transcribed from DNA: following addition of [^{3}H]-adenosine to vegetative cells, radioactive poly(A)$_{100}$ sequences, attached to mRNA, appear in the cytoplasm after only a 2 min. lag period. By contrast, labeled poly(A)$_{25}$ sequences and labeled nonpoly(A) segments of mRNA (i.e., cytoplasmic polyadenylated RNA) are found in the cytoplasm only after a 4 min. lag. These results mean that it takes only 4 min. for an mRNA precursor molecule, containing a poly(A)$_{25}$ sequence, to be processed and transported from the nucleus. The poly(A)$_{100-150}$ sequence is added during the final 2-min. period in the nucleus.

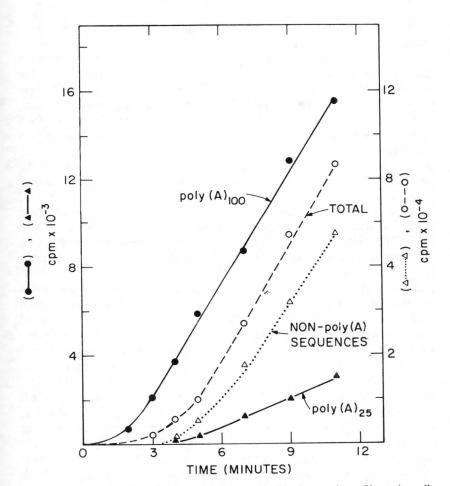

Fig. 3. Kinetics of appearance of poly(A)$_{100}$ and poly(A)$_{25}$ in the cytoplasm. Vegetative cells were labeled with [³H]-adenosine; at various times cytoplasmic RNA was isolated by the proteinase K method (Firtel and Lodish, 1973). Poly(A)-containing RNA was purified by chromatography on poly(U)-Sepharose. Total poly(A) was determined by the fraction of the [³H]-adenosine label that was resistant to RNases A and T1; the fraction of poly(A) radioactivity representing poly(A)$_{100}$ and poly(A)$_{25}$ sequences was determined by electrophoresis on 10% polyacrylamide gels as in Jacobson et al (1974b). Non-poly(A) sequences were the fraction of [³H]-radioactivity that was sensitive to the RNases. All samples were normalized for a given amount of rRNA present in the extracted samples. Open circles = total poly(A)-containing RNA; open triangles = non-poly(A) sequences; solid circles = poly(A)$_{100}$; solid triangles = poly(A)$_{25}$.

It is of interest to point out that mammalian mRNA does not contain poly(A)$_{25}$ sequences. Such sequences are, however, found in the large nuclear heterogeneous RNA, the presumed precursor to mammalian mRNA (Nakazato et al., 1974).

Many cellular and viral mRNAs in mammalian cells contain an unusual sequence of nucleotides at the 5' end (Adams and Cory, 1975; Furuichi et al., 1975a; 1975b; Perry et al., 1975; Wei, Gershowitz, and Moss, 1975). A general formula for these sequences is $m^7G^{5'}$ ppp$^{5'}$ XmpYpZp. . . . The nucleoside 7-methyl guanosine is linked by a 5'5' triphosphate to the nucleoside X at the 5' end of the RNA. X also contains a 2'0-methyl substituent, and in many RNAs the second nucleoside, Y, also contains a 2'0-methyl group. In mRNA from HeLa, L, or murine plasmacytoma cells, X can be any of the four nucleosides. In the case of reovirus or vesicular stomatitis virus, the 7-methyl guanosine and 2'0-methyl groups are added by virion transcriptases, and the 5' nucleoside X is either A or G (Furuichi et al., 1975a). Mammalian cell mRNA also contains one or more 6-methyl adenine residues, although the position of the m^6A residue in the mRNA is not clear (Furuichi et al., 1975b; Perry et al., 1975; Wei, Gershowitz, and Moss, 1975).

It is of interest that *Dictyostelium* mRNA contains some, but not all, of the methyl groups characteristic of mammalian mRNA. Some of these results are shown by the experiments in figure 4. [^{32}P]-labeled mRNA (cytoplasmic RNA purified by chromatography on oligo(dT)-cellulose) was digested with alkali and then chromatographed on a column of DEAE cellulose using a linear gradient of NaCl (0.05 M to 0.4 M) in 7 M urea. Over 99% of the label eluted, as expected, with mononucleotides containing a charge of -2. But a small fraction (0.5%) eluted at a position indicating it had 4 negative charges (fig. 4A). A smaller fraction appears to have 5 negative charges. mRNA can also be labeled with [^{3}H]-methyl methionine (fig. 4C); when [^{3}H]-methyl-labeled RNA was digested with alkali and chromatographed, 60% of the material eluted at the -4 and -5 peaks coincident with the [^{32}P] (compare fig. 4A and 4C). A charge of -5 but not -4 is consistent with a structure of the general formula written above. Methyl-labeled rRNA yielded no such peaks (fig. 4B); all of the material eluted at -2 (mononucleotides) or -3 (dinucleotides) containing presumably a 2'0-methylated nucleotide. No [^{3}H]-labeled material eluted at -2 when mRNA was analyzed.

Fig. 4 (opposite). Column chromatography pattern of nucleotides from *Dictyostelium* RNA. Vegetative cells were starved for 2 hrs. in suspension (2 × 10^8 cells in 20 ml MES-PDF [Firtel and Lodish, 1973]) prior to pulse labeling for 1 hr. (30 mCi [^{32}P]-phosphoric acid or 1 mCi [^{3}H]-methyl-methionine). RNA from the cytoplasm was extracted with cold phenol, precipitated with ethanol, and applied to oligo(dT)-cellulose to purify poly(A)-containing mRNA from rRNA and tRNA. RNA was reprecipitated and then digested in alkali (200 µl 0.5 M NaOH for 16 hrs. at 37°), neutralized, and chromatographed on 1 × 20 cm DEAE cellulose column with a gradient of NaCl (0.05 to 0.4 M in 7 M urea, 50 mM Tris, pH 8.0). Yeast RNA digested with RNase A was included as marker in order to determine the positions of oligonucleotides with charges of -2 to -5. Fractions (2 ml) were collected and counted. (A) dT-binding [^{32}P] mRNA; (B) dT column flow-through of [^{3}H]-methyl-methionine-labeled RNA containing mainly rRNA and tRNA; (C) dt-binding [^{3}H]-methyl-methionine-labeled RNA (mRNA).

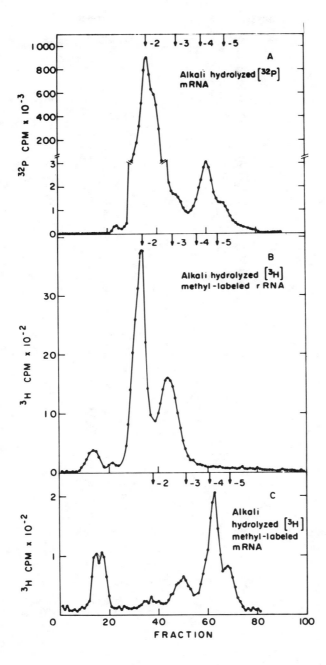

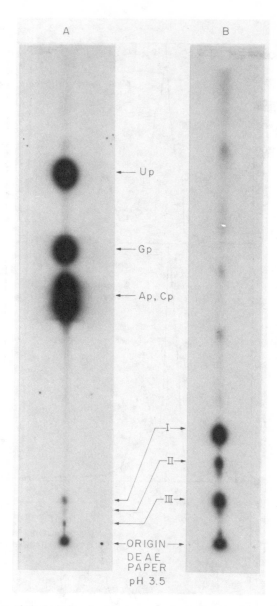

Fig. 5. Separation of blocked 5′ nucleotides by paper electrophoresis. A sample of [^{32}P]-labeled mRNA (fig. 4) was digested with a mixture of RNases A (50 μg/ml), T1 (200 units/ml), and T2 (5 units/ml) in 50 mM ammonium acetate, pH 4.5. The resulting digest was analyzed by electrophoresis on DEAE paper at pH 3.5 in 5% acetic acid acid, 2 mM EDTA, and 0.5% pyridine (left panel). The electrophoresis in the right panel used more [^{32}P] RNA and was done for a longer period of time, so that the mononucleotides ran off the end of the paper. The paper was exposed to Kodak Royal Blue X-ray film, and shown here is a photograph of this radioautogram.

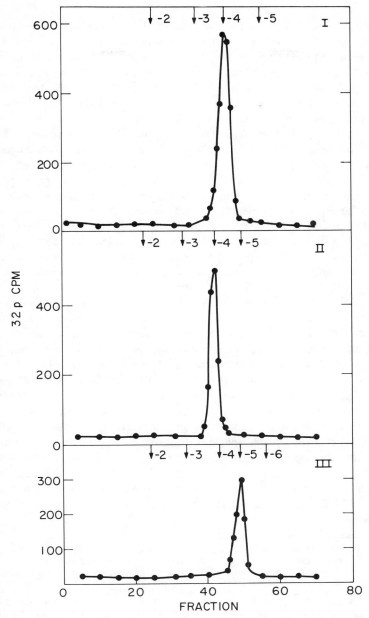

Fig. 6. Column chromatography of 5' structures purified by electrophoresis. The material in spots labeled I, II, III in figure 5 was eluted with 30% triethylamine bicarbonate, pH 8, and chromatographed on a DEAE column and analyzed as in figure 4.

The oligonucleotides on the −4 and −5 peaks from alkali digestion of mRNA can also be resolved into three well-separated spots, tentatively called I, II, and III, by electrophoresis on DEAE paper at pH 3.5 (fig. 5). In this case the RNA was digested with a mixture of ribonucleases A, T1, and T2, instead of by alkali. Structure I contains 60–65% of the [^{32}P]-label in the three spots, and structures II and III contain 10% and 20% respectively. The identity of these structures with the material of charges −4 and −5 was confirmed by elution of the nucleotides from DEAE paper and chromatography on the DEAE column as before. Figure 6 shows that structures I and II have charges of −4. The material from the structure labeled III has a charge of −5. This latter material, but not that from I or II, can be further resolved by ionophoresis at pH 3.5 on Whatman 3mm paper into two structures called III and IV of equal radioactivity (data not shown). Discrete spots migrating between structure I and the mononucleotides in figure 5B are sensitive to spleen phosphodiesterase and are therefore oligonucleotides containing 2′0-methyl substituents. They probably are low-level rRNA contaminants.

The nucleotide sequences of these 5′ structures have been determined to be: I, m^{7}G$^{5'}$ ppp$^{5'}$ Ap; II, m^{7}G$^{5'}$ ppp$^{5'}$ Gp; III, m^{7}G$^{5'}$ ppp$^{5'}$ AmpAp; and IV, m^{7}G$^{5'}$ ppp$^{5'}$ AmpUp. The sequences of I and II are consistent with structures of charge −4, and that of III and IV with structures of charge −5. Simple structures such as I and II have not yet been found in higher eukaryotes.

Our analysis of the sequence of spot I was based on the observation that digestion of spot I with either bacterial alkaline phosphatase (BAP) or Pl nuclease gave identical products. Nuclease P1, like BAP, has a 3′ phosphatase activity, but it is also a phosphodiesterase that releases nucleoside 5′ monophosphates. The products of digestion of spot I were analyzed by ionophoresis on Whatman 3mm paper and localized by autoradiography (see fig. 7). With BAP, free phosphate and a resistant fragment migrating more slowly than the undigested material were produced. The ratio of radioactivity in phosphate to that in the fragment was 1 to 3. With P1 the result was identical, with no indication that a nucleoside 5′ monophosphate was also produced by digestion. Therefore, structure I probably contains no XmpYp sequence.

Fig. 7 (opposite). Electrophoretic separation of digestion products of 5′ structure I. Structure I was purified by electrophoresis in a second dimension on Whatman 3mm paper at pH 3.5 (now shown). It was localized by autoradiography (see fig. 5), eluted with water, and lyophilized. Aliquots of 5 μl containing 2,000-3,000 cpm [^{32}P] were digested for 1 hr. at 37° in capillary tubes. One sample contained 100 μg/ml of nuclease P1 from *Penicillium citrinum* (Yamosa Shoyu Co.), 50 mM MES, pH 6.5, and 2 mg/ml yeast RNA. A second aliquot was digested for 1 hr. at 37° in 100 μg/ml bacterial alkaline phosphatase (Worthington) in 5 μl, 10 mM Tris HCl, ph 7.2, and applied to Whatman 3mm paper. Undigested material (labeled 0) and the blue dye xylene cyanol were also applied to the origin, and electrophoresis was performed in ph 3.5 buffer until the dye had migrated 10 cm. The radioactive products were localized by autoradiography, cut, and counted for Cerenkoy radiation.

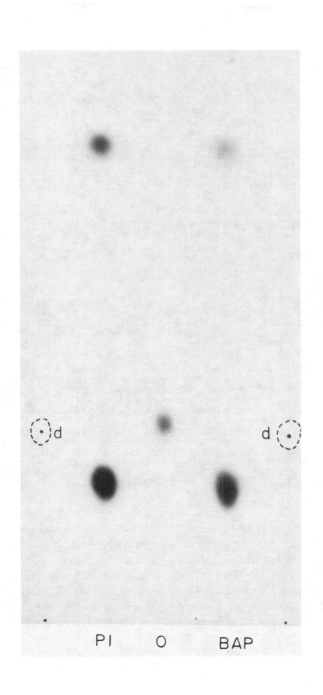

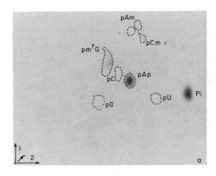

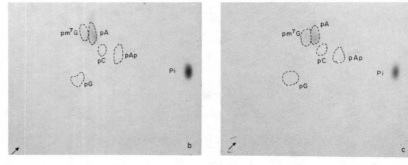

Fig. 8. Two-dimensional thin layer chromatographic separation of digestion products of 5′ structure I and its derivatives. Samples (5μl) were digested 3 hrs. at 37°C in 50μl/ml snake venom phosphodiesterase, 10 mM Tris HC1, pH 7.4, and a mixture of the nucleotides pG, pm⁷G, pU, pAp, and pC at 1 mg/ml each. Ten to thirty micrograms of each of the above nucleotides as well as pAm, pCm, and pA were spotted at the origin of a glass-backed thin-layer cellulose plate (Brinkman). The solvent system used in the first dimension was isobutyric acid; ammonia; water (58; 3.8; 38.2); and for the second dimension t-butanol; HC1; water (70;15;15). Panel "a" shows the autoradiogram of the digestion products from structure I. Panels "b" and "c" show those from the fragment that was resistant to further digestion by P1 or BAP respectively. The diagonal arrow indicates the origin and arrows 1 and 2 indicate the first and second dimensions respectively.

Next, the P1 or BAP-resistant fragments from spot I and the undigested material were treated with snake venom phosphodiesterase. This enzyme is a 3′ exonuclease that releases 5′ mononucleotides (pN) from standard phosphodiesterase bonds in RNA or DNA, nucleoside 3′-5′ diphosphates from a 3′ phosphorylated terminus, and phosphate from pyrophosphates (Barrell, 1971). The products were analyzed by two-dimensional chromatography on thin-layer cellulose with appropriate UV absorbing markers and localized by autoradiography (fig. 8). When structure I was digested with snake venom phosphodiesterase without prior treatment, the products were pAp, pm⁷G, and P_i (fig. 8A). When it was first treated with P1 or BAP and the resistant fragment digested with snake venom phosphodiesterase, the products in both cases were pA, pm⁷G and P$_i$ (fig. 8B, C). No. 2′0-methylated nucleotide (pNm) was obtained. These data establish the sequence of spot I, m⁷G⁵′ppp⁵′ Ap. Similar analyses established the sequence of spots II-IV. The recovery of spots I-IV is such that each mRNA appears to have one of the blocked 5′ structures (Dottin, Weiner, and Lodish, in preparation).

The mRNA of *Dictyostelium* has several significant differences from that of higher eukaryotes; all of the 5′ nucleotides are purines; 75% of the 5′

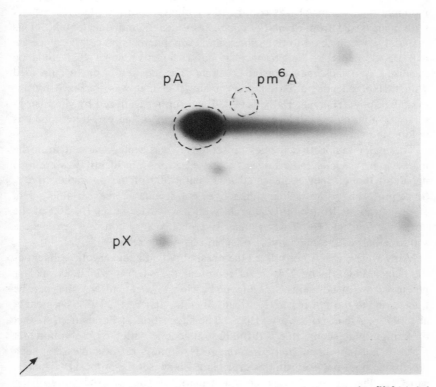

Fig. 9. Two-dimensional thin layer chromatographic separation of pA and pm⁶A. [³²P]-labeled mRNA (10⁶ cpm) of *Dictyostelium* and 20 μg pm⁶A (Terra Marine Bioresearch) were incubated in 5 μl nuclease P1 (as in fig. 7) and subjected to two-dimensional electrophoresis at pH 3.5. The first dimension was done on cellulose acetate paper saturated with pH 3.5 buffer (see fig. 5) that also contained 7 M urea (Adams and Cory, 1975). The second dimension was done on DEAE paper. The paper was incubated in an atmosphere of ammonia to facilitate visualization of pm⁶A by UV light. The nucleotide pA, localized by autoradiography, coincided with pm⁶A in this system. These nucleotides were eluted with 30% triethylammonium bicarbonate, pH 8, and lyophilized. Aliquots were further analyzed by two-dimensional chromatography, as in figure 8 except that the solvent system for the first dimension was isobutyric acid; ammonia; water (66; 1; 33).

structures lack 2'0-methyl substituents, and, as shown in the following experiments, N^6-methyl-adenosine does not occur in its mRNA.

The absence of $[^3H]$-methyl-labeled material eluting at -2 in figure 4C was the first indication that N^6-methyl-adenosine is absent from *Dictyostelium* mRNA. This base-methylated nucleoside has been located in the mRNA of both murine plasmacytoma and HeLa cells at a frequency of one per mRNA molecule. Its exact location in the RNA molecule is not known, but it is not at the 5' end of mRNA; therefore, in such mRNAs, $[^3H]$-methyl-labeling does not uniquely label the 5' end. The absence of N^6-methyl-adenosine 5' monophosphate (pm^6A) was confirmed by digestion of $[^{32}P]$-labeled mRNA with nuclease P1 from *Penicillin citrinum* to yield 5' mononucleotides. This material was subjected to two-dimensional ionophoresis on cellulose acetate and DEAE paper in the presence of non-radioactive pm^6A that could be localized by its absorbance under UV light. The location of pm^6A coincided with that of adenosine 5' monophosphate (pA) that was localized by autoradiography. This material was eluted and further analyzed by chromatography on thin-layer cellulose; the locations of pm^6A and pA, determined as before, are shown in figure 9.

The major radioactive species present, pA, was well separated from the marker pm^6A. Other radioactive species (e.g., pX) not identified were also apparent, though they represented less than 1/500 of the pA radioactivity. Since pm^6A shows no visible radioactive spot, it must be present in less than 1/500 of the nucleotides that migrate with pA and less than 1/1,500 of the nucleotides in mRNA. This estimate is probably very conservative since a spot one-half of the intensity of pX could be easily seen.

Many workers have considered the possibility that in eukaryotic cells modified nucleotides in mRNA might represent the sites at which its nuclear precursor might be cleaved during processing to yield mRNA that can be transported to the cytoplasm (Rottman, Shatkin, and Perry, 1974; Furuichi et al., 1975b; Adams and Cory, 1975). The suggestion of Fuiuichi et al. that m^6A might play such a role is difficult to reconcile with the observation that pm^6A is not present in *Dictyostelium* mRNA unless one assumes that such processing does not occur in this organism. Likewise, the proposal of Adams and Cory that ribose methylation might mark the site for processing of the nuclear precursor does not explain the fact that 75% of the 5' structures lack these sites unless one postulates that the mRNAs are not processed.

The mechanism of biogenesis of messenger RNA in *Dictyostelium* indeed appears to be much simpler than in mammalian cells. Nuclei of *Dictyostelium* cells labeled *in vivo* or *in vitro* under a variety of conditions do not contain material analogous to the larger nuclear heterogeneous RNA found in mammalian cells (Firtel and Lodish, 1973). Mammalian mRNA is thought to be derived from the 3′ terminal portions of a precursor 2–30 times the size of mRNA, and over 90% of the HnRNA is degraded within the nucleus. Apparently a small amount of HnRNA is the precursor to mRNA (Darnell, Jelinek, and Molloy, 1973). By contrast, the majority of pulse-labeled *Dictyostelium* nuclear RNA that is not a precursor to rRNA has an average weight of 500,000 daltons, only 20% longer than cytoplasmic mRNA (Firtel and Lodish, 1973). These RNAs contain at least the shorter sequences of polyadenylic acid, poly(A)$_{25}$, (Jacobson, Firtel, and Lodish, 1974a, 1974b). Pulse-labeling experiments showed that a large fraction of the nuclear poly(A)-containing RNA is a material precursor to cytoplasmic mRNA (Firtel and Lodish, 1973; Lodish, Firtel, and Jacobson, 1973). When intact cells are labeled for short periods of time, these nuclear poly(A)-containing molecules do not contain a triphosphate group at the 5′ terminus. However, full length poly(A)$_{25}$-containing pre-mRNAs can be synthesized in isolated nuclei, as

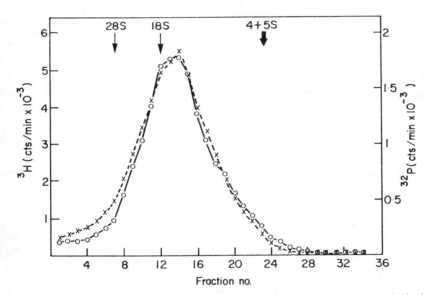

Fig. 10. Dimethyl sulfoxide (DMSO)-sucrose gradient analysis of mRNA precursor synthesized in isolated nuclei. Messenger RNA precursor was labeled in isolated nuclei (Jacobson, Firtel, and Lodish, 1947a) or in whole cells and purified by poly(U)-Sepharose chromatography (Firtel, Jacobson, and Lodish, 1972; Firtel and Lodish, 1973). *In vitro* labeling was with [α^{32}P]-UTP; *in vivo* labeling was with [^{3}H]-uracil (Jacobson, Firtel, and Lodish, 1974a; Firtel and Lodish, 1973). Aliquots of the [^{32}P]- and [^{3}H]-labeled molecules were mixed and centrifuged on a 0 to 8% sucrose gradient containing 99% dimethylsulfoxide, 0.001 M sodium EDTA, and 0.00025 M TES, pH 6.8. Constant volume fractions were collected from the bottom of the tube after centrifugation. Radioactivity was determined by adding 1.5 ml water and 10 ml aquasol to each sample. Dashed line (×) = mRNA precursor labeled with [^{3}H]-uracil in whole cells; solid line (O) = mRNA precursor labeled with [α^{32}P]-UTP in isolated nuclei.

shown in figure 10 (Jacobson, Firtel, and Lodish, 1974b), and an appreciable fraction of the labeled poly(A)-containing RNA molecules do possess a 5' triphosphate residue (A. Jacobson, personal communication). This is strong evidence that these nuclear poly(A)-containing RNAs represent a primary transcript of the nuclear DNA and are not derived from a longer RNA precursor.

Of the polynucleotide sequences in cytoplasmic mRNA, over 90% are complementary to, and thus transcribed from, single-copy DNA, i.e., DNA sequences present in only one copy per genome; less than 10% of the cytoplasmic RNA is transcribed from repetitive DNA. By contrast, 25–30% of the sequences in nuclear poly(A)-containing RNA are complementary to DNA sequences that are present in 100–300 copies per genome (repetitive DNA). The remainder of the sequences are complementary to single-copy DNA. Most of the repetitive sequences in nuclear poly(A)-containing RNA are localized near the 5' ends of the molecules. These same RNAs contain, at the 3' end, a sequence of poly(A)$_{25}$ that is presumably transcribed from the poly(T)$_{25}$ sequences in the nuclear DNA (Firtel and Lodish, 1973; Jacobson, Firtel, and Lodish, 1974a). The presence in the same primary RNA transcript of RNA sequences transcribed from repetitive DNA, single-copy DNA, and poly(T) is in agreement with the length and interspersion of these sequences within the nuclear DNA genome: approximately 60–70% of the *Dictyostelium* genome consists of interspersed reiterated and single-copy DNA sequences. The interspersed repetitive DNA sequences have an average length of 250–400 nucleotide pairs, whereas the average length of the interspersed single-copy sequences is between 1,000 and 1,200 nucleotide pairs (fig. 2). (Approximately 20% of the single-copy DNA sequences is found in tracts 3,000 nucleotides long without interspersed reiterated DNA sequences, and about 35% of the repetitive DNA sequence is found in long tracts without interspersed single-copy DNA sequences [Firtel and Kindle, 1975].)

Fig. 11 (opposite). Protein synthesis throughout development. (A) Wild-type AX3 cells; (B) *agg* 2, a mutant unable to aggregate; (C) JM 94, a mutant able to aggregate but not to form slugs. Exponentially growing cells were harvested and washed; 5×10^6 cells were plated on each of many 13 mm diameter black Millipore filters supported by Millipore pads saturated with PDF (Tuchman, Alton, and Lodish, 1974). For labeling, one filter was transferred to a 10 μl drop of [^{35}S]-methionine solution (1 mCi per ml) in PDF and incubated 30 min. The incorporation was stopped by immersing the filter in Laemmli's sample buffer (Laemmli, 1970), vortexing, and boiling for 3 min. Aliquots were then electrophoresed through a 7.5% SDS polyacrylamide gel by the method of Laemmli (1970). An equal amount of acid-insoluble radioactivity was applied to each slot in the slab. Cell streaming was visible at 8 hrs., slug formation at 15 hrs., and culmination was complete by 24 hrs., in the case of AX3.

The mutant *agg* 2 (obtained from D. McMahon) was analyzed by the same method as was the wild type with the addition of a labeling point between 0.5 to 1.0 hrs.

The mutant JM 94 was induced in the strain AX3 by mutagenesis with N-methyl-N'-nitro-N-nitrosoguanidine and was analyzed by the same method as was the wild type. This mutant shows cell streaming at 8 hrs. and forms discrete flat aggregates by 10 hrs. These flat aggregates never differentiate further.

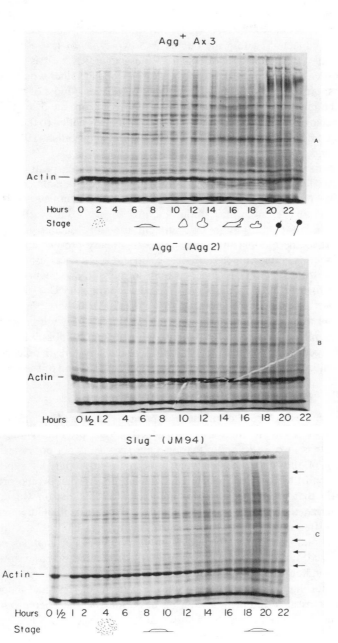

Agg⁺ Ax3

Actin —

Hours 0 2 4 6 8 10 12 14 16 18 20 22
Stage

Agg⁻ (Agg 2)

Actin —

Hours 0 ½ 1 2 4 6 8 10 12 14 16 18 20 22

Slug⁻ (JM94)

Actin —

Hours 0 ½ 1 2 4 6 8 10 12 14 16 18 20 22
Stage

Several years ago we proposed a model for biogenesis of mRNA; this model assumes that each molecule of nuclear poly(A)-containing RNA generates one molecule of mRNA. According to this model, nuclear poly(A)-plus RNA is subjected, within the nucleus, to two types of processing reactions before they exit into the cytoplasm as messenger RNA. It is not known in what order these might occur, nor is it clear whether either would be coupled to transport from the nucleus. First, about 300 bases—most of the transcripts from the repetitive DNA—appear to be removed from the 5' end. Second, a sequence of about 100–150 adenylic acid residues is added to the 3' end of the RNA (Lodish, Firtel, and Jacobson, 1973; Firtel and Lodish, 1973; Jacobson, Firtel, and Lodish, 1974b).

Recent experiments have called into question certain aspects of this model. We have discovered that nuclear polyadenylated RNAs isolated after a short (15 min.) pulse with [^{32}P] contains only the 5' end structures I and II. All four structures are present in the cytoplasmic mRNA of the same cells. Therefore, attachment of the 2'0-methyl substituent probably occurs during or after transport to the cytoplasm. Since pm^{7}G is already present after such short pulse labeling, either processing of the repeated sequence at the 5' end does not occur or else pm^{7}G is attached both to the mRNA precursor and to the product formed after its cleavage (Weiner, Dottin, and Lodish, in preparation). Further experiments are necessary to distinguish these possibilities. It is important to emphasize that our work, to date, deals only with mixed populations of mRNA and pre-mRNA. This work raises the possibility that some mRNA species are synthesized directly without any longer precursor at all, and possibly others have repetitive transcripts at the 5' end of their precursors.

PROTEIN SYNTHESIS DURING DIFFERENTIATION

The synthesis of none of the developmentally regulated enzymes studied to date represents more than 1% of the cell's total protein synthesis at any instant. It is also well known that enzyme activity is not necessarily a valid measure of the amount of enzyme protein. In any study of synthesis and translation of mRNA, it is easier to focus on those proteins (and presumably mRNAs) that are made in larger amounts; for this reason we decided to characterize the predominant species of polypeptides that are synthesized during different developmental stages (Tuchman et al., 1974). Figure 11A shows a radioautogram of an SDS polyacrylamide gel analysis of protein synthesized during 30 min. pulses of [^{35}S]-methionine given at hourly intervals throughout development of wild-type cells.

As determined by the difference in the patterns of [^{35}S]-met incorporation into proteins at different times during development, the *Dictyostelium* morphogenic sequence can be divided into at least four general stages: preaggre-

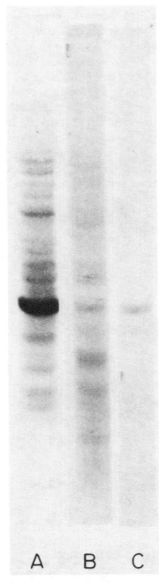

A B C

Fig. 12. SDS-polyacrylamide gels of various *Dictyostelium* samples. (A) Autoradiograph of 0 to 2 hrs. labeled sample; (B) Coomassie blue stain of *Dictyostelium* membrane fraction from developing cells; (C) Coomassie blue stain of purified *Dictyostelium* actin. Conditions for gel electrophoresis and for purification of actin were given in Tuchman, Alton, and Lodish (1974).

gation (0 to 7 hours), aggregation (8 to 12 hours), postaggregation (13 to 18 hours), and culmination (19 to 24 hours). During the preaggregation stage, as much as 30% of the [^{35}S]-met incorporated by the cells represents a single species that we have shown to be *Dictyostelium* actin.

As one example, figure 12 shows that the predominant polypeptide synthesized during early development comigrates on SDS polyacrylamide gels with authentic *Dictyostelium* actin. This labeled polypeptide also co-polymerizes with authentic actin and also contains the unusual amino acid 3-methylhistidine, characteristic of *Dictyostelium* and vertebrate actins (Tuchman et al., 1974).

The percentage of total cell protein synthesis that is actin rises from 8% in growing cells to over 30% at 3 hours of development (fig. 13). During the aggregation state the synthesis of actin declines relative to total cell protein synthesis; only 7% of protein synthesized by 14 hr. cells is actin, and this percentage drops further at later stages (cf. fig. 11A). During the aggregation stage other major changes occur in the pattern of proteins synthesized. The

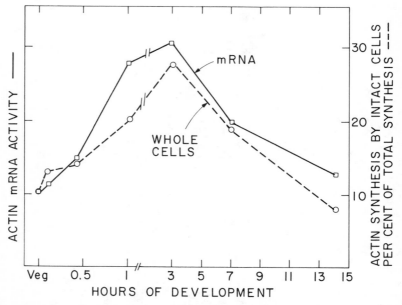

Fig. 13. Content of actin mRNA and rate of actin synthesis. Dashed line = Actin synthesis by whole cells. Radioautograms similar to those of figure 11 were scanned, and the fraction of the total area which was under the actin peak was determined. Solid line = Content of actin mRNA. The amount of actin mRNA, relative to ribosomal RNA, was estimated from the slopes of the curves in figure 16.

synthesis of two other predominant "preaggregation" proteins decreases significantly, while the synthesis of at least four new "aggregation stage" polypeptides increases.

Much of our work to date has focused on the regulation of actin synthesis during differentiation. We have shown that *Dictyostelium* actin mRNA can be translated faithfully in cell-free extracts from rabbit reticulocytes or wheat germ, and we take the amount of actin synthesized in these extracts as a measure of the amount of actin mRNA (Alton and Lodish, in preparation). As an example, figure 14 shows that RNA isolated from the cells of age 2 hrs.

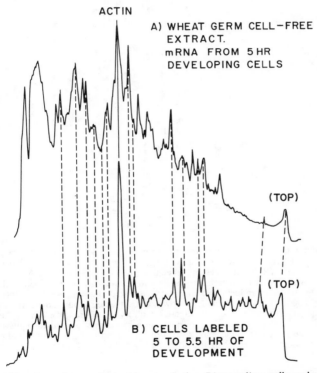

ACTIN

A) WHEAT GERM CELL–FREE
EXTRACT.
mRNA FROM 5 HR
DEVELOPING CELLS

(TOP)

(TOP)

B) CELLS LABELED
5 TO 5.5 HR OF
DEVELOPMENT

Fig. 14. Profile of proteins synthesized by developing *Dictyostelium* cells and wheat germ extracts programmed with slime mold RNA. (A) From whole *Dictyostelium* cells plated for 5 hrs. of development, RNA was isolated by lysis with phenol-chloroform-SDS, followed by precipitation with ethanol. The RNA was translated in the wheat germ extract as described by Roberts and Patterson (1973) except that the reaction contained 800 μM spermidine and 1.5 mM Mg^{++}. (B) Each 50 μl reaction contained 16 μg of whole-cell RNA. Whole cells were labeled from 5 to 5.5 hrs. of development as described in figure 11A. The reaction products and the *in vivo* proteins were subjected to electrophoresis on SDS-polyacrylamide gels containing an exponential gradient of acrylamide as described by Van Blerkom and Manes (1974). Autoradiograms were scanned with a Joyce-Loebl microdensitometer.

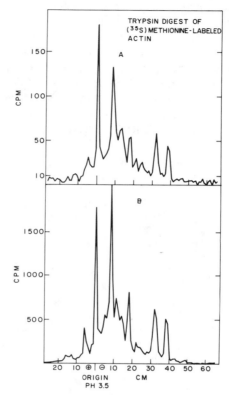

Fig. 15. Tryptic peptides of actin synthesized *in vivo* and in wheat germ extracts programmed with slime mold RNA. (A) Synthesized in wheat germ extract directed by mRNA isolated from 5 hr. developing cells. (B) Synthesized by vegetative *Dictyostelium* cells. RNA from whole cells plated 5 hrs. was prepared and translated in wheat germ extract as described in the legend to figure 14. Translation products and *in vivo*-synthesized proteins were separated on SDS-polyacrylamide gels that were fixed, dried down, and subjected to autoradiography. The heavily labeled bands (actin) were excised and digested with trypsin as described by Tuchman, Alton, and Lodish (1974). The resulting tryptic peptides were then subjected to high-voltage paper ionophoresis at pH 3.5 (40 V/cm, 3 hrs.), the dried paper cut into 1 cm strips, and radioactivity determined by scintillation counting in a Toluene-POPOP cocktail.

directs the synthesis, in wheat germ extracts, predominatly of a single polypeptide that comigrates on SDS polyacrylamide gel electrophoresis with *Dictyostelium* actin. Analysis of tryptic peptides of this *in vitro*-produced protein by paper electrophoresis shows that it is indeed actin (fig. 15). As shown by the dashed lines in figure 14, it appears that other authentic *Dictyostelium* polypeptides are made in this cell-free system, but we have not yet confirmed their identity by peptide mapping.

The amount of translatable actin mRNA at the different developmental stages, relative to the amount of rRNA, is shown in figure 13 and figure 16. The amount of rRNA per cell gradually declines during differentiation; at 24 hours each cell contains only about one-third the initial amount of RNA. Hence, the values in figure 13 should have to be corrected in order to give the value of actin mRNA per cell. Nonetheless, it is clear that the amount of translatable actin mRNA per cell increases threefold during the first three hours of development and then declines. The apparent half-life of actin mRNA after 3 hours is about 6–8 hours. It should be pointed out that we do not yet know the absolute rate of actin synthesis per cell, only the rate relative to other cell proteins. But figure 13 does indicate that there is a good correlation between the relative rate of actin synthesis and the amount of translatable actin mRNA per cell.

Although direct evidence is lacking, we surmise that the increased level of translatable actin mRNA during the first three hours is a result of *de novo* synthesis of new actin mRNA.

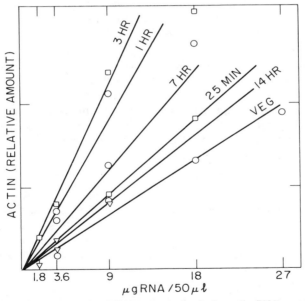

Fig. 16. Relative amount of actin mRNA present in developing cells. RNA was prepared from whole cells, at stages indicated, as described in figure 14 and translated in the wheat germ extract. Products were analyzed on SDS-polyacrylamide gels that were fixed, dried, and autoradiographed (see figs. 11 and 14). The autoradiograms were then scanned and the actin peak determined. Plotted is the area under the actin peak relative to the amount of input RNA. The slopes of these curves are a measure of the content of actin mRNA.

Further insight into the regulation of protein synthesis during the early phases of differentiation has come from a study of mutants that are unable to aggregate normally. We have studied ten independently isolated aggregation-deficient mutants. These mutants either fail to aggregate at all or form flat, diffuse aggregates that never become spherical or progress into slugs.

Mutants that fail to aggregate at all show essentially the same patterns of protein synthesis as the wild type for the first 6 hours after plating (fig. 11B). However, these mutants continue making most of the "early" proteins, including actin, for at least 24 hours after plating. They show no induction of the polypeptides synthesized in wild-type cells during aggregation. As measured by the incorporation of [^{35}S]-methionine into protein during a 30 min. label, the rate of protein synthesis by these cells declines by no more than twofold during the first 24 hours (data not shown). We conclude that both the reduction in synthesis of certain early proteins and the increase in synthesis of late proteins after aggregation require selective gene expression during differentiation (Margolskee and Lodish, in preparation). We do not know how these genes affect protein synthesis. Nor do we know at what level this control is exerted. One possibility is that cell-cell contact, or some excreted cell product that accumulates during aggregation, is responsible for induction of synthesis of new "aggregation-specific" mRNAs and for cessation of synthesis of "early" mRNAs. Whether, in addition, mRNA stability is developmentally controlled also remains for future work.

It is of interest that mutants that show some aggregation, but do not form proper pseudoplasmodia, do show increases in synthesis of some, but not all, of the "aggregation-stage" proteins (fig. 11C). However, these mutants, in contrast to wild-type cells, continue to synthesize these proteins for up to 24 hours after initiation of development.

SUMMARY

It is clear that further progress requires exact measurement of the absolute rates of synthesis, per cell, of several developmentally significant proteins, such as actin. Also, it is essential to purify mRNAs for many of these proteins, and also complementary DNA or RNA to use as hybridization probes for these mRNAs. Only then will it be possible to quantitate the rates of synthesis and destruction of specific mRNAs during differentiation. We will have to analyze protein and mRNA synthesis in a much larger number of aggregation-defective mutants, particularly mutants that are known to be in different complementation groups.

Finally, it is worth emphasizing that detailed understanding of even one Agg⁻ mutant will require the coordinated efforts of many laboratories. It is clear that differentiation in this relatively simple organism, *Dictyostelium,* is extremely complex. This realization emphasizes the importance of understanding simple model systems as a prelude to understanding the more complex systems of higher forms.

ACKNOWLEDGMENTS

We thank Mr. Martin Brock for expert technical assistance. This work was supported by grants GB-42597 and BMS74-04869 from the National Science Foundation. Harvey F. Lodish is a recipient of a Research Career Development Award GM50175 from the U.S. National Institutes of Health; Tom Alton and Jeanne P. Margolskee have predoctoral fellowships from the N.S.F.; Robert Dottin is a Centennial Postdoctoral Fellow of the Canadian Medical Research Council; and Allan M. Weiner is a Helen Hay Whitney Postdoctoral Fellow.

LITERATURE CITED

Adams, J., and S. Cory. 1975. Modified nucleosides and bizarre 5'-termini in mouse myeloma mRNA. Nature 255:28–33.

Ashworth, J. M. 1971. Cell development in the cellular slime mould *Dictyostelium discoideum.* Symp. Soc. Exp. Biol. 25:27–49.

Barrell, B. 1971. Fractionation and sequence analysis of radioactive nucleotides. *In* G. L. Cantoni and D. R. Davies (eds.). Proceedings in nucleic acid research 2:775–79.

Bishop, J. W., M. Rosbash, and D. Evans. 1974. Polynucleotide sequences in eukaryotic DNA and RNA that form ribonuclease-resistant complexes with polyuridylic acid. J. Mol. Biol. 85:75–86.

Brody, T., and K. L. Williams. 1974. Cytological analysis of the parasexual cycle in *Dictyostelium discoideum.* J. Gen. Micro. 82:371–83.

Bonner, J. T. 1971. Aggregation and differentiation in the cellular slime molds. Ann. Rev. Microbiol. 25:75–79.

Darnell, J. E., W. R. Jelinek, and G. R. Molloy. 1973. Biogenesis of mRNA: Genetic regulation in mammalian cells. Science 181:1215–21.

Durston, A. 1974. Pacemaker activity during aggregation in *Dictyostelium discoideum.* Devel. Biol. 37:225–35.

Dimond, R., M. Brenner, and W. F. Loomis, Jr. 1973. Mutations affecting N-acetyl-glucosaminidase in *Dictyostelium discoideum.* Proc. Nat. Acad. Sci. USA 70:3356–60.

Erodos, G. W., K. B. Raper, and L. K. Vogen. 1973. Mating types and macrocyst formation in *Dictyostelium discoideum.* Proc. Nat. Acad. Sci. USA 70:1828–30.

Erdos, G. W., K. B. Raper, and L. K. Vogen. 1975. Sexuality in the cellular slime mold *Dictyostelium giganteum.* Proc. Nat. Acad. Sci. USA 72:970–973.

Firtel, R. A. 1972. Changes in the expression of single-copy DNA during development of the cellular slime mold *Dictyostelium discoideum.* J. Mol. Biol. 66:363–77.

Firtel, R. A., L. Baxter, and H. F. Lodish. 1973. Actinomycin D and the regulation of enzyme biosynthesis during development of *Dictyostelium discoideum.* J. Mol. Biol. 79:315–27.

Firtel, R. A., and J. T. Bonner. 1972. Characterization of the genome of the cellular slime mold *Dictyostelium discoideum*. J. Mol. Biol. 66:339–61.

Firtel, R. A., and K. Kindle. 1975. Structural organization of the genome of the cellular slime mold *Dicytostelium discoideum:* Interspersion of repetitive and single-copy DNA sequences. Cell 5:401–11.

Firtel, R. A., A. Jacobson, and H. F. Lodish. 1972. Isolation and hybridization kinetics of messenger RNA from *Dictyostelium discoideum*. Nature New Biol. 239:225–28.

Firtel, R. A., and H. F. Lodish. 1973. A small nuclear precursor of messenger RNA in the cellular slime mold *Dictyostelium discoideum*. J. Mol. Biol. 79:295–314.

Francis, D. W. 1962. The movement of pseudoplasmodia of *Dictyostelium discoideum*. Ph.D. thesis. University of Wisconsin, Madison, Wis.

Franke, J., and M. Sussman. 1973. Accumulation of uridine diphosphoglucose pyrophosphorylase in *Dictyostelium discoideum* via preferential synthesis. J. Mol. Biol. 81:173–85.

Freeze, S. J., and W. F. Loomis, Jr. 1974. Isolation of mutation in *Dictyostelium discoideum* affecting α-mannosidase. Biochimie 56:1525–28.

Furuichi, Y., M. Morgan. S. Muthukrishnan, and A. Shatkin. 1975a. Reovirus messenger RNA contains a methylated, blocked 5′-terminal structure: m^{7}G(5′)ppp(5′) CmpCp. Proc. Nat. Acad. Sci. USA 72:362–66.

Furuichi, Y., M. Morgan, A. J. Shatkin, W. Jelinek, M. Salditt-Georgieff, and J. E. Darnell. 1975b. Methylated, blocked 5′-termini in HeLa cell mRNA. Proc. Nat. Acad. Sci. USA 72:1904–8.

Garrod, D. R. 1969. The cellular basis of movement of the migrating apex of the slime mould *Dictyostelium discoideum*. J. Cell Sci. 4:781–98.

Gerisch, G., D. Malchow, and B. Gess. 1974. pp. 279–298. *In* L. Jaenicke (ed.). Biochemistry of sensory Functions. Pp. 279–98. Berlin, Springer-Verlag.

Gingold, E. B., and J. M. Ashworth. 1974. Evidence for mitotic crossing-over during the parasexual cycle of the cellular slime mold *Dictyostelium discoideum*. J. Gen. Microbiol. 84:70–78.

Gustafson, G. L., W. Y. Kong, and B. E. Wright. 1973. Analysis of uridine diphosphate-glucose pyrophosphorylase during differentiation in *Dictyostelium discoideum*. J. Biol. Chem. 248:5188–96.

Hohl, H. R., and S. T. Hamamoto. 1969. Ultrastructure of spore differentiation in *Dictyostelium:* the prespore vacuole. J. Ultrastr. Res. 26:442–53.

Jacobson, A., R. A. Firtel, and H. F. Lodish. 1974a. Synthesis of messenger and ribosomal RNA precursors in isolated nuclei of the cellular slime mold *Dictyostelium discoideum*. J. Mol. Biol. 82:213–30.

Jacobson, A., R. A. Firtel, and H. F. Lodish. 1974b. Transcription of poly(dT) sequences in the genome of the cellular slime mold *Dictyostelium discoideum*. Proc. Nat. Acad. Sci. USA 71:1607–11.

Jacobson, A., and H. F. Lodish. 1975. Genetic control of development of the cellular slime mold *Dictyostelium discoideum*. Ann. Rev. Genetics 9:145–85.

Katz, E., and L. Bourguignon. 1974. The cell cycle and its relationship to aggregation in the cellular slime mold *Dictyostelium discoideum*. Dev. Biol. 36:82–87.

Katz, E. G., and V. Kao. 1974. Evidence for mitotic recombination in the cellular slime mold *Dictyostelium discoideum*. Proc. Nat. Acad. Sci. USA 71:4025–26.

Kessin, R. H., K. L. Williams, and P. C. Newell. 1974. Linkage analysis in *Dictyostelium discoideum* using temperature-sensitive growth mutants selected with bromodeoxyuridine. J. Bacteriol. 119:776–83.

Killick, K. A., and B. E. Wright. 1974. Regulation of enzyme activity during differentiation in *Dictyostelium discoideum*. Ann. Rev. Microbiol. 28:139–66.

Laemmli. U. K. 1970. Cleavage of structural proteins during the assembly of the head of bacteriophage T4. Nature 227:680–85.

Lodish, H. F., R. Firtel, and A. Jacobson. 1974. Transcription and structure of the genome of the cellular slime mold *Dictyostelium discoideum*. Cold Spring Harbor Symp. Quant. Biol. 38:899–907.

Lodish, H. F., A. Jacobson, R. Firtel, T. Alton, and J. Tuchman. 1974. Synthesis of messenger RNA and chromosome structure in the cellular slime mold. Proc. Nat. Acad. Sci. USA 71:5103–8.

Loomis, W. F., Jr. 1969. Temperature-sensitive mutants of *Dictyostelium discoideum*. J. Bacteriol. 99:65–69.

Loomis, W. F., Jr. 1975. *Dictyostelium discoideum,* a developmental system. Academic Press, New York.

Loomis, W. F., Jr., and J. M. Ashworth. 1968. Plaque-size mutants of the cellular slime mold *Dictyostelium discoideum*. J. Gen. Microbiol. 53:181–86.

Nakazato, H., M. Edmonds, and D. W. Kopp. 1974. Differential metabolism of large and small poly(A) sequences in the heterogeneous nuclear RNA of HeLa cells. Proc. Nat. Acad. Sci. USA 71:200–204.

Newell, P. C., J. S. Ellingson, and M. Sussman. 1969. Synchrony of enzyme accumulation in a population of differentiating slime mold cells. Biochim. Biophys. Acta 177:610–14.

Newell, P. C. 1971. The development of the cellular slime mould *Dictyostelium discoideum:* A model system for the study of cellular differentiation. *In* P. N. Campbell and F. Dickens (eds.). Essays in biochemistry. 7:87–126. Academic Press, New York and London.

Perry, R. P., D. E. Kelley, K. Friderici, and F. Rottman. 1975. The methylated constituents of L-cell messenger RNA: Evidence for an unusual cluster at the 5′-terminus. Cell 4:387–94.

Raper, K. B. 1940. Pseudoplasmodium formation and organization in *Dictyostelium discoideum*. J. E. Mitchell Sci. Soc. 56:241–82.

Roberts, B. E., and B. M. Paterson. 1973. Efficient translation of tobacco mosaic virus RNA and rabbit globin 9S RNA in a cell-free system from commercial wheat germ. Proc. Nat. Acad. Sci. USA 70:2330–34.

Robertson, A., and M. H. Cohen. 1972. Control of developing fields. Ann. Rev. Biophys. Bioeng. 1:409–64.

Rosen, S., J. A. Kafka, D. L. Simpson, and S. H. Barondes. 1973. Developmentally-regulated carbohydrate binding protein in *Dictyostelium discoideum*. Proc. Nat. Acad. Sci. USA 70:2554–57.

Rossomando, E. I., and M. Sussman. 1973. A 5′-adenosine monophosphate-dependent adenylate cyclase and an adenosine 3′:5′-cyclic monophosphate-dependent adenosine triphosphate pyrophosphohydrolase in *Dictyostelium discoideum*. Proc. Nat. Acad. Sci. USA 70:1254–57.

Rottman, F., A. J. Shatkin, and R. P. Perry. 1974. Sequences containing methylated nucleotides at the 5′ termini of messenger RNAs: Possible implications for processing. Cell 3:197–99.

Sussman, R. R. 1961. A method for staining chromosomes of *Dictyostelium discoideum* myxamoebae in the vegetative stage. Exp. Cell Res. 24:154–55.

Sussman, M. 1966. Biochemical and genetic methods in the study of cellular slime mold development. *In* D. Prescott (eds.). Methods in cell physiology. Pp. 397-410. Academic Press, New York.

Sussman, R. R., and M. Sussman. 1967. Cultivation of *Dictyostelium discoideum* in axenic medium. Biochem. Biophys. Res. Comm. 29:53–55.

Sussman, M., and E. P. Rayner. 1971. Physical characterization of deoxyribonucleic acids in *Dictyostelium discoideum*. Arch. Biochem. Biophys. 144:127–37.

Tuchman, J., T. Alton, and H. F. Lodish. 1974. Preferential synthesis of actin during early development of the slime mold *Dictyostelium discoideum*. Devel. Biol. 40:116–29.

Van Bleikom, J., and C. Manes. 1974. Development of preimplantation rabbit embryos *in vivo* and *in vitro* 11: A comparison of qualitative aspects of protein synthesis. Devel. Biol. 40:40–51.

Van Tiegham, P. 1880. Sur quelques myxomycètes à plasmode agrégé. Bull. Soc. Biol. Fr. 27:317–22.

Watts, D. J., and J. M. Ashworth. 1970. Growth of myxamoebae of the cellular slime mould *Dictyostelium discoideum* in axenic culture. Biochem. J. 119:171–74.

Wei, C. M., A. Gershowitz, and B. Moss. 1975. Methylated nucleotides block 5′ terminus of HeLa cell messenger RNA. Cell 4:379–86.

Williams, K. L., R. H. Kessin, and P. C. Newell. 1974. Parasexual genetic in *Dictyostelium discoideum:* Mitotic analysis of acriflavin resistance and growth in axenix medium. J. Gen. Micro. 84:59–69.

TOM HUMPHREYS AND KENNETH C. KLEENE

Regulation of RNA and Protein Synthesis During Early Animal Embryology

9

INTRODUCTION

During embryogenesis the relatively simple egg must be reconstructed into a much more complex, functional organism. Regulatory reactions at tissue, cellular, and molecular levels are known to participate in guiding this extraordinarily complex and intricate unfolding. At the center of the cellular reactions controlling differentiation lie the mechanisms that control the expression of the genetic information encoded in the zygote nucleus. Molecular studies over the past decade have elucidated the general patterns of RNA and protein synthesis in embryos and have identified many changes that provide insight into the interrelationships of macromolecular synthesis and embryogenesis. Even though our knowledge is still rudimentary, the literature on this is already quite extensive and leads to many interesting considerations (Davidson, 1968; Humphreys, 1973). Rather than try in this paper to provide a summary review of these studies of macromolecular synthesis during embryogenesis, we have chosen to concentrate on three examples of regulation of RNA and protein synthesis in embryogenesis that are currently the subject of especially successful and interesting analysis. These are (1) activation of maternal messenger RNA; (2) regulation of histone synthesis during the rapid cell divisions of cleavage; and (3) regulation of the synthesis and accumulation of informational RNA during early development.

ACTIVATION OF MATERNAL MESSENGER RNA IN SEA URCHIN EMBRYOS

Protein synthesis increases rapidly after fertilization of sea urchin eggs without a concomitant synthesis of RNA. This result suggests that there is a

Kewalo Marine Laboratory, University of Hawaii, Honolulu, Hawaii 96822.

store of maternal mRNA molecules that have accumulated in the egg during oogenesis and that may serve some specific and important function in early development. At present the activation of messenger RNA seems established, but its developmental significance remains obscure.

Elucidation of this activation began with Hultin's observation (1952) that isotopically labeled amino acids were incorporated into protein much more rapidly after fertilization of sea urchin eggs. Some of the increased incorporation was due to increased transport of the labeled amino acid, but appropriate controls showed a 5- to 20-fold increase in the absolute rate of protein synthesis (Nakano and Monroy, 1958; Epel, 1967; McIntosh and Bell, 1969b; Humphreys, 1969). We showed that the increased protein synthesis was not based on a more efficient use of mRNA (Humphreys, 1969). Polysomes were the same size before and after fertilization, showing that the rate of initiation of nascent protein chains per message did not change. The rate of movement of the ribosomes along the mRNA also did not change. It appeared to take 2 to 3 minutes to complete an average protein at both stages (Humphreys, 1969). The number of polysomes increased about 30-fold during the first two hours after fertilization, when protein synthesis was also increasing (Humphreys, 1971). Thus the increase in protein synthesis depended upon the use of messenger RNA molecules that were not previously active or associated with polysomes.

The idea that these newly active messenger RNA molecules come from a store of mRNA accumulated during oogenesis was first suggested by the observation that inhibition of RNA synthesis with Actinomycin D had no effect on the activation of protein synthesis (Gross, Malkin, and Moyer, 1963). Subsequent quantitative studies of incorporation of radioactive precursor into newly synthesized RNA confirmed that there was not enough newly synthesized messenger RNA to account for the increase in polysomes (Humphreys, 1971). In those measurements we used adenosine as a precursor, determined the specific activity of the ATP pool, and determined the incorporation of isotope into polysomal RNA. These results permitted the calculation that newly synthesized messenger RNA was sufficient to account for only about 15% of the message needed to make the polysomes. With the discovery that poly (A) is added to maternal mRNA after fertilization (Slater et al., 1973; Wilt, 1973), this 15% newly synthesized RNA can, actually, be equated quantitatively with this added poly (A) sequence. Thus significant amounts of mRNA coding sequences are not synthesized for the first two hours after fertilization, and it is evident that the messenger RNA entering polysomes during this period must be present before fertilization but maintained in an inactive state.

What is the developmental significance of the stored or maternal mRNA? The mRNA is not a special set of sequences for a few selected proteins, but is a general population of mRNA, probably rather similar to those active in the egg before fertilization or active in other kinds of cells. The general cell proteins, tubulin (Raff et al., 1972) and histones (Gross et al., 1973; Ruderman and Gross, 1974), have been identified among the proteins produced from egg RNA translated *in vitro,* and they are also synthesized in actinomycin D-treated embryos that have only maternal RNA. These mRNA molecules thus are already present in the egg but used after fertilization. They may be present in larger amounts than found in the "average" cell, but rigorous quantitation is not available to establish this point. Several studies have attempted to define the diversity of the proteins synthesized on the maternal mRNA by extensively fractionating proteins that were labeled *in vivo* with radioactive amino acids (McIntosh and Bell, 1969; Terman, 1970; Brandhorst, 1976). The most extensive study, accomplished with two-dimensional electrophresis, has defined more than 150 major bands of proteins (Brandhorst, 1976). Recent studies (Anderson, et al., 1976, with RNA:DNA hybridization using egg RNA indicate that the complexity of maternal mRNA may be similar to mRNA in sea urchin gastrulae, where there are 10,000 to 15,000 different kinds of mRNA molecules (Galau et al., 1974). Most of these different kinds of mRNA molecules are present in very small numbers per egg and thus produce undetectably small amounts of the protein.

Even if the population of maternal mRNA is very diverse and includes sequences for a number of general cellular proteins, there may be a special subset of these mRNA molecules that are developmentally important and possibly are specifically activated by a translational-level control mechanism.

A comparison of radioactive bands on acrylamide gels of proteins synthesized before and after fertilization indicates little, if any, change (McIntosh and Bell, 1969; Brandhorst, 1975). Similar studies on embryos treated with actinomycin D to stop synthesis of all new mRNA indicate that a few of the proteins being synthesized change with development (Terman, 1970; Ruderman and Gross, 1974). One of these proteins has been identified. The H_1 histone protein only begins to be synthesized at about the blastula stage, and its synthesis occurs in actinomycin-treated embryos (Ruderman and Gross, 1974). This well-documented change is apparently the result of differential timing of the activation of specific mRNA species and indicates a specificity for different messengers by the translational control mechanism. (Note added in proof: Recent evidence shows that this change in H_1 histone is due to a transcriptional rather than a translational change [Arceci, Senger, and Gross, 1976].) Further analysis of the regulation of this specific mRNA should be fascinating.

More than twenty papers dealing directly with the regulatory mechanisms involved in activating the maternal mRNA have been published over the last decade (see Humphreys, 1973a). These studies have led to interesting ideas, but they have been diverse and conflicting. No one has yet been able to elucidate the actual activation mechanism. Several years ago we attempted to delineate the characteristics required of the regulatory mechanism based on the parameters of protein synthesis in eggs and embryos and the kinetics of activation of protein synthesis at fertilization (Humphreys, 1969, 1971). From our studies we concluded that completely inactive mRNA molecules had to become active after fertilization. This activation occurred over a 2-hour period in which the ribosomes in polysomes increased from 0.75% to 20% of the total ribosomes of the egg (Humphreys, 1971). We reasoned that at the mid-point of the 2-hour transition either all the mRNA molecules were activated half-maximally or half of them were maximally activated. This distinction is important because it distinguishes two main classes of hypotheses. The former possibility suggests that activation occurs through some general component of the protein synthetic machinery, whereas the latter case indicates that the activity of the mRNA is controlled directly. We measured the size of the polysomes during the transition after fertilization; they were always the same size, and only their number increased (Humphreys, 1971). If ribosomes, tRNAs, or other such components of the protein synthesis machinery were limiting, then the size of polysomes during the transition period would be expected to change. Rather, the results imply that the regulatory mechanism must act directly to control the activity of the mRNA (Humphreys, 1969; 1971).

There are three general classes of mechanisms that could regulate the translatability of the maternal mRNA directly: (1) the mRNA could be compartmentalized, (2) it could interact with a repressor or activator molecule, or (3) its structure could be altered. At present, data are not available to evaluate these possibilities rigorously. After gentle homogenization the maternal histone mRNA sediments more slowly than ribosomal subunits, suggesting that this maternal mRNA is not sequestered but free in the cytoplasm as ribonucleo-protein particles (Skoultchi & Gross, 1973). In our opinion there is no good evidence for activator or inhibitor molecules associated with the mRNA. Ideas that have recently received the widest interest involve alteration of the structure of the mRNA. The poly (A) segment of maternal mRNA is increased from 100 to 200 nucleotides upon fertilization (Slater et al., 1972; Wilt, 1973). It seemed reasonable that this change in structure might be involved in activation of the mRNA. However, protein synthesis increased even when poly (A) synthesis was inhibited with the drug 3' deoxyadenosine, which terminates growing RNA chains (Mescher and Humphreys, 1974). This newly added poly (A) is not necessary for the activation of the maternal mRNA. Since the maternal mRNA is believed to be stable (Gross et al., 1974), it has been postulated that the poly (A) might be involved in stabilizing the maternal mRNA after it was activated (Wilt, 1973; Mescher and Humphreys, 1974). This, however, seems unlikely. Using quantitative pool-labeling procedures (Humphreys, 1973b), we found that all of the poly (A) in the embryo rapidly incorporates radioactive adenosine at a rate that is consistent with a 30-minute half-life (Dolecki and Humphreys, in preparation). This incorporation into the poly (A) occurs soon after fertilization when total poly (A) is doubling and at two and one-half hours after fertilization when total poly (A) is no longer increasing. The poly (A) of mRNA located in cytoplasmic polysomes becomes labeled after very short times, suggesting that turnover occurs on mRNA while it is being translated. The poly (A) on maternal mRNA thus turns over rapidly, and it is difficult to maintain that unstable poly (A) stabilizes the mRNA moleculem The relationship of poly (A) to maternal mRNA activation and/or function remains obscure.

The recent realization that the 5' end of mRNA is capped by methylated nucleotides that are necessary for translation has aroused speculation that this may be the mechanism of activation of maternal mRNA (Both et al., 1975). At present no data have been published on this possibility.

SYNTHESIS OF HISTONES FOR CLEAVAGE

A series of interesting regulatory phenomena are exhibited in the strategies that are employed by embryos to synthesize the large amounts of histone proteins needed within the nuclei that are formed very rapidly in cleavage stage. These are special mechanisms in addition to those exhibited in the usual cell cycle and are required when nuclei are doubling every 15 to 60 minutes as occurs in cleavage. They involve synthesizing a store of histone proteins during oogenesis to add to nuclei during cleavage, accumulating a store of histone mRNA molecules during oogenesis to be translated during cleavage, and replicating the complement of histone genes manyfold so histone mRNA can be formed rapidly during cleavage.

In amphibian oocytes the usual coupling of histone synthesis with DNA synthesis observed in other cells (Robbins and Borun, 1967) is broken, and these oocytes synthesize histones without synthesizing DNA. Radioactive amino acids are incorporated into authentic histone proteins, identified by acrylamide gel electrophoresis and confirmed by peptide analysis (Adamson and Woodland, 1974). Calculation of absolute rates of histone formation from measurements of the amino acid pool specific radioactivity and the rate of incorporation of isotope into individual protein species indicate that up to 80% of the total histones needed for cleavage could be formed during oogenesis. This store of histone proteins has not yet been identified or measured directly as a physical component of the amphibious oocytes or eggs, and its location in the cell poses interesting questions. The histones appear to be in the germinal vesicle (Adamson and Woodland, 1974), because radioactive histones injected into oocytes localize there (Gurdon, 1970). It has been assumed that the reason for the usual close coupling of DNA and histone synthesis is to neutralize their opposite charges to prevent problems that would otherwise be created by such highly charged molecules. The presence of enough histone for almost 10^5 nuclei in one nucleus must require interesting special adaptations. Synthesis or accumulation of histone proteins has not been demonstrated in other oocytes. However, appropriate experiments have not been carried out, and other oocytes may also accumulate histone proteins.

Histones are also synthesized very rapidly during cleavage. In amphibians, calculations from rates of incorporation of radioactive amino acids and amino acid pool specific activity suggest 10 to 20% of the total histone required during cleavage is synthesized after fertilization (Adamson and Woodland, 1974). Similar quantitative data are not available for sea urchins, but it is generally believed that most of the histones for cleavage are synthesized after fertilization. Histone synthesis after fertilization is also not coordinated with DNA synthesis in amphibians. Histone synthesis is 500 times faster than DNA synthesis at first cleavage, and there is no cyclic synthesis of histone correlated with cyclic DNA synthesis (Adamson and Woodland, 1974). Equivalent direct measurements of rates of histone protein synthesis are not available for other embryos, although a certain coordination of DNA and histone synthesis does occur in sea urchins (Kedes and Gross, 1969). The nature and extent of this coordination will be discussed more fully below.

Rapid histone synthesis during sea urchin cleavage is achieved by activating a store of maternal mRNA (Gross et al., 1973; Skoultchi and Gross, 1973; Ruderman and Gross, 1974) and by synthesizing new histone mRNA (Kedes and Gross, 1969) on a complement of reinterated histone genes (Kedes and Birnstiel, 1971). Direct evidence for both of these mechanisms is available only for the sea urchin embryo, but other embryos probably employ them also.

The presence of a significant store of histone mRNA in mature sea urchin eggs has been demonstrated by two rigorous criteria. First, egg RNA translated in a Krebs II ascites cell *in vitro* system produces the 5 classes of histones, identified by acrylamide gel electrophoresis and confirmed by tryptic peptide analysis (Gross et al., 1973). Second, egg RNA competes in the hybridization reaction between authentic radioactive histone mRNA and sea urchin DNA (Skoultchi and Gross, 1973). The amount of histone mRNA in eggs was estimated from this competition experiment and amounted to about 25% of the total histone mRNA accumulated during cleavage. This histone mRNA in eggs is utilized for histone synthesis after fertilization, since extensive histone synthesis occurs even when histone mRNA formation after fertilization has been stopped with actinomycin D (Johnson and Hnilca, 1971; Ruderman and Gross, 1974).

Normally there is extensive synthesis of new histone mRNA after fertilization in sea urchins. This was first recognized as an accumulation of radioactive RNA on small polysomes that incorporate more lysine than tryptophan, as is characteristic of histone polysomes (Lindsay and Nemer, 1969; Kedes et al., 1969; Moav and Nemer, 1971). This newly synthesized mRNA sedimented as a broad band at 9 to 12S and separated into 5 bands of acrylamide gels (Kedes and Gross, 1969; Weinberg et al., 1973). Probably, mRNA sequences for all the major classes of histone proteins are synthesized (Grundstein et al., 1973). The synthesis and stability of these histone mRNA molecules are coordinated with the cell cycle. Inhibition of cleavage with the DNA synthesis inhibitor, hydroxyurea, inhibits the formation of 9 to 12S RNA and causes degradation of the small polysomes already formed (Kedes and Gross, 1959; Kedes et al., 1969).

Use of 9 to 12S radioactive RNA in DNA:RNA hybridization reactions revealed that many copies of the histone genes were present in the genome. When radioactive histone RNA was hybridized with a great excess of DNA so that the rate of reaction is determined by the concentration of the genes in the DNA, the radioactive RNA hybridized at a rate consistent with 400 to 1,000 copies of each histone gene per genome (Kedes and Birnstiel, 1971). These genes appear as a cluster, each containing one copy of each histone mRNA sequence, and the clusters occur as tandem repeats in the DNA. This organization was first deduced from the fact that all histone genes banded together in a CsCl density gradient (Kedes and Birnstiel, 1971; Birnstiel et al., 1974) and has been confirmed by isolation of individual repeats of the histone genes by cloning on bacterial plasmids (Kedes et al., 1975a, 1975b). The histone genes are apparently reiterated to provide for the rapid synthesis of histone mRNA during cleavage. Evidence suggests that the histone genes may also be highly reiterated in *Xenopus* (Kedes and Birnstiel, 1971) and *Drosophila* (Birnstiel et al., 1973) where cleavage is rapid, but are reiterated only 10 to 20 times in mammals (Wilson et al., 1974) where cleavage is slow. Histone mRNA synthesis has not been studied in any of these other embryos.

The observations with sea urchins raise a number of interesting regulatory problems that should be examined more fully. The synthesis and translation of histone mRNA during cleavage depends on continuing DNA synthesis, since inhibiting DNA synthesis stops mRNA synthesis and translation. This is similar to cultured cells where histone polysomes appear at the beginning of the DNA synthesis phase and decay when DNA synthesis ends or is inhibited (Robbins and Borun, 1967). The formation and activity of the newly synthesized histone mRNA during cleavage could be similarly coordinated with the S phase of the cell cycle. This raises questions about the maternal histone mRNA that has been stored during oogenesis. Is it also subject to cyclical use, and possibly degradation, as the cells enter mitosis? In amphibians, histone mRNA seems to be activated before first cleavage, and its translation is not coordinated with DNA synthesis (Adamson and Woodland, 1974). Does the same occur in sea urchins? If so, the use and metabolism of the maternal histone mRNA would presumably be different from the newly synthesized histone mRNA. An alternative is that the activation, synthesis, and translation of histone mRNA is somehow coupled to the rapid cleavage state rather than to the individual cell cycles of the cleaving cells. Then it would be only at the end of cleavage that the histone mRNA synthesis is shut off and histone mRNA decays. Such possibilities could be easily distinguished by measuring the kinetics of synthesis and decay of histone mRNA and of histone protein synthesis during cleavage and when cleavage is stopped with hydroxyurea. Histone mRNA synthesis in other cleaving embryos should also be studied more fully.

REGULATION OF HETEROGENEOUS NUCLEAR AND MESSENGER RNA SYNTHESIS

The developmental processes of determination and differentiation during embryogenesis must involve the most complex and important regulation of gene expression that occurs in the life cycle of an organism. Although in fact it is not known, one assumes that many of the large number of genes in an animal genome (potentially enough information to code for 10^6 proteins) function only during development. Analysis of the RNA synthesized from these genes would provide insight into the regulation of genetic expression in development. Another major group of genes, dubbed the "housekeeping genes," are those necessary for general cellular functions. The products of these two groups of genes make up the heterogeneous nuclear RNA and messenger RNA, (hnRNA, and mRNA) of the cell. Consequently, and presumably operationally, these genes are distinguished respectively as genes that are expressed only in specific cells at specific developmental times and genes that are expressed in most cells. Present studies on RNA synthesis in early embryos are just beginning to compare the populations of RNA sequences present at different stages so as to establish the extent of gene regulation associated with developmental changes. Much prior work has laid the foundation for current studies with sea urchins, which have been paralleled by studies on other animal cells to define and establish the characteristics of heterogenous nuclear and messenger RNA. Such studies on embryos have advanced furthest in sea urchins and illustrate the important conclusions now available.

Early studies on sea urchin and other embryos (Nemer, 1963; Wilt, 1964; Brown and Littna, 1964) showed that heterogenous, DNA-like RNA was the predominant RNA synthesized until gastrulation when ribosomal RNA synthesis begins to predominate. Subsequent quantitative analysis of these changes has led to two conclusions. (1) There is a 10- to 20-fold coordinate reduction in the accumulation of newly synthesized hnRNA and mRNA per nucleus between cleavage and pluteus stage (Kijima and Wilt, 1969; Roeder and Rutter, 1970; Emerson and Humphreys, 1970, 1971; Brandhorst and Humphreys, 1971, 1972). (2) Ribosomal RNA synthesis is repressed to a rate of 300 copies of ribosomal RNA per cell per hour, or about one molecule per gene per hour, throughout early sea urchin development (Emerson and Humphreys, 1970; 1971). Activation of the ribosomal RNA genes does not occur until pluteus larvae begin to feed (Humphreys, 1973a). This negligible rate of ribosomal RNA synthesis in sea urchin embryos has greatly facilitated studies on the synthesis of hnRNA and mRNA because they are uncomplicated by ribosomal RNA synthesis. The developmental significance of the considerable reduction of the amount of hnRNA and mRNA accumulating during development remains unknown; but the reduction is the result of slowing the rate of production of transcripts from the active genes and not due to a change in the number of genes that are active or in stabilities of gene products (see below).

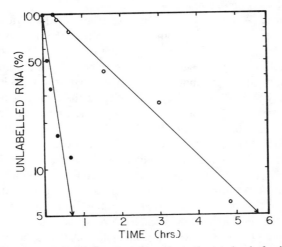

Fig. 1. First-order decay plot of the accumulation to a steady-state level of radioactive RNA in pure nuclear (represented by solid circles) and cytoplasmic (open circles) fractions of sea urchin mesenchyme blastulae. The nuclear RNA has an apparent half-life of about 10 minutes. Accumulation of RNA in the cytoplasm does not begin until 15 minutes, and then RNA accumulates consistent with a 70- to 90-minute half-life. (Adapted from Brandhorst and Humphreys, 1972.)

Rates of synthesis and decay of hnRNA and mRNA have been determined in sea urchin embryos from the kinetics of incorporation of exogenous radioactive nucleosides into nucleotide triphosphate precursor pools and into RNA to calculate actual amounts of RNA synthesized (Kijima and Wilt, 1969; Roeder and Rutter, 1970; Brandhorst and Humphreys, 1971; 1972). Accumulation curves of both classes of RNA show a rapid initial increase that slows with time until a steady-state plateau is achieved. This pattern of accumulation is typical of the labeling of a steady-state population of rapidly decaying molecules. At first, accumulation of radioactive RNA is equal to synthesis; but as radioactive RNA accumulates, its decay reduces net accumulation of radioactive RNA and its level finally approaches a steady state. This accumulation curve of radioactive RNA is the inverse of the decay of the unlabeled RNA that made up the steady-state level when isotope was added; to maintain this steady state, labeled RNA had to replace unlabeled RNA as the latter decayed. This inverse curve for the decay of unlabeled RNA can be plotted as a standard first-order decay curve, as shown for purified nuclear and cytoplasmic RNA of sea urchin blastulae in figure 1. The slope of the decay curve gives the half-life of the RNA. It is 7–10 minutes for nuclear RNA and about 90 minutes for cytoplasmic mRNA (Brandhorst and Humphreys, 1972). Comparisons of accumulation curves from different stages of development indicate that the rates of synthesis of hnRNA and mRNA decrease coordinately throughout development while the rates of decay of these classes of RNA do not change.

The nuclear RNA that decays with a 7- to 10-minute half-life accounts for about 90% of the total RNA synthesized, whereas the mRNA, with a 90-minute half-life, accounts for only 10 percent of the RNA synthesized. Because of the difference in half-life, the more stable mRNA accumulates more extensively and makes up about 65% of the steady-state level of unstable RNA, and nuclear RNA makes up only 35% of the steady-state level. The steady-state level of mRNA amounts to 2% of the ribosomal RNA in polysomes. This level is similar to the 2% mRNA found in hemoglobin polysomes (Labrie, 1969) and suggests that the 90-minute half-life of RNA accounts for much of the mRNA of the embryo. The possibility of a longer-lived mRNA population exists because the data are complicated by accumulation of significant ribosomal RNA during long labeling periods. Such possibilities have not been rigorously dealt with in experiments published to date. However, our data indicate that it is unlikely that such RNA can account for much of the mRNA. The poly (A) component of both nuclear and cytoplasmic RNA also appears to turn over with similar decay rates (Wu and Wilt, 1973). Estimates of slower decay of hnRNA and mRNA in sea urchins (Kijima and Wilt, 1969; Aronson and Wilt, 1970; Nemer, Dubroff, and Graham, 1975) have been presented. The overestimates of the half-life of nuclear RNA probably derive from contamination of the nuclear fraction with cytoplasm, which gives a composite decay rate averaging hnRNA and mRNA decay and yielding an apparent longer half-life. For accurate measurement it is necessary to use procedures that eliminate cytoplasmic contamination of the nuclear fraction; our nuclear fraction contained less than 1% of the ribosomal RNA (Brandhorst and Humphreys, 1972). The estimate of a longer half-life for mRNA is a maximum estimate that was not corrected for actual pool specific activity (Nemer et al., 1975). When we recalculate the data taking into account incorporation into stable ribosomal RNA, the half-life of the mRNA appears to be under 2 hours.

The genome of sea urchins, like all other eukaryotes, contains DNA sequences that appear only once in each haploid DNA complement and other sequences that are repeated 20 to 10,000 times (Graham et al., 1974). The repetition of DNA sequences that are transcribed as hnRNA or mRNA has been identified by DNA:RNA hybridization in which trace amounts of labeled RNA were reacted with an excess of DNA. Eight percent of hnRNA from gastrulae hybridizes with repetitive DNA sequences, and 92% hybridizes with nonrepetitive DNA sequences (Smith et al., 1974). A large percentage of the hnRNA molecules have repetitive elements interspersed with the nonrepetitive elements. In contrast, greater than 97% of the mRNA in gastrulae hybridizes with nonrepetitive DNA (Goldberg et al., 1973). In the ultimate of sophistication of these kinds of studies, it has been shown that 80–100% of mRNA is transcribed from nonrepetitive DNA sequences that are contiguous to short repeated DNA sequences (Davidson et al., 1975).

The earliest studies using RNA:DNA hybridization of RNA in early sea urchin development were probably concerned only with transcripts of repeated DNA (Glissen et al., 1966; Whiteley, McCarthy, and Whiteley, 1966). These studies suggested that the expression of repeated DNA sequences changes during development. However, these results cannot be interpreted in terms of actual active sequences because transcripts of a single repeated sequences will hybridize with all of the members of a family of related sequences that resemble the original sequence that was transcribed. Moreover, these early studies did not detect hybrids with nonrepetitive DNA from which the vast majority of heterodisperse RNA molecules and the vast majority of the diversity of RNA molecules are transcribed.

The numbers of nonrepetitive genes being transcribed into hnRNA and mRNA in gastrulae have been measured recently (Hough et al., 1975; Gaulau, Britten, and Davidson, 1974). These measurements were obtained by determining the percentage of radioactive tracer DNA, consisting of pure nonrepetitive sequences, which forms RNA-DNA hybrids in a reaction carried to completion by high concentrations of either purified hnRNA or mRNA. When the radioactive nonrepetitive DNA is reacted with gastrula hnRNA, about 12% forms hybrids with hnRNA (Hough et al., 1975) and about 1% forms hybrids with mRNA (Galau et al., 1974). Since the RNA is transcribed from a single strand of DNA, and some of the radioactive DNA tracer is too small to hybridize, these data indicate that 28% of the nonrepetitive DNA is transcribed into hnRNA and 2.7% of the nonrepetitive DNA appear as mRNA. Thus about 90% of the transcribed DNA sequences appear only in the nucleus, and 10% are transported to the cytoplasm and function as mRNA. This division is very similar to the ratios of the mass of the total RNA synthesized that becomes hnRNA or mRNA and indicates that the hnRNA and mRNA sequences are transcribed at about the same rate per active gene.

The characterization of these RNA populations is still incomplete. Most of the sequences in the hnRNA and mRNA appear very infrequently. The rate of the hybridization reactions indicates that less than 10% of the hnRNA and mRNA are included in the population that is reacting with the majority of the nonrepetitive DNA. In HeLa and other cells (Bishop et al., 1974; Getz et al., 1975) it has been shown, using enzymatically produced DNA copies of purified poly (A) containing RNA, that some RNA sequences occur much more frequently in the hnRNA and mRNA than other sequences. Most of the different kind of RNA molecules occur infrequently while the majority of the mass of the RNA is made up of a much smaller number of sequences that are present in larger numbers. Similar analysis has not been performed on sea urchin RNA populations. The sequence complexity found in sea urchin gastrula mRNA indicates the presence of about 14,000 different kinds of average-sized mRNA molecules. Most of these different mRNA molecules are probably present at about 300 to 400 copies per gastrula embryo of 600 cells and account for only a few percent of the RNA. Presumably, some mRNA sequences are present in much larger numbers and account for the bulk of the mRNA. Studies to more fully define these parameters in the RNA populations are needed.

Study of the developmental regulation of sequences expressed as RNA in sea urchins is just beginning. We have been comparing the sequences found in hnRNA of hatching blastula and pluteus stage of embryos of *Tripnesutes gratilla* (Kleene and Humphreys, 1975). Using the basic procedures developed in Britten and Davidson's laboratory (Galau et al., 1974; Hough et al., 1975), we have prepared tritium-labeled nonrepetitive DNA sequences of high specific activity, and determined the percent of radioactive DNA that reacts with hnRNA. The reactions followed the pseudo–first order kinetics expected of RNA:DNA hybridization reactions in RNA excess, and at completion about 16% of the labeled DNA formed hybrids with both blastula and pluteus RNA (figure 2). Apparently, the number of genes that are expressed at the two stages is about the same.

The sequences represented in blastula and pluteus hnRNA were compared by two experiments. A 1:1 mixture of hnRNA from blastula and pluteus stages was reacted with labeled nonrepetitive DNA (figure 2). The kinetics and plateau level of the reaction of labeled DNA with the mixture were

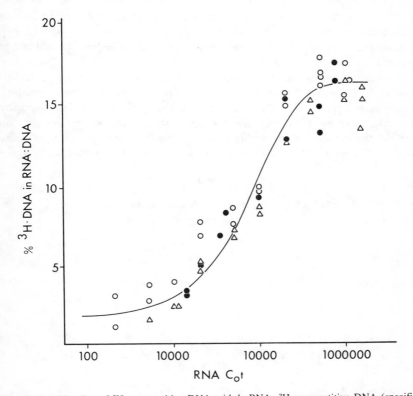

Fig. 2. Hybridization of ^{3}H-nonrepetitive DNA with hnRNA. ^{3}H-nonrepetitive DNA (specific activity: 2.2 × 10[6] dpm/μg) was prepared from *Tripneustes* embryos labeled through cleavage stage with ^{3}H-adenosine and ^{3}H-Thymidine. The nonrepetitive DNA sequences were purified as described by Galau et al. (1974). Reassociation of the ^{3}H-nonrepetitive DNA with an excess of whole *Tripneustes* DNA and chromatography on hydroxylapatite showed that, at most, 2% repetitive sequences remained and that 85% of the ^{3}H-DNA would form duplexes. hnRNA from hatching blastulae and early plutei was purified from isolated nuclei (Brandhorst and Humphreys, 1972; Hough et al., 1975), and dissolved at 10–20 mg/ml in 0.41 M phosphate buffer, 0.1% SDS and 0.01 M ETA. 10–40 μg of hnRNA was combined with 0.01 μg ^{3}H-DNA, denatured by boiling and incubated to the desired equivalent Cot. The RNA Cot points were analyzed for total ^{3}H-DNA as duplex and ^{3}H-DNA as DNA:DNA duplex using hydroxylapatite as described by Galau et al., 1974. Open circle = blastula RNA; open triangle = pluteus RNA; solid circle = blastula and pluteus RNA.

identical to the individual preparations, indicating that there is little difference in the sequences represented in the two populations. In the second experiment, RNA from each stage was reacted with the labeled DNA to remove those sequences represented in the RNA of that stage. The non-hybridized labeled DNA that had been depleted of the sequences complementary to hnRNA were repurified, and each was then reacted with hnRNA from both blastula and pluteus stages. In each case, the reaction of labeled DNA with hnRNA was about 10% of the original reaction, and there was no difference depending on the source of the RNA (table 1). The results of both experiments, therefore, indicate that the sequences transcribed by blastulae and plutei are essentially the same.

Currently there are little published data on changes in mRNA populations during development. Mouse brain mRNA appears to be much more complex than mouse liver mRNA (Ryffel and McCarthy, 1975), and the brain-specific sequences are mostly present in low frequency. In the absence of data on mRNA populations in sea urchin development (Note added in proof: Galau et al. (1976) have shown that low-frequency class of mRNA changes by about

TABLE 1

³H-DNA ISOLATED AS SINGLE STRAND AFTER REACTION
WITH BLASTULA RNA TO COT 40,000*

Driver	DNA or RNA Cot	%H³-DNA DNA-DNA	RNA-DNA
Tripuneustes DNA	20,000	71.0	......
		60.0	......
		63.0	......
Blastula RNA	30,000	6.1	1.1
		6.4	2.2
		6.4	2.1
Pluteus RNA	30,000	6.4	1.2
		6.6	2.5
		6.5	1.5

³H-DNA ISOLATED AS SINGLE STRAND AFTER REACTION WITH
PLUTEUS RNA TO COT 40,000*

Driver	DNA or RNA Cot	%³H-DNA DNA-DNA	RNA-DNA
Tripneustes DNA	20,000	72.0	......
		75.0	......
Pluteus RNA	30,000	4.1	4.2
		4.2	2.0
Blastula RNA	30,000	4.1	2.8
		4.5	2.5

*³H-nonrepetitive DNA was mixed with blastula or pluteus hnRNA and incubated to RNA Cot 40,000. The single-strand ³H-DNA was separated from H³-DNA in duplexes by chromatography on hydroxylapatite. The ³H-DNA was treated with RNAse to destroy any remaining RNA, digested with proteinase K, and extracted with phenol:chloroform. The ³H-DNA was concentrated, mixed with either blastula hnRNA, pluteus hnRNA, or whole *Tripneustes* DNA, denatured, and incubated to the desired Cot. The amount of ³H-DNA in DNA:RNA hybrids was measured as described in fig. 2.

50% between blastula and pluteus stages of sea urchin development.), it is difficult to interpret our finding that hnRNA does not change during development. However, it seems obvious that mRNA populations must change with development; and based on this assumption, there are a number of possible interpretations of our results. (1) The vast majority of hnRNA may not be a precursor of mRNA, and the transcription of hnRNA is not regulated in development. The mRNA sequences that are regulated in early embryos account for too small a percentage of the total nuclear RNA sequences to be resolved by current techniques. (2) hnRNA is a precursor of mRNA. However, there is little control of hnRNA synthesis, and regulation is accomplished at a post-transcriptional level. (3) Regulation of hnRNA synthesis does occur at the transcriptional level, but every sequence is still produced in some tissue, and our studies used RNA from whole embryos. These possibilities leave a wide latitude for speculation and experimentation, and it is obvious that we are at an early stage of exploration. However, we believe that it should not be long until a basic description of the patterns of regulation of hnRNA and mRNA during early sea urchin development is complete.

ACKNOWLEDGMENTS

The work from our laboratory has been supported by grants from the National Institute of Child Health and Human Development. Kenneth C. Kleene is an NIH Postdoctoral Fellow.

REFERENCES

Adamson, E. D., and H. R. Woodland. 1974. Histone synthesis in early amphibian development: Histone and DNA synthesis are not coordinated. J. Mol. Biol. 88:263–85.

Anderson, D., G. A. Galau, R. J. Britton, and E. H. Davidson. 1976. Sequence complexity of the RNA accumulated in oocytes of *Arbacia punctulata*. Devel. Biol. 51:138–45.

Arceci, R. J., D. R. Senger, and P. R. Gross. 1976. The programmed switch in lysine-rich histone synthesis at gastrulation. Cell 9:171–78.

Aronson, A. I., and F. H. Wilt. 1969. Properties of nuclear RNA in sea urchin embryos. Proc. Nat. Acad. Sci. USA 62:186–93.

Bishop, J. O., J. G. Morton, and M. Rosbash. 1974. Three abundance classes of HeLa cell messenger RNA. Nature 250:199–204.

Birnstiel, M. L., E. S. Weinberg, and M. L. Pardue. 1973. Evolution of 9S mRNA sequences. *In* B. A. Hamkalo and J. Papaconstantinou (eds.). Molecular cytogenetics. Pp. 75–94. Plenum Press, New York.

Birnstiel, M. J. Telford, E. Weinberg, and D. Stafford. 1974. Isolation and some properties of the genes coding for histone proteins. Proc. Nat. Acad. Sci. USA 71:2900–04.

Both, G. W., A. K. Banerjee, and A. J. Shatkin. 1975. Methylation-dependent translation of viral mRNA *in vitro*. Proc. Nat. Acad. Sci. USA 72:1189–93.

Brandhorst, B. P. 1976. Two-dimensional gel patterns of protein synthesis before and after fertilization of sea urchin eggs. Devel. Biol. 52:310–17.

Brandhorst, B. P., and T. Humphreys. 1971. Synthesis and decay rates of major classes of DNA-like RNA in sea urchin embryos. Biochem. 10:877–81.

Brandhorst, B. P., and T. Humphreys, 1972. Stabilities of nuclear and messenger RNA molecules in sea urchin embryos. J. Cell Biol. 53:474–82.

Brown, D. D., and E. Littna. 1964. RNA synthesis during the development of *Xenopus laevis*, the South African clawed toad. J. Mol. Biol. 8:669–87.

Davidson. E. 1968. Gene activity in early development. Academic Press, New York.

Davidson, E. H., B. R. Hough, W. H. Klein, and R. J. Britten. 1975. Structural genes adjacent to interspersed repetitive DNA sequences. Cell 4:217–38.

Emerson, C. P., and T. Humphreys. 1970. Regulation of DNA-like RNA and the apparent activation of ribosomal RNA synthesis in sea urchin embryos: Quantitative measurements of newly synthesized RNA. Develop. Biol. 23:86–112.

Emerson, C. P., and T. Humphreys. 1971a. Ribosomal RNA synthesis and the multiple, atypical nucleoli in cleaving embryos. Science 171:891–901.

Emerson, C. P., and T. Humphreys. 1971b. A simple and sensitive method for quantitative measurement of cellular RNA synthesis. Anal. Biochem. 40:254–66.

Epel, D. 1967. Protein synthesis in sea urchin eggs: A "late" response to fertilization. Proc. Nat. Acad. Sci. USA 57:899–906.

Galau, G. A., R. J. Britten, and E. H. Davidson. 1974. A measurement of the sequence complexity of polysomal messenger RNA in sea urchin embryos. Cell 2:9–20.

Galau, G. A., W. H. Klein, M. M. Davis, B. J. Wold, R. J. Britten, and E. H. Davidson. 1976. Structural gene sets active in embryos and adult tissues of the sea urchin. Cell 7:487–505.

Getz, M. J., G. D. Birnie, B. D. Young, E. MacPhail, and J. Paul. 1975. A kinetic estimation of base sequence complexity of nuclear poly(A) containing RNA in mouse friend cells. Cell 4:121–29.

Glisen, V. R., M. V. Glisen, and P. Doty. 1966. The nature of messenger RNA in the early stages of sea urchin development. Proc. Nat. Acad. Sci. USA 56:285–89.

Goldberg, R. B., G. A. Galau, R. J. Britten, and E. H. Davidson. 1973. Non-repetitive DNA sequence representation in sea urchin embryo mRNA. Proc. Nat. Acad. Sci. USA 70:3516–20.

Gross, K. W., J. V. Ruderman, M. Jacobs-Lorena, C. Baglioni, and P. R. Gross. 1973. Cell-free synthesis of histones directed by messenger RNA from sea urchin embryos. Nature New Biology 241:272–74.

Gross, P. R., L. I. Malkin, and W. A. Moyer. 1964. Templates for the first proteins of embryonic development. Proc. Nat. Acad. Sci. USA 51:407–14.

Grundstein, M., S. Levy, P. Schedl, and L. Kedes. 1973. Messenger RNAs for individual histone proteins: Fingerprint analysis and *in vitro* translation. Cold Spring Harbor Symp. Quant. Biol. 38:717–24.

Hough, B. R., M. J. Smith, R. J. Britten, and E. H. Davidson. 1975. Sequence complexity of heterogenous nuclear RNA in sea urchin embryos. Cell 5:291–99.

Hultin, T. 1952. Incorporation of ^{15}N-labeled glycine and alanine into the proteins of developing sea urchin eggs. Exptl. Cell Res. 3:494–96.

Humphreys, T. 1969. Efficiency of translation of messenger RNA before and after fertilization in sea urchins. Develop. Biol. 20:435–58.

Humphreys, T. 1971. Meaurements of mRNA entering polysomes upon fertilization of sea urchin eggs. Develop. Biol. 26:201–8.

Humphreys, T. 1973a. RNA and protein synthesis during early animal embryogenesis. *In* S. J. Coward (eds). Developmental regulation: Aspects of cell differentiation. Pp. 1–22. Academic Press, New York.

Humphreys, T. 1973b. Quantitative meaurement of RNA synthesis. *In* M. Chrispeels (ed.). Molecular techniques and approaches in developmental biology. Pp. 141–163. Wiley & Sons, New York.

Johnson, A. W., and L. S. Hnilca. 1971. Cytoplasmic and nuclear basic protein synthesis during early sea urchin development. Biochem. Biophys. Acta. 246:141–54.

Kedes, L. H., and M. Birnstiel. 1971. Reiteration and clustering of DNA sequences complementary to histone mRNA. Nature New Biol. 230:165–69.

Kedes, L. H., and P. R. Gross. 1969. Identification in cleaving embryos of three RNA species serving as templates for the synthesis of nuclear proteins. Nature 223:1335–39.

Kedes, L. H., P. R. Gross, G. Cognetti, and A. L. Hunter. 1969. Synthesis of nuclear and chromosomal proteins on light polyribosomes during cleavage in the sea urchin embryo. J. Mol. Biol. 45:337-51.

Kedes, L. H., A. C. Y. Chang, D. Houseman, and S. N. Cohen. 1975. Isolation of histone genes from unfractionated sea urchin DNA by subculture cloning in *E. coli*. Nature 255:533–38.

Kedes, L. H., R. H. Cohen, J. D. Lowry, A. C. Y. Chang, and S. N. Cohen. 1975. The organization of sea urchin histone genes. Cell 6:359–69.

Kijima, S., and F. H. Wilt. 1969. Rate of nuclear RNA turnover in sea urchin embryos. J. Mol. Biol. 40:235–46.

Kleene, K. C., and T. Humphreys. 1975. Complexity of nuclear RNA in blastula and pluteus stage sea urchin embryos. J. Cell Biol. 67:214a.

Labrie, F. 1969. Size of hemoglobin mRNA. Nature 221:1217.

MacKintosh, F. R., and E. Bell. 1969a. Proteins synthesized before and after fertilization in sea urchin eggs. Science 164:961–63.

MacKintosh, F. R., and E. Bell. 1969b. Regulation of protein synthesis in sea urchin eggs. J. Mol. Biol. 41:365–80.

Mescher, A., and T. Humphreys. 1974. Activation of maternal mRNA in the absence of poly(A) formation in fertilized sea urchin eggs. Nature 249:138–39.

Moav, B., and M. Nemer. 1971. Histone synthesis: Assignment to a special class of polyribosomes in sea urchin embryos. Biochem. 10:881–88.

Nakano, E., and A. Monroy. 1958. Incorporation of ^{35}S-methionine in the cell fractions of sea urchin eggs and embryos. Exptl. Cell Res. 14:236–43.

Nemer, M. 1963. Old and new RNA in embryogenesis of the purple sea urchin. Proc. Nat. Acad. Sci. USA 50:217–21.

Nemer, M., L. M. Dubroff, and M. Graham. 1975. Properties of sea urchin embryo mRNA containing and lacking poly(A). Cell 6:171–78.

Nemer, M., and D. T. Lindsay. 1967. Evidence that the S-polysomes of early sea urchin embryos may be responsible for the synthesis of chromosomal histones. Biochem. Biophys. Res. Comm. 35:156–60.

Raff, R. A., H. V. Colot, S. E. Selvig and P. R. Gross. 1972. Oogenetic origin of mRNA for embryonic synthesis of microtubule protein. Nature 235:211–14.

Robbins, E., and T. W. Borun. 1968. The cytoplasmic synthesis of histones in HeLa cells and its temporal relationship to DNA replication. Proc. Nat. Acad. Sci. USA 57:409–16.

Roeder, R. G., and W. J. Rutter. 1970. Multiple RNA polymerases and RNA synthesis during sea urchin development. Biochem. 9:2543–53.

Ruderman, J. V., and P.R . Gross. 1974. Histones and histone synthesis in sea urchin development. Develop. Biol. 36:286–98.

Ryffel, G. V., and B. J. McCarthy. 1975. Complexity of cytoplasmic RNA in different mouse tissues measured by hybridization of poly(A) RNA to complementary DNA. Biochem. 14:1379–85.

Skoultchi, A., and P. R. Gross. 1973. Maternal histone mRNA: detection by molecular hybridization. Proc. Nat. Acad. Sci. USA 70:2840–44.

Slayter, I., D. Gillespie, and D. W. Slayter. 1973. Cytoplasmic adenylation and processing of maternal mRNA. Proc. Nat. Acad. Sci. USA 70:406–11.

Smith, M. J., B. R. Hough, M. E. Chamberlain, and E. H. Davidson. 1974. Repetitive and non-repetitive sequences in sea urchin hnRNA. J. Mol. Biol. 85:103–126.

Terman, S. A. 1970. Relative effect of transcriptional level control of protein synthesis during early development of the sea urchin. Proc. Nat. Acad. Sci. USA 65:985–92.

Weinberg, E. S., M. L. Birnsteil, J. P. Purdom, and R. Williamson. 1972. Genes coding for polysomal 9S RNA of sea urchins: Conservation and divergence. Nature 240:225–28.

Whitely, A. H., B. J. McCarthy, and H. R. Whitely. 1966. Changing populations of messenger RNA during sea urchin development. Proc. Nat. Acad. Sci. USA 55:519–25.

Wilson, M. C., M. Melli, and M. L. Birnsteil. 1974. Reiteration frequency of histone coding sequences in man. Biochem. Biophys. Res. Comm. 61:404–9.

Wilt, F. H. 1964. RNA synthesis during sea urchin embryogenesis. Develop. Biol. 9:299–313.

Wilt, F. H. 1973. Polyadenylation of maternal RNA of sea urchin eggs after fertilization. Proc. Nat. Acad. Sci. USA 70:2345–49.

Wu, R. S., and F. H. Wilt. 1973. Poly(A) metabolism in sea urchin embryos. Biochem. Biophys. Res. Comm. 54:704–14.

Abstracts of Contributed Papers

EDITORS' NOTE: Contributed papers were presented during the colloquium. Since these presentations added significantly to the meeting, we felt that inclusion of abstracts of these papers in this volume would make the reader aware of this work and the scope of the colloquium.

J. D. KARAM AND M. G. BOWLES

Transcription of T4 Phage Genes 44 and 62

The protein products of T4 genes 45, 44, and 62 are required for phage DNA replication. Some evidence suggests that in T4-infected *E. coli* these three genes are cotranscribed in the 45 to 44 to 62 direction. We have isolated a phage mutation, named H6, that results in hyperproduction of the protein products of genes 44 and 62, without affecting the level of synthesis of the gene 45 protein. The hyperproduction of 44- and 62-proteins is more pronounced at 42°C than at 30°C. This mutation maps between genes 45 and 44, is *cis*-dominant, does not affect the temporal order of T4 gene expression except that it appears to cause continued expression of genes 44 and 62 throughout the phage growth cycle. These effects of H6 are being studied by the use of SDS-polyacrylamide slab-gel electrophoretic assays. H6 appears to be an up-promoter mutation for the genes 44 and 62. It is possible that these two genes are normally transcribed in at least two modes: one mode being initiated at the promoter for gene 45 and a second mode being initiated at a gene 44 promoter. Alternatively, H6 might represent the mutational creation of a secondary promoter for genes 44 and 62. In either case, it appears that the H6 alteration leads to a T4 promoter site that is efficiently recognized by most, if not all, of the T-4 induced alterations of host RNA polymerase.*

Department of Biochemistry, Medical University of South Carolina, Charleston, South Carolina 29401

*Supported by U.S.P.H.S. Grant GM18842 and RCDA GM-70-725.

GERALD R. GALLUPPI AND JOHN P. RICHARDSON

RNA-Dependent Nucleoside Triphosphatase Activity of Rho Factor Is Required for Rho-Mediated Termination of Transcription

The rho transcription termination factor has an RNA-dependent nucleoside triphosphate phosphohydrolase activity. In order to determine whether this phosphate cleavage is necessary for rho to terminate RNA synthesis, we compared in vitro T7 RNA transcripts formed in the presence of the normal nucleoside triphosphates (NTPs) with the RNA made using β-γ-methylene (NMPPCH$_2$P) analogues of the triphosphates. These analogues can be incorporated into RNA, but their γ-phosphates cannot be hydrolized.

Analysis of the transcripts made with the normal NTPs on 1M formaldehyde-sucrose gradients indicates that the RNA transcribed in the absence of rho sediments at 18s (2×10^6 daltons), whereas if rho is present during transcription, the RNA is much smaller, sedimenting around 6s. However, when the analogue NTPs are used, the RNAs made in the presence and in the absence of rho both sediment around 14s. Additon of normal GTP to the analogue reaction mixture restores rho factor's termination activity. Under these conditions the RNA synthesized without rho sediments at 15s, and with rho sediments at 6s. We conclude that the RNA-dependent NTPase activity is essential for rho factor to terminate transcription.

Department of Chemistry, Indiana University, Bloomington, Indiana 47401.

FRED SIEGMAN and GEORGE GUTHRIE

Evidence for Post-Transcriptional Regulation of T4 Bacteriophage Early Gene Expression

Bacteriophage T4 "early genes" are transcribed and translated from immediately after infection until approximately the time of initiation of DNA synthesis in a normal infection cycle. In some abnormal cycles this regulation is lost, and early gene products continue to accumulate over a longer period and to a higher level of activity. This loss of control on gene expression can be observed in mutants that fail to synthesize DNA or in infections with wild-type phage inactivated with ultraviolet light. From such studies it has been suggested that "shut off" of early genes requires the synthesis of one or more specific regulatory proteins whose synthesis does not occur in the mutant or irradiated viruses.

We have studied the effects of rifampicin on early gene expression in infections with normal phage. This system permits the translation of initiated mRNA molecules but prevents molecules that would have been initiated later from competing in the protein-synthesizing system of the host.

The general effect of rifampicin on early gene expression was to cause excessive production of enzymes from mRNA molecules being translated after the addition of rifampicin compared with untreated cells. In further studies an appropriate concentration and time of addition of rifampicin was determined that led to selection of the mRNA of at least two early enzymes for continuous translation even beyond the time that control cells had completed the entire multiplication cycle. Thus the functional lifetime of this mRNA appeared to have been indefinitely extended. Additional data suggested that the extended synthesis was caused by protection of the mRNA from degradation rather than prevention of synthesis of a specific protein for terminating

School of Medicine, Evansville Center, Indiana University, Evansville, Indiana 47712.

the expression of these two genes. These studies suggest that, in the normal multiplication cycle, gene expression may be limited by competition between existing and newly synthesized mRNA for available ribosomes. Rifampicin treatment, by preventing the initiation of new mRNA molecules, created an excess of free ribosomes that protects some of the mRNA molecules present at the time of its addition and thereby extends their functional lifetime. Thus functional lifetime may reflect extrinsic factors related to translation rather than an intrinsic instability of mRNA molecules or obligatory synthesis of proteins that cause termination of translation of specific early genes.

R. L. SOMERVILLE AND A. McPARTLAND

New High-Efficiency Promoters within the *trp* Operon of *Escherichia coli*

In *E. coli* strains where the *lac* structural genes are fused to the *trp* operon (Reznikoff et al., 1974, J. Bacteriol. 117:1213), β-galactosidase synthesis is subject to the control of the *trp* repressor-operator system. Selection for elevated levels of β-galactosidase in such fusion strains leads mainly to the isolation of derivatives lacking functional *trp* repressor. A minority class is due to mutations within *trp* DNA. Several properties of the latter group support the idea that simple structural changes in DNA may confer promoter activity upon regions that had previously been inert with respect to the initiation of transcription. In media containing excess tryptophan the production of β-galactosidase and appropriate downstream *trp* enzymes was *cis*-dominant, at a level from 3- to 16-fold higher than that of the controls. Auxotrophic promoter mutations, eight in number, were localized within *trp* structural genes E, D, C, and A. Prototrophic promoter mutations were localized at several regions within the *trp* operon by analysis of the levels of the tryptophan biosynthetic enzymes: genes on the operator-proximal side of the new promoter were expressed at a low level characteristic of wild type, whereas genes on the operator-distal side were expressed at a high rate. Each auxotrophic promoter gave rise to Trp$^+$ revertants devoid of promoter activity. Reversion was stimulated by base analog mutagens such as 2AP, EMS and NG. One promoter site in *trpD* is an *ochre* mutation, as shown by response to known suppressors and reversion analysis. Considering the size of the *trp* operon and the number of promoter precursor sites so far identified, it is predicted that transcription initiation requires a specific sequence of 6–8 base pairs in DNA.

Department of Biochemistry, Purdue University, West Lafayette, Indiana 47907.

R. J. DOWNEY, I. M. KANNO, and M. E. STAMBAUGH

Control of the NADPH-Nitrate Reductase in *Aspergillus*

Synthesis of the NADPH-nitrate reductase in *Aspergillus nidulans* is induced by nitrate and repressed by ammonium. Since protein degradation contributes significantly to regulation in certain eukaryotic systems, we have examined the disposition of newly synthesized nitrate reductase following removal of its inducer as well as addition of a repressor. Detectable induced synthesis of nitrate reductase is evident within 2 min of nitrate addition. Once the induction has begun, withdrawal of inducer does not abruptly halt synthesis. The half-life of the enzyme following removal of inducer was determined to be about 55 min. Induction and formation of nitrate reductase requires protein synthesis since cycloheximide, puromycin, or chloramphenicol quickly inhibits formation of the enzyme. When fully induced mycelia are subsequently shifted to a condition of full repression by ammonium, the enzyme is degraded at a rate similar to that occurring upon removal of inducer and is three times faster than the doubling time of the culture. If the intracellular concentration of ammonium is greater than 2.0 mM, repression of nitrate reductase occurs independently of the nitrate concentration inside the cell. Measurement of *de novo* synthesis during enzyme induction and repression suggests that nitrate reductase, a co-repressor of its own synthesis, affects translation.

Department of Zoology and Microbiology, Ohio University, Athens, Ohio 45701.

ARTHUR L. KOCH

Does the Initiation of Chromosome Replication Regulate Cell Division?

The control of cell division and chromosome replication is still very obscure. Ultimately, the ability of the organism to produce protoplasm from the resources of the environment limits growth and must time the initiation of chromosome replication, nuclear division, and cell division. Here arguments based on the variability of these processes within cultures of bacteria in balanced growth are made to try to perceive a hierarchy of those processes. The results of this paper are based largely on autoradiographic data of Chai and Lark (1970) and Forro (unpublished).

The analysis excludes models in which initiation of replication takes place only when cells achieve a precise size. It also shows that variation in cell size at initiation can be no smaller than the variation in cell size at division. So either these two processes are unconnected events with similar variation, or are connected by a total C and D period, from initiation to division, that is so constant that it introduces little random additional variation to the size at division. Arguments are presented that make the constancy of C + D in the population unlikely.

Division of Biological and Medical Research, Argonne National Laboratory, Argonne, Ill., 60439.

HELEN H. EVANS, SANDRA LITTMAN, AND THOMAS E. EVANS

Studies on the Inhibition of DNA Replication by Cycloheximide in *Physarum polycephalum*

Inhibitors of protein synthesis have been shown to interfere with DNA replication in many eukaryotic cells, but whether the inhibition is due to a decrease in the rate of chain elongation or to a decrease in the number of replicating units being elongated is a subject of some controversy (Gautschi, 1974, J. Mol. Biol. 84:223). In this study treatment of naturally synchronous plasmodia of *P. polycephalum* with cycloheximide was found to cause a decrease in the specific activity of TTP (determined according to Walters, Tobey, and Ratliff, 1973, Biochim. Biophys. Acta 319:336). During the first 15 minutes after drug addition, the amount of DNA synthesis—determined by ^{3}H-thymidine incorporation into DNA corrected for the change in the specific activity of TTP—was 70% of the control level. Similarly, the molecular weight of progeny strands pulse-labeled during the first 15 minutes of the S period in the presence of cycloheximide was approximately 70% of the control, as determined by sedimentation in alkaline sucrose density gradients. Our previous results have indicated that this drug has no effect on either the initiation of replication units or on the ligation of DNA fragments produced by ionizing radiation (Evans, Evans, and Brewer, in Proceedings of the 1975 ICN-UCLA Symposium on DNA synthesis and its regulation, ed. M. Goulian and P. Hanawalt; W. A. Benjamin, Menlo Park, Calif.) It appears, therefore, that cycloheximide inhibits the elongation of progeny strands within replication units, presumably by affecting the synthesis of short-lived proteins necessary for this process.*

Division of Radiation Biology, Case Western Reserve University, Cleveland, Ohio 44106.

*Supported by NIH Grant GM 19484, U.S.A.E.C. Contract W-31-109-ENG-78, and U.S.E.R.D.A. Contract AT (11-1)2486.

WILLIAM G. McGUIRE

Binding of Aryl Sulfatase to Cell Walls of *Neurospora*

The mural enzyme aryl sulfatase is one of a group of proteins whose synthesis is regulated by *cys-3* locus and derepressed under conditions of sulfur limitation. Cell walls prepared from derepressed cultures bind partially purified aryl sulfatase in a reaction that is rapid, specific, occurs within a narrow pH range, and is eliminated by treatments that remove peptide material from the cell wall. The type and/or location of binding sites within the cell wall is influenced by the chemical form of the external sulfur source. Cell walls prepared from sulfate-grown mycelia possess enzyme-binding ability only when growth was on limiting sulfate concentrations. Aryl sulfatase bound to such sites *in vitro* is extremely labile to heat inactivation. By contrast, methionine-grown hyphal walls possess binding sites irrespective of the external methionine concentration and enzyme bound *in vitro* to these sites is only slightly more heat labile than unbound enzyme. In addition, growth of vegetative hyphae in medium containing low concentrations of both sulfate and methionine yields cell walls that have both types of binding sites.

The presence of binding sites in cell walls from methionine-grown cultures is independent of the function of either the structural gene for aryl sulfatase (*ars*) or the *cys-3* regulatory gene. While the binding site found in walls of sulfate-grown mycelia is also independent of the *ars* function, cell walls isolated from a temperature-sensitive *cys-3* revertant that can utilize sulfate slowly at 25°C could only bind about half as much enzyme as those of a similar *cys-3*+ culture. Other types of control mechanisms also appear to influence the presence of aryl sulfatase binding sites during development; aerial hyphae

Department of Biology, Univeristy of California—Los Angeles, Los Angeles, California 90024.

isolated from methionine-grown pads had far less enzyme-binding ability than the vegetative hyphae upon which they had formed, whereas the reverse was true for aerials produced from pads grown on high sulfate medium.*

*This work was supported by an NSF grant to R. W. Siegel.

Post-Transcriptional Regulation of mRNA Production In Resting and Growing Fibroplasts

The regulation of RNA content appears to be an important aspect of the control of cell growth. It has been long known that growing cells contain significantly more ribosomes than do resting cells. In our studies on the cultured mouse fibroblast line 3T6, we found that per unit of DNA growing cells contain 1.6 times as much rRNA and tRNA, and 2.3 times as much poly(A) + mRNA as resting cells. When expressed as amounts per cell, the differences are even greater (Johnson, Abelson, Green, and Penman, 1974, Cell 1:95).

The cell uses a variety of mechanisms to increase its content of the different classes of cytoplasmic RNA during a serum-induced transition from the resting to the growing state. The increases in rRNA and tRNA content are the result of increases in the rate of synthesis (Mauck and Green, 1973, Proc. Nat. Acad. Sci. USA 70:2819) as well as increases in the stability of the RNA species (Abelson, Johnson, Penman, and Green, 1974, Cell 1:161). The content of mRNA must be regulated by a different mechanism since both the over-all rate of synthesis of hnRNA and the half-life of mRNA appear to be the same in resting and stimulated cells. The rate of mRNA production, and therefore content, is apparently regulated by controlling the efficiency of conversion of hnRNA into cytoplasmic mRNA.

Evidence supporting such a mechanism comes from two different types of experiments. First, in both continuous labeling and in pulse-chase experiments, we found that the efficiency of export of poly(A) from the nucleus to the cytoplasm is about twice as high in growing cells as in resting cells. The efficiency was found to increase from the resting level to the growing level

Department of Biochemistry, Ohio State University, Columbus, Ohio 43210.

within 3 hours after serum stimulation of resting 3T6 cells. We also found that there is no detectable difference between resting and growing cells in the content of nuclear poly(A) per unit of DNA or the ratio of polyadenylated to non-polyadenylated hnRNA (Johnson, Williams, Abelson, Green, and Penman, 1975, Cell 4:69).

Second, we have determined directly the proportion by weight of hnRNA that is converted to cytoplasmic poly(A) + mRNA by measuring the initial rates of labeling of these RNA species. We found that this proportion is 2–3 times greater for growing or serum-stimulated cells than for resting cells. Despite the altered efficiency, the kinetics of nuclear processing are identical in resting and growing cells.*

*This work was completed while the author was a post-doctoral fellow in the laboratory of Dr. H. Green at M.I.T., and was done in collaboration with Drs. S. Penman, H. T. Abelson, and J. G. Williams.

LAURENCE D. ETKIN

Gene Regulation in Transferred Somatic Cell Nuclei

Results of previous experiments have shown that in amphibians the general type of nucleic acid synthesized by transferred somatic cell nuclei is directed by the cytoplasm of the host cell (Gurdon, 1974, The control of gene expression in animal development, Harvard University Press, Cambridge). Differentiated brain cell nuclei that are synthesizing RNA begin to synthesize DNA when transferred into unfertilized eggs, but continue RNA synthesis when transferred into oocytes (Gurdon, 1967, Proc. Nat. Acad. Sci. USA 58:102, J. Embryol. Exp. Morph. 20:54). The question still remains whether the products synthesized by these nuclei are characteristic brain cell products or oocyte products.

The answer to this question is being sought by examining the regulatory effect of oocyte cytoplasm on the synthetic activity of transferred liver cell nuclei, using an interspecific hybrid combination of *Ambystoma texanum* and *Ambystoma mexicanum* (axolotl). The enzymes lactate dehydrogenase (LDH) and alcohol dehydrogenase (ADH) are used as markers of gene activity since the enzymes of the two species migrate differently upon starch gel electrophoresis. LDH is synthesized in both liver and oocytes, while ADH is tissue-specific, being found in the liver of both species.

A. texanum liver nuclei were transferred into both nucleated and enucleated axolotl oocytes. The recipient oocytes were cultured in modified amphibian Ringers solution for three weeks. During this period groups of recipient oocytes were homogenized and analyzed by starch gel electrophoresis for the presence of *A. texanum* LDH and ADH. In most cases the results showed that after one to two weeks in culture no *A. texanum* enzymes were detected;

Department of Zoology, Indiana University, Bloomington, Indiana 47401.

however, after three weeks *A. texanum* LDH but not ADH was detected. The presence or absence of the maternal axolotl nucleus did not appear to effect the expression of the transferred liver nuclei. In one experiment *A. texanum* LDH was detected after one week in culture, but oocytes that had received *A. texanum* liver cell cytoplasm injections intead of nuclei did not show the presence of any detectable *A. texanum* LDH or ADH.

These results indicate that the transferred *A. texanum* liver nuclei continue to synthesize a product (LDH) produced in both liver cells and oocytes, but fail to synthesize the liver-specific product (ADH). Thus in the case of ADH and LDH the oocyte cytoplasm appears to be able to regulate the synthetic activity of the transferred somatic cell nuclei so as to conform to the oocytes' normal synthetic output.

T. J. BYERS, M. C. KUHNS, L. E. KING,
J. J. SEILHAMER, AND E. A. NIES

A Model for Inhibitor-Induced Amoebic Encystment

A large number of chemical agents either stimulate or inhibit cyst formation by amoebas of the genus *Acanthamoeba,* but studies in different laboratories have been performed under sufficiently different conditions to make the results confusing. Therefore, we have reexamined a number of the inhibitor effects in a single system and have obtained results that begin to fit a more consistent pattern. In general, the effects have been tested by treating unagitated log phase cells (LM) during active growth in nutrient medium or postlog phase cells (PGD) that have been diluted in nutrient medium to log phase concentrations. The methods are similar to those used by Neff and Neff (1972, Compt. Rend. Lab. Carlsberg 39:111).

In examining inhibitors of protein and nucleic acid synthesis, we found four categories of effects that are represented by the following: (1) ethidium bromide and mitomycin c can induce high levels of encystment in both LM and PGD cells; (2) hydroxyurea and fluorodeoxyuridine induce low levels of encystment in LM cells, but considerably higher levels in diluted PGD cells; (3) actinomycin blocks encystment by LM cells, but induces encystment in diluted PGD cells; and (4) cycloheximide and emetine block encystment by both LM and PGD cells. These results are interpreted in terms of a model in which cells are presumed to reversibly initiate encystment in the G_1 phase of the cell cycle. The data are consistent with the assumption that the initiation of encystment by LM cells requires RNA and protein synthesis. Since diluted PGD cells in our system immediately revert to multiplication in the absence of inhibitors, the induction of encystment by agents in categories 1, 2, and 3

Department of Microbiology and Developmental Biology Program, Ohio State University, Columbus, Ohio 43210.

suggests that reversion depends at least on RNA synthesis and probably also on protein and DNA synthesis. It is presumed that only those PGD cells that have already completed the RNA synthesis necessary for encystment encyst upon dilution in the presence of inhibitors. PGD cells apparently still require protein synthesis for encystment and, therefore, do not encyst in the presence of cycloheximide or emetine. Low levels of LM encystment induced by category 2 inhibitors may be attributed to an accumulation of cysts resulting from the inhibitors having a stronger blocking effect on the reversion pathway than the initiation pathway. The high levels of LM encystment induced by category 1 inhibitors may be due to a stimulatory effect on the initiation pathway. The nature of the stimulation is unknown, but work with several agents suggests that mitochondrial protein synthesis may be involved.

J. C. BAGSHAW AND J. M. D'ALESSIO

RNA Polymerase Activity in Developing Brine Shrimp Embryos: Here It Comes, There It Goes

Postgastrula development of the brine shrimp *Artemia salina* offers two transcriptional "switches" for biochemical studies. The cryptobiotic encysted gastrulae are metabolically inert. Thus, renewed RNA synthesis upon breaking dormancy represents an "on" switch. Between 36 and 72 hours after development resumes, an "off" switch reduces RNA synthesis *in vivo* by more than 90%. By definition, RNA polymerases must be involved in some manner, active or passive, in these transcriptional switches. Nuclei isolated from encysted gastrulae not only fail to yield soluble RNA polymerase activity but also adsorb or inactivate RNA polymerases from larvae. However, soluble extracts of cyst nuclei do not inhibit larval RNA polymerases. In fact, these extracts contain a protein factor that stimulates RNA synthesis by *Artemia* RNA polymerase II, but not by other eukaryotic RNA polymerases. After one hour of development, this stimulatory activity has virtually disappeared, and soluble RNA polymerases can be obtained from the nuclei. The "off" switch is accompanied by a decrease in total RNA polymerase activity and an increase in the relative amount of RNA polymerase II. RNA polymerase II from 72 hr larvae comprises four subunits with molecular weights of approximately 170,000, 130,000, 34,000, and 25,000. Comparison by SDS gel electrophoresis of RNA polymerase II from 36 hr and 72 hr larvae suggests that the "off" switch does not require the physical disappearance of the enzyme.*

School of Medicine, Wayne State University, Detroit, Michigan 48201.
*Work supported by NIH Research Grant GM21376-01.

Index